Oral Cancer

Sol Silverman, Jr. M.A., D.D.S.
Professor and Chairman of Oral Medicine
University of California, San Francisco

Third Edition

The American Cancer Society • Atlanta

Published 1981. Third edition 1990.
Printed in the United States of America.

Library of Congress Cataloging in Publication Data

Oral cancer / edited by Sol Silverman, Jr. — 3rd ed.
p. cm.
Includes bibliographical references.
ISBN 0-944235-05-0
1. Mouth—Cancer. I. Silverman, Sol, 1916- II. American Cancer Society.
[DNLM: 1. Head and Neck Neoplasms. 2. Mouth Neoplasms. WU 280 0621]
RC280.M6067 1990
616.99'431—dc20
DNLM/DLC
for Library of Congress 90-199
CIP

Oral Cancer

Contributors

John Beumer III, D.D.S., M.S.
Professor and Director
Hospital Maxillofacial Dentistry
University of California, Los Angeles

Roger Boles, M.D
Professor of Otolaryngology
School of Medicine
University of California, San Francisco

Thomas A. Curtis, D.D.S.
Professor of Removable Prosthodontics
School of Dentistry
University of California, San Francisco

Herbert H. Dedo, M.D.
Professor of Otolaryngology
School of Medicine
University of California, San Francisco

William P. Dillon, M.D.
Associate Professor of Radiology and Neurology
School of Medicine
University of California, San Francisco

Karen K. Fu, M.D.
Professor of Radiation Oncology
School of Medicine
University of California, San Francisco

Maurice Galante, M.D.
Professor of Surgery
School of Medicine
University of California, San Francisco

Theodore L. Phillips, M.D.
Professor and Chairman
Department of Radiation Oncology
School of Medicine
University of California, San Francisco

Mark Schubert, D.D.S., M.S.D.
Assistant Professor
Department of Oral Medicine
University of Washington, Seattle

Edward J. Shillitoe, B.D.S., Ph.D.
Professor and Chairman
Department of Microbiology
Dental Branch, University of Texas
Health Science Center at Houston

Ivan J. Silverberg, M.D.
Associate Clinical Professor of Medicine and Radiation Oncology and Research Associate in Cancer Research
School of Medicine
University of California, San Francisco

Ian M. Zlotolow, D.M.D.
Chief of Dental Service
Department of Surgery
Memorial Sloan Kettering Cancer Center, New York, NY

Acknowledgments

Appreciation is expressed to Margaret R. Hall for her invaluable contributions in editing this book and in coordinating its publication and production. Special thanks also to Robert Eustachy, graphic designer, and to Georgette Salazar of the University of California Printing Services, Berkeley, for their painstaking work and exceptional efforts in putting the book together.

Contents

Introduction

All multicellular animals, and certainly all vertebrates, can develop cancer. The ability to develop cancer is a characteristic of all cells that are capable of reproduction and growth. By its very nature—an abnormal, seemingly unrestricted growth of body cells—cancer is distinguished from other forms of illness.

There are many differences in the occurrence of cancer types and sites among human populations. Two examples are the high incidence of nasopharyngeal cancer among Chinese as compared with other ethnic groups, and the low (less than one-fourth) incidence of skin cancer among blacks as compared with whites.

Although cancer may occur at any age, it is preponderantly a disease of aging, and it can be both acute and chronic in its course. Whereas many types of cancer are perceptible only when they are extensive or involve organs difficult to treat, others may be detected early, treated, and cured.

This complex disease is one of the nation's major causes of morbidity and disability. It is second only to heart disease as the leading cause of death. Approximately one in every three Americans will have cancer in his or her lifetime, and more than one in every five deaths is due to a malignant tumor.

Oral cancer accounts for about 4% of all cancers and 2.2% of all cancer deaths. Mortality is high. In the United States, fewer than half the patients with oral cancer are cured. However, when mouth cancers are detected early (i.e., when lesions are less than 3 cm in size and show no evidence of deep invasion or metastasis), survival rates increase dramatically. Unfortunately, over the past decade, there has not been a dramatic improvement in earlier diagnosis of oral cancer: over half of all oral cancers at the time of diagnosis are extensive, late-stage malignancies. Hence, treatment is more aggresssive, which creates more morbidity and has led to only a slight improvement in survival rates. Therefore, early diagnosis of a lesion during the localized stage, combined with adequate treatment, appears to be the most effective way to further improve oral cancer control. Thus, professional and public education regarding early signs and symptoms is a most important and critical activity. In addition, as our knowledge of cancer initiators and promotors increases, prevention seems to be a realistic goal. Certainly the increased risks of tobacco and alcohol must be recognized.

Optimal cancer control calls for a diversity of approaches among many health professionals. The dental profession shares an important responsibility in the management of oral cancer, from diagnosis through rehabilitation. Dentists have a unique opportunity in the routine mouth examination to detect malignant neoplasms while they are still asymptomatic, innocuous, and unsuspected. In addition, the dentist is most often the first clinician consulted for general oral complaints and, therefore, has the initial responsibility of differentiating benign from malignant conditions.

Treatment of oral cancer often produces certain dysfunctions and distortions in speech, appearance, mastication, swallowing, saliva control and consistency, emotional stability, and dental health. Therefore, rehabilitation becomes a major consideration in patient management.

In preparing for their participation in cancer control, health professionals must acquire knowledge of the biologic and epidemiologic aspects of cancer, its prevention, early detection, diagnosis, treatment, and rehabilitation, and an understanding of the psychosocial and economic aspects of the disease.

This third edition of *Oral Cancer* updates the entire problem of oral cancer control: epidemiology, etiology, premalignant factors and prevention, diagnosis, treatment, rehabilitation, and survival. The chapters "Etiology," "Diagnosis," and "Treatment" focus mainly on squamous cell carcinoma because it is by far the most common type of oral cancer. The etiology, diagnosis, and treatment of certain other head and neck cancers are covered in a separate chapter. Also treated separately are the leukemias and lymphomas, malignancies that often have oral manifestations and require special dental management.

SOL SILVERMAN, JR.
January 1990

1

Epidemiology

SOL SILVERMAN, JR.

Epidemiology is that branch of science which is concerned with the study of disease as it appears in its natural surroundings and as it affects a community of people. Epidemiologic studies yield important information such as the origin, relative prevalence, and trends of certain diseases which can also furnish etiologic clues. These data, in turn, aid in determining appropriate and optimal direction of health care services, prevention strategies, research, and resources.

INCIDENCE

Approximately one million new cancers of all sites (excluding skin) will be diagnosed in the United States this year. Cancers of the lips, tongue, floor of the mouth, palate, gingiva and alveolar mucosa, buccal mucosa, and oropharynx will account for almost 31,000 of these cases (3.1%). About 10% of all malignancies in the U.S. occur in California, and oral cancer comprises about 3.4% of all cancers in this state. If the nasopharynx, hypopharynx, larynx, sinuses, and major salivary glands are included with the oral sites, then cancers of these sites combined will account for more than 5% of all cancers in the U.S. Cancer now strikes approximately one person in every three, and three families of every four. An estimated 75 million Americans now living can be expected some day to have cancer.

HISTOLOGIC TYPES

Carcinomas account for about 96% of all oral cancers and sarcomas for about 4%. Since the most common type of oral cancer is squamous cell carcinoma, which accounts for approximately nine out of every ten oral malignancies, the oral cancer problem primarily concerns the diagnosis, biology, and management of squamous cell carcinoma.

AGE AND SEX

Of all the factors that may contribute to the development of cancer, age is the factor which incurs the highest risk. Oral cancer, like most cancers, is a disease of older age. About 95% of all oral cancers occur in persons over 40 years of age, and the average age at the time of diagnosis is about 60. The importance of this factor in cancer prevalence is augmented by the fact that the "over-65" population in the United States now exceeds 30 million, or about 13% of the population. Furthermore, the increase in the population over age 65 has far exceeded that of the rest of the population in the last decade and, at present, more than one-third of the American people are over the age of 45. The average life expectancy of Americans is at an all-time high, exceeding 74 years, and the age-adjusted death rate is at an all-time low. White women have the longest life expectancy (79 years), followed by black women (73 years), white men (72 years), and black men (64 years). A study of 3,535 consecutive autopsied patients over 65 years of age showed that 1,149 (32.5%) had one or more cancers.[1]

The older age of oral cancer patients suggests that a time factor may be operating which involves predetermined changes in the biochemical-biophysical processes (nuclear, enzymatic, metabolic, immunologic) of aging cells—changes which may be influenced by chemicals, viruses, hormones, nutrients, or physical irritants.

Of the one million new cancers estimated for Americans this year, the occurrence in men and women will be about equal. Oral cancer occurs more frequently in males, but the male-female ratio, which in 1950 was about 6:1, is now about 2:1. One explanation for this reduced ratio is thought to be the great increase in smoking among women. In addition, considering cancer is an age-related disease, it should be noted that in the over-65 age group in the general population, the number of women exceeds the number of men by 45%.

Data obtained by the National Cancer Institute in its Surveillance, Epidemiology, End Results Program (SEER) covering the years 1973–1984, demonstrate the age- and sex-related distribution of oral cancer (Table 1-1).[2] During this period there were no significant differences when comparing the time interval 1973–1978 with that of 1979–1984. The impact of age was reflected by the fact that 44% of all the oral cancers occurred in persons over 65 years of age while this group accounted for less than 13% of the total population.

Table 1.1 AGE/SEX DISTRIBUTION OF ORAL CANCER* (Based on 20,115 Cases)

	Distribution by Percentage of Cases	
Age	Male (71%)	Female (21%)
≤19	<1	<1
20–39	3	2
40–49	10	8
50–64	44	44
≥65	43	46

*Cancers diagnosed and/or treated during 1973–1984 according to biostatistical information from 9 population-based tumor registries in Connecticut, Hawaii, Iowa, New Mexico, Utah, Atlanta, Detroit, San Francisco-Oakland, and Seattle-Puget Sound. (Source: National Cancer Institute: Surveillance, Epidemiology and End Results Program, SEER.[2])

SITES

The tongue is the most common site for oral cancer in both men and women. Data from the SEER Program showed that 85% of all oral cancers diagnosed between 1973 and 1984 occurred in the tongue, oropharynx, mouth floor, and lips (Table 1-2). Oral cancer incidence has remained stable relative to the occurrence of all newly diagnosed cancers, with absolute numbers increasing each year. The only site contrary to this trend was lip, where a 5% reduction occurred. This trend may reflect public education regarding the dangers of ultraviolet exposure and the use of sunscreens. The greatest increase in cancer of the four most frequent oral cancer sites was in the tongue. Oral tongue malignancies (located in the anterior two-thirds) accounted for 53% of tongue cancers. Since 47% occur in the base of the tongue, the problems regarding recognition of signs and symptoms and early diagnosis are apparent.

Table 1-2. ORAL CANCER, SEER DATA 1973–1984*

Site	All Cases 1973–1984 Total	1973–1978 Cases	(%)	M:F	Mean Age†	1979–1984 Cases	(%)	M:F	Mean Age‡	Interval Change (%)
1. Tongue	5037§	2197	(23.8)	1.9	61	2840	(26.1)	1.9	62	+29
2. Oropharynx	4450	2008	(21.7)	2.0	61	2442	(22.5)	2.0	61	+22
3. Lip	4395#	2257	(24.4)	12.2	64	2138	(19.7)	9.0	66	− 5
4. Floor	3288	1493	(16.1)	2.2	61	1795	(16.5)	2.2	62	+20
5. Gingiva	1676¶	715	(7.7)	1.8	66	961	(8.8)	1.5	67	+34
6. Buccal	577	277	(3.0)	1.0	69	300	(2.8)	1.1	69	+ 8
7. Hard Palate	376	172	(1.9)	1.0	66	204	(1.9)	1.5	66	+19
8. Mouth	316	132	(1.4)	2.2	64	184	(1.7)	2.0	66	+39
Total	20,115	9,251	(100)	2.5	63	10,864	(100)	2.3	63	+17

*Source: Data from National Cancer Institute: Surveillance, Epidemiology and End Results Program (SEER), 1973–1984.[2]
† Range = 10–103 Years
‡ Range = 17–102 Years
§ Oral Tongue = 53%
# Lower Lip = 94%
¶ Mandibular gingiva = 86%

Table 1-3. ORAL CANCER IN CALIFORNIA, 1974–1985*

Site	Cases (%)	M:F	Mean Age†
Tongue	1226 (26.9)	1.6	62
Oropharynx	1224 (26.8)	1.6	62
Floor	807 (17.7)	1.7	61
Lips	700 (15.3)	7.2	64
Gingiva	397 (8.7)	1.2	65
Buccal	119 (2.6)	0.8	70
Hard Palate	64 (1.4)	1.0	67
Mouth, Unspecified	25 (0.6)	1.5	68
Total	4,562 (100)	1.8	63

*Data from Northern California Cancer Program
† Range = 11–103 years

Table 1-3 shows 12-year oral cancer data (1974–1985) collected from the Northern California Cancer Program which represents 67 hospitals from five San Francisco Bay Area counties with a population base of 7.2 million. Ethnic backgrounds of patients recorded included 83% whites and 10% blacks. Squamous carcinomas accounted for 90% of all malignancies. Ninety-seven percent of the oral cancers occurred in patients over 40 years of age, with 43% of all oral cancers developing in persons over 65.

Data from a previous study at the University of California, San Francisco reveal certain associations between oral cancer sites, patient characteristics, and diagnostic patterns.[3] The study group comprised 595 patients with oral cancer who were seen in the university's Oral Medicine Clinic between 1968 and 1982. The most frequent site was the tongue, which accounted for 30% of all the malignancies. Closely follow-

Table 1-4. OCCURRENCE OF ORAL CARCINOMA IN 595 PATIENTS: ASSOCIATION OF SITE, SEX, AGE, AND TOBACCO HABITS*

Carcinoma				Age of Onset (yr)		Tobacco Users
Site	No.	(%)	M:F	Mean	Range	(%)
Tongue†	181	(30)	1.4	57	19-90	82
Oropharynx	159	(27)	2.2	60	35-86	85
Floor of mouth	137	(23)	1.4	60	39-91	90
Gingiva‡	51	(8)	1.0	60	26-88	67
Buccal mucosa	29	(5)	0.5	63	27-85	69
Lip§	23	(4)	2.3	59	20-89	63
Hard palate	15	(3)	0.9	49	15-76	55
All Sites	595	(100)	1.4	59	15-91	82

*Data from Silverman et al.[3]
† Oral tongue = 76%
‡ Mandibular gingiva = 84%
§ All lower lip

Table 1-5. CHARACTERISTICS OF ORAL CARCINOMAS IN 595 PATIENTS: ASSOCIATION OF SITE, STAGE, AND DIAGNOSTIC PATTERNS*

	Stage at Diagnosis (%)				First Professional Visit (%)	
Site	Localized	Spread	Mean Delay Time (mo)†	Pain as First Complaint (%)	Dentist	Physician
Tongue	51	49	4.2	66	36	64
Oropharynx	43	57	3.0	56	16	84
Floor of mouth	64	36	3.4	59	44	56
Gingiva	56	44	3.5	64	52	48
Buccal mucosa	79	21	3.4	52	50	50
Lip	88	12	5.0	27	46	54
Hard palate	75	25	4.5	50	57	43

*Data from Silverman et al.[3]
† Time from patient's recognition of first sign or symptom to diagnosis.

ing sites were the oropharynx and floor of mouth. Together, these three sites accounted for 80% of the malignancies seen in the clinic (Table 1-4). Male patients outnumbered female 352 to 243 (59% to 41%). The male preponderance existed for all sites except the buccal mucosa and hard palate. Although the age at onset of tumor ranged between 15 and 91 years, the mean age was 59, with more than 95% of tumors occurring in individuals over 40 years of age. Tobacco usage far exceeded national estimates for both men and women. At the time of diagnosis more than half of the tumors found at each site were localized, except for those in the oropharynx where more than half of the lesions already showed regional lymph node metastases (Table 1-5). However, when the tongue was subdivided into oral (anterior two-thirds) and base, a significant difference emerged: 73% of oral-tongue carcinomas were localized, whereas 78% of the malignancies found in the base of the tongue already had regional metastases at the time of diagnosis.

When the localized lesions were compared with those associated with lymph node involvement, it was found that the more advanced lesions had a longer delay time before diagnosis. Pain was by far the most frequent first complaint, with the second most common complaint being that of a "lump."

In the U.S., the increased male prevalence of oral cancer appears due to the proportionately higher number of lip cancers that occur in men, approximating a ratio of ten to one. The preponderance of cases in men may also be partly accounted for by out-of-doors occupations and recreational activities and histories of heavier daily tobacco and alcohol consumption by the male patients.

In all of the studies cited here the tongue was the most frequent oral cancer site. But, unlike the University of California study in which the oropharynx and floor of the mouth were the second and third leading sites, the SEER national data indicated the lip as the third leading (but decreasing in frequency) site. A report by Szpak et al. has confirmed the varying frequencies of lip cancer in metropolitan centers.[4] They report the Dallas-Fort Worth area as having the highest incidence of lip cancer, although the cause of this was not evident. The decreasing frequency of lip cancer may reflect public education about the dangers of sunlight exposure and the use of sunscreens and lubricants.

STAGE AT DIAGNOSIS

In comparing various tumor registry data, there was uniform agreement that about 90% of all oral cancers were squamous cell carcinomas. Based on 12,425 cases recorded in the SEER program for which there was adequate information, advanced lesions (staged as "spread") outnumbered localized lesions by more than two to one (Table 1-6). The lip was the only site where localized cancers were more frequently found than those that were advanced. If only the three leading oral cancer sites were considered (tongue, oropharynx, floor of mouth), the number of localized tumors at diagnosis would be reduced to 22% for the 1973–1978 period and 26% for 1979–1984. It becomes obvious at the present time that earlier diagnosis is a key factor in oral cancer control. (See Chapter 7 on prognosis and survival.)

Table 1-6. ORAL CANCER: STAGE AT DIAGNOSIS*

Cancer Site	No. of Cases	1973–1978 (5,394) Percentage		1979–1984 (7,031) Percentage	
		Localized	Spread	Localized	Spread
Tongue	3715	29	71	32	68
Oropharynx	3612	21	79	21	79
Mouth Floor	2017	11	89	20	80
Lip	1822	75	25	87	13
Gingiva	657	10	90	14	86
Buccal	320	12	88	24	76
Hard Palate	282	35	65	34	66
	12,425	29	71	34	66

*Source: Data from National Center Institute: Surveillance, Epidemiology and End Results Program (SEER), 1973–1984.[2]

RACE AND GENETICS

Ethnic background is known to influence many types of cancer. For example, cancer in American blacks is increasing at a faster rate than in whites. Blacks have proportionately higher rates of oropharyngeal cancer than do other racial groups. This finding suggests a genetic factor, although habits or living differences have also been implicated.[5] As another example, cancer of the nasopharynx is 20 to 30 times more prevalent in Chinese than in whites. The rate of nasopharyngeal carcinoma is highest in Chinese who have remained in Asia, for example those in Southeast Asia, where it is one of the most common cancers. (See Chapter 9.)

Studies of human cancer of certain specific sites (breast, lung, colon, stomach, liver, and skin) have shown that these neoplasms tend to occur in families, implying a genetic influence.[6] However, as yet no inheritance patterns have been identified, and it seems likely that the increased risk for first-degree relatives is due to environmental factors. No such evidence of familial grouping has been presented for oral cancer.

Most human tumors show chromosome aberrations which are usually proportional to the degree of malignancy and vary with each tumor and patient (Fig. 1-1). It is not known whether the chromosomal abnormalities are the cause or the result of malignancy.

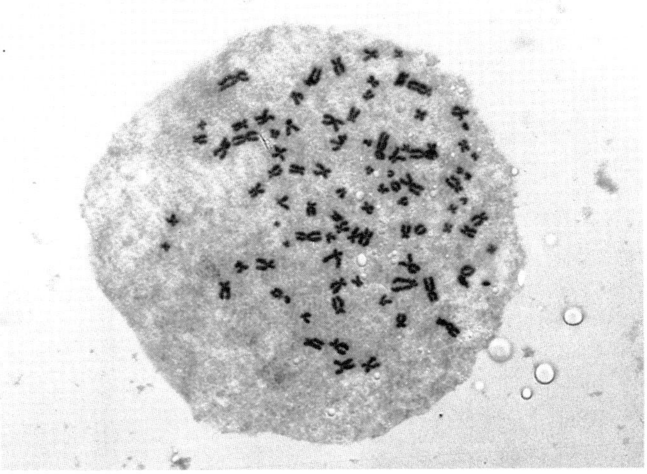

Fig. 1-1. Chromosome preparation from a malignant cell; note aneuploidy. Karyotyping is used to characterize aberrations of malignant cells.

MULTIPLE CANCERS

The data unequivocally show that persons with oral cancer are at an increased risk for developing subsequent additional malignancies.

A study of the smoking habits of oral cancer patients at the University of California, San Francisco found that of 160 patients observed for more than one year after treatment, 18% developed second primary oral cancers.[7] The risk was greater for those whose tobacco habits remained unchanged (30%) than for those who quit (13%).

In a study of 153 patients with carcinoma of the mouth floor who were treated and observed at the University of California, San Francisco between 1957 and 1973, it was found that 36% of the patients had at least one second primary cancer.[8] Twenty-three patients (15%) had a second primary oral cancer. In a similar follow-up study involving 204 patients with carcinoma of the oral tongue who were observed between 1940 and 1971, 19% had second primary cancers; 61% of these were second oral primary malignancies (12% of the total group).[9]

In a 1969 review of 1,250 patients with cancers of the mouth, pharynx, or larynx, it was found that 104 (8.3%) developed second primary cancers within the same anatomic areas.[10] In a 1970 study of 9,415 patients with squamous carcinomas of the respiratory or upper digestive tract, second primary cancers occurred at a rate that was twice the expected incidence.[11] The observed-expected ratio for oral cancer patients was 1.9:1.

The increased risk for additional new oral cancers in patients also has been confirmed in three other studies.[12–14] One study[13] of 377 patients treated for cancer in the floor of the mouth reported that 18% developed new cancers of the respiratory and upper digestive tracts, and 9% had second primary cancers occurring in the mouth. Another of these studies suggested an increased risk of subsequent oropharyngeal carcinoma in women with already diagnosed primary carcinomas of the breast or uterus.[14] The increased risk for multiple head and neck primary carcinomas is further accentuated in tobacco and alcohol users.[15]

MORTALITY

Worldwide, cancer of various forms accounts for more than 2 million deaths each year. In the United States cancer is a leading killer, second only to cardiovascular disease (Table 1-7). It is responsible for more than one out of every five American deaths—about 500,000 deaths each year, more than 1,300 each day. Someone in the United States dies of cancer almost every minute.

The cancer death rate has risen almost without interruption in the United States (over 200/100,000 currently). Oral cancer accounts for about 9,000 yearly deaths (1.7% of all cancer-caused deaths). The relative survival rate for black patients is lower than that for white patients, and in recent years there does not appear to be an improvement in these figures (Table 1-8). This may be due to socioeconomic disadvantages in the health care system as well as to the known greater prevalence of smoking and alcohol consumption in that population. Table 1-9 shows the estimated incidence of selected cancers by site for 1990, as well as male-female ratios and numbers of patients dying of cancer according to site. Most discouraging is that about half of all oral cancer patients die of their disease and neither earlier detection nor survival has shown improvement during the past decade.

Table 1-7. LEADING CAUSES OF DEATH IN THE UNITED STATES

Rank	Cause of Death	Percentage of Total Deaths*
1	Heart disease	36.4
2	Cancer	22.3
3	Stroke	7.1
4	Lung diseases	6.9
5	Accidents	4.5
6	Diabetes mellitus	1.8
8	Cirrhosis of the liver	1.2
13	AIDS	0.7

*Total number of deaths: 2,105,361 (1986).

Table 1-8. RELATIVE 5-YEAR SURVIVAL RATES, ORAL CAVITY AND PHARYNGEAL CANCER BY RACE*

	1960–1973	1977–1979	1980–1985
Whites	44%	53%	54%
Blacks	—	36%	31%

*Source: *CA: A Cancer Journal for Clinicians*, 40: 26, 1990.

Table 1-9. CANCER IN USA: ESTIMATES FOR SELECTED SITES, 1990*

Site	New Cases	M:F	Deaths
All sites	*1,040,000*†	*1.0*	*520,000*
Lung	155,000	1.9	142,000
Colorectal	151,000	0.9	61,300
Lymphoma	51,800	1.1	27,400
Oral (3.1%)	30,600	2.1	8,650
Leukemia	27,300	1.3	18,100
Larynx	12,300	4.3	3,700

*Source: Data from *CA: A Cancer Journal for Clinicians* 40:18-19, 1989. (Values for selected sites are shown.)
†Carcinoma in situ and non-melanoma skin cancers are not included in totals.

ACQUIRED IMMUNODEFICIENCY SYNDROME

The current epidemic of the acquired immunodeficiency syndrome (AIDS) continues unabated. Hundreds of thousands of AIDS cases have been reported thoughout the world and untold millions of individuals are now infected with the human immunodeficiency virus (HIV). Because infectivity appears to be lifelong with variable and prolonged incubation periods, asymptomatic carriers pose a common and complex problem.

HIV infection has a predilection for the helper-inducer T lymphocytes (T4) which modulate the immune system. As the viruses multiply and reduce the number of T4 lymphocytes, the immunocompromised host becomes susceptible to opportunistic infections and malignancies.

The most common of these malignancies is Kaposi's sarcoma which occurs in more than 15% of all reported AIDS patients and in over 25% of homosexual males with AIDS.[16–19] Lymphomas and carcinomas also occur more frequently than would be expected in a similar segment of the general population. The AIDS epidemic has implications regarding oral cancer because the malignancies associated with HIV infection do occur in the mouth, making diagnosis as well as treatment an important consideration for all health professionals. (See Chapter 8.)

REFERENCES

1. Sven KC, Lau LL, Yermakov V: Cancer and old age. An autopsy study of 3535 patients over 65 years old. *Cancer* 33:1164, 1974.
2. National Cancer Institute: Surveillance, Epidemiology and End Results Program (SEER), 1973–1984. Bethesda, MD (computer tape).
3. Silverman S Jr, Gorsky M, Greenspan D: Oral cancer: Part I. Current trends in the occurrence of oral cancer. *J Dermatol Allergy* 6:26, 1983.
4. Szpak CA, Stone MJ, Frenkel EP: Some observations concerning the demographic and geographic incidence of carcinoma of the lip and buccal cavity. *Cancer* 40:343, 1977.
5. Mahboubi E: The epidemiology of oral cavity, pharyngeal and esophageal cancer outside of North America and Western Europe. *Cancer* 40:1879, 1977.

6. Albert S, Child M: Familial cancer in the general population. *Cancer* 40:1674, 1977.
7. Silverman S Jr, Gorsky M, Greenspan D: Tobacco usage in patients with head and neck carcinomas: A follow-up study on habit changes and second primary oral/oropharyngeal cancers. *J Am Dent Assoc* 106:33, 1983.
8. Fu KK, Lichter A, Galante M: Carcinoma of the floor of the mouth: An analysis of treatment results and the sites and cause of failures. *Int J Radiat Oncol Biol Phys* 1:829, 1976.
9. Fu KK, Ray JW, Chan EK et al: External and interstitial radiation therapy of carcinoma of the oral tongue. *Am J Roentgenol Radium Ther Nucl Med* 126:107, 1976.
10. Wynder EL, Dodo H, Bloch DA et al: Epidemiologic investigation of multiple primary cancer of the upper alimentary and respiratory tracts. I. A retrospective study. *Cancer* 24:730, 1969.
11. Berg JW, Schottenfeld D, Ritter F: Incidence of multiple primary cancers. III. Cancers of the respiratory and upper digestive system as multiple primary cancers. *JNCI* 44:263, 1970.
12. Cahan WB, Castro EB, Rosen PP et al: Separate primary carcinomas of the esophagus and head and neck region in the same patient. *Cancer* 37:85, 1976.
13. Tepperman BS, Fitzpatrick PJ: Second respiratory and upper digestive tract cancers after oral cancer. *Lancet* 2:547, 1981.
14. Newell GR, Krementz ET: Multiple malignant neoplasms in the Charity Hospital of Louisiana Tumor Registry. *Cancer* 40:1812, 1977.
15. Wynder EL, Mushinski MH, Spivak JC: Tobacco and alcohol consumption in relation to the development of multiple primary cancers. *Cancer* 40:1872, 1977.
16. Lozada F, Silverman S Jr, Migliorati CA et al: Oral manifestations of tumor and opportunistic infections in the acquired immunodeficiency syndrome (AIDS): Findings in 53 homosexual men with Kaposi's sarcoma. *Oral Surg* 56:491, 1983.
17. Lozada-Nur F, Silverman S Jr, Migliorati CA et al: The diagnosis of AIDS and AIDS-related complex in the dental office: Findings in 171 homosexual males. *J Calif Dent Assoc* 12:21, 1984.
18. Silverman S Jr: AIDS Update: oral findings, diagnosis, and precautions. *J Am Dent Assoc* 115:559, 1987.
19. Ficarra G, Berson T, Silverman S Jr et al: Kaposi's sarcoma of the oral cavity: A study of 134 patients. *Oral Surg Oral Med Oral Pathol* 66:551, 1988.

2

Etiology and Predisposing Factors

SOL SILVERMAN, JR.
EDWARD J. SHILLITOE · Viruses

The exact cause of oral cancer is unknown. Because time is needed for the cellular events involved in the development of neoplasia to accumulate, the most prominent factor determining susceptibility to cancer is age. Variations in incidence rates among different groups or populations can be explained by differences in exposure to carcinogenic initiators or promoters.[1] For example, the use of tobacco or alcohol significantly increases the risk of cancer, indicating an etiologic role. The role of factors such as immunologic susceptibility and enzyme action in promoting human cancer remains unclear. The known fact is that at a certain time, a cell or group of cells may undergo uncontrolled growth. This capacity for disorderly division continues in daughter cells, producing a malignancy through subsequent spread and destruction of other tissues and organs whose integrity and function are necessary for life. In 20 generations, one cell, whose progeny maintain the ability to duplicate themselves, becomes the source of more than one million cells. However, since some of the cells comprising a malignant tumor do not maintain the ability to divide and generation times vary considerably, growth patterns of tumors are highly irregular and unpredictable.

Humans are exposed continually and simultaneously to a broad spectrum of biological, chemical, and physical forces. To complicate matters even more, each individual reacts somewhat differently to these forces. Everyone's reactions are conditioned by heredity, age, sex, and by a multitude of other factors. If the evidence now in hand suggests one conclusion more strongly than any other, it is that there probably are multiple causes for every type of cancer.

Death rates from around the world (Table 2-1) suggest marked differences in the occurrence of oral cancer which may reflect different combinations of ethnic and environmental factors. Occurrence rates also reflect differences according to geographic location. The data from the National Cancer Institute's SEER Program, 1973–1984, from nine population base areas, indicated the average yearly incidence rate of oral cancer cases for this period in the U.S. was about 11/100,000 population. This incidence rate was exceeded in several countries and was highest in one state in India where the rate was 21/100,000. In Asia, oropharyngeal cancer is the leading cancer in men, and in Africa and Asia it is the third most frequent cancer site in women.

Table 2-1. AGE-ADJUSTED DEATH RATES FOR ORAL CANCER PER 100,000 POPULATION, 1982–83*
(Selected from 50 nations studied)

Area	Males	(Rank)†	Females	(Rank)
France	18.6	(1)	1.6	(20)
Singapore	16.0	(2)	6.9	(1)
Hungary	11.4	(3)	1.6	(20)
Puerto Rico	9.2	(4)	2.0	(10)
Switzerland	8.9	(5)	1.2	(29)
Cuba	8.5	(6)	2.3	(5)
Australia	5.6	(18)	1.7	(17)
Canada	5.6	(18)	1.8	(13)
Ireland	5.6	(18)	1.6	(20)
Germany	5.5	(21)	1.1	(35)
United States	5.3	(22)	1.8	(13)
Kuwait	4.3	(28)	5.0	(2)
Denmark	4.1	(30)	1.7	(17)
England	3.7	(33)	1.6	(20)
Sweden	3.4	(36)	1.2	(29)
Venezuela	3.1	(38)	2.5	(4)
Japan	2.5	(43)	0.9	(42)
Greece	2.3	(46)	0.7	(46)
Mexico	2.2	(47)	0.9	(42)
Israel	2.1	(48)	1.1	(35)

*Source: *CA: A Cancer Journal for Clinicians,* 38: 14–15, 1988.
†Rank = relative ranking.

THE IMMUNE SYSTEM

Immune competence and immune cell surveillance diminish with age. This fact undoubtedly contributes to the association between age and malignancy. Furthermore, studies have shown that there are increased risks of cancer developing in individuals whose immune systems are either congenitally defective or have been suppressed by chemotherapy for various diseases. The association between increased cancer occurrence and immunosuppression has been demonstrated dramatically in the acquired immunodeficiency syndrome (AIDS). In AIDS patients, there has been a high frequency of oral Kaposi's sarcoma, as well as a higher-than-expected occurrence of oral squamous carcinoma (see Chapter 9). However, for persons in the general population who develop oral cancers and who are not otherwise known to have or be at risk of immunodeficiency, it is not clear whether differences found in some immunologic variables are a result or a cause of the malignancy.[2,3] The role of cellular transforming genes, or oncogenes, at this time remains unclear for human cancers.[4]

TOBACCO

Smoking may be viewed as a worldwide epidemic, causing serious diseases and immense health problems. Apart from its effect on mortality, smoking results in a considerably increased morbidity rate with consequent losses in working days and productivity, excessive demand on medical services, and increased health expenditures.

Tobacco was first introduced to Western civilization by the Spanish explorers of America in the early 16th century. At first it was simply smoked in pipes, but as it became more popular it was also chewed and snuffed. Cigarettes were first made in Spain in the mid-17th century, and in the 20th century they became the most popular form of the tobacco habit. Cigars were introduced at the beginning of the 19th century.

Suspicion of an association between the use of tobacco and oral cancer dates back to the early 18th century when cancer of the lip was noted among tobacco users. Several other serious diseases, among them lung cancer, emphysema, bronchitis, laryngeal cancer, and heart disease, affect smokers more often than nonsmokers. For heavier smokers, the risks are greatest.

TOBACCO COMPONENTS

Thousands of substances have been identified in tobacco. In the combustion mainstream of one cigarette, there are approximately 500 mg of gas (92%) and particulate matter (8%). Eighty-five percent of the gaseous phase is carbon dioxide, oxygen, and nitrogen. Even though the percentage of carbon monoxide is low, it is enough to raise blood levels of this gas significantly, in turn influencing the hemoglobin exchange system. "Tars" (aromatic hydrocarbons) range from less than 1 to 35 mg. The most potent carcinogens are in this group of compounds. Nicotine, which contributes to habituation, platelet adhesion associated with cardiovascular disease, ulcer susceptibility from decreased pancreatic bicarbonate, and hypertension, ranges from less than 1 to 3 mg.[5] Effective filtering can reduce these substances.[6] However, reductions in nicotine (the habituation factor) and tars (the basis for tobacco "taste") often lead to increased smoking, negating the potential advantage. In addition, many filters do not effectively "filter." Tobacco substitutes (i.e., vegetable and wood products) and "smokeless" cigarettes have not been popular and have therefore been financial as well as therapeutic failures.

TOBACCO USE AND HEALTH

Reports from the U.S. Surgeon General and others[7–9] conclude that cigarette smoking is the main single cause of cancer mortality in the United States, contributing to an estimated 30% of all cancer deaths and substantially to cancers of the head and neck. A federal law requires that one of the following four warnings be printed in rotation on all cigarette packages sold in the U.S.:

"Surgeon General's Warning: Smoking causes lung cancer, heart disease, emphysema and may complicate pregnancy.

"Surgeon General's Warning: Quitting smoking now greatly reduces risk to your health.

"Surgeons General's Warning: Smoking by pregnant women may result in fetal injury, premature birth, and low birth weight.

"Surgeon General's Warning: Cigarette smoke contains carbon monoxide."

Despite intensified warnings about the health hazards of smoking, American consumption continues at substantial rates, exceeding 600 billion cigarettes annually. Approximately 43 million Americans have quit smoking, however, most of these are older persons, and the habit among persons in the younger age group continues to be a problem.

About 30% of adult Americans smoke regularly (Table 2-2). Although smoking habits tend to decrease after middle age, smoking among school children is consistently increasing. A recent federal report describing smoking trends among Americans aged 12 to 18 years indicated that 19% of both the boys and the girls smoked regularly. The percentage of dentists and physicians who smoke has dropped from more than 30% to about 20% during the past two decades.

Table 2-2. SMOKERS, USA, 1988: PERCENTAGE OF PERSONS WHO SMOKE REGULARLY ACCORDING TO SEX AND AGE*

	Adults (%)	Under 18 (%)
Males	33	15
Females	28	21
Mean	30	19

*Source: Statistical data from U.S. Center for Disease Control, Atlanta, GA.

CANCER RISK AND SMOKING

The association between cigarette use and oral carcinoma appears to have been established from epidemiologic studies[10–12] revealing that there are more than twice as many smokers among oral cancer patients as among control populations. A study of oral cancer patients at the University of California, San Francisco (UCSF), found that more than eight out of ten of them were smokers (Table 2-3), demonstrating the very high risk for tobacco users[13] In addition, the smoker who has oral cancer has been found, on the average, to be a much heavier user of tobacco than the smoker who does not have cancer.

Numerous laboratory studies have shown that some hydrocarbons isolated from tobacco products have induced buccal carcinomas in animals under certain experimental conditions. Benzo(a)pyrene, the most potent of these carcinogens, binds to nucleoproteins and is mutagenic as well as carcinogenic. The association between tobacco use and oral malignancies also appears to include cigars, pipes, and chewing preparations.

Certain enzymes can metabolize tobacco hydrocarbons into more potent carcinogenic forms. Aryl hydrocarbon hydroxylase (AHH), an enzyme produced principally in human leukocytes in varying amounts, increases the carcinogenicity of benzo(a)pyrene.[14] Therefore, smokers who produce large amounts of this enzyme may have a very high risk of developing malignancies in "tobacco zone" sites. These findings indicate that persons likely to develop cancer if they smoke might be identified prospectively.[15]

At the University of California, San Francisco, the pretreatment tobacco habits of patients with oral carcinoma were analyzed in order to assess the relationships between tobacco use and the oral cancer site (Table 2-3). Another study at UCSF on 277 patients with head and neck carcinomas was carried out to assess the association between tobacco usage and the development of second primary oropharyngeal multiple carcinomas (Table 2-4). Almost 68 percent had smoked. This rate of smoking is more than double the current rate found in the general population and indicates that, for cigarette smokers, the risk of developing oral carcinoma exceeds about five times that for nonsmokers.

In almost one in five patients (17.7%) second primary oral/oropharyngeal cancers developed in a mean time of five years. Those who did not change their original tobacco habits incurred the greatest risk, as a second primary cancer developed in 25.6% of that group. Discontinuing smoking appeared to have the same beneficial effect as found in nonsmokers. There was also an increased risk for multiple cancers in males, probably because they smoked more per day than women.

A similar degree of correlation between smoking and second primaries has been reported in other studies.[16–18] One concerned a group of 203 oral and laryngopharyngeal cancer patients in whom the disease had been eradicated for more than three years.[16] Of 120 patients who continued to smoke, 37% developed second primary cancers, while only 6% of 81 ex-smokers developed second primaries.

Table 2-3. NUMBER OF TOBACCO USERS AMONG ORAL CANCER PATIENTS TREATED AT THE UNIVERSITY OF CALIFORNIA, SAN FRANCISCO*

Cancer Site	No. Patients	Percentage Smokers
Soft palate	26	96
Floor of mouth	127	90
Oropharynx	73	85
Tongue	163	82
Buccal mucosa	26	69
Gingiva, alveolar mucosa	42	67
Lip	19	63
Hard palate	11	55
Total	487	82

*Data from Silverman, Gorsky and Greenspan, 1983.[13]

Table 2-4. SMOKING HABITS AMONG 277 ORAL CANCER PATIENTS, ORAL MEDICINE CLINIC, UNIVERSITY OF CALIFORNIA, SAN FRANCISCO, 1989*

Smoking Status			Cancer Status
Tobacco Usage	At Time of Cancer Diagnosis	One Yr. Post Treatment	Second Primary Oropharyngeal Cancer†
Yes	187 (67.5%)	90 (48%)	23 (25.6%)
Discontinued		97 (52%)	13 (13.4%)
No‡	90 (32.5%)	90 (100%)	13 (14.4%)

*Source: Unpublished data, Oral Medicine Clinic, University of California, San Francisco.
†Follow-up mean = 5 years.
‡Never smoked or stopped > 1 year.

The combined effects of tobacco and alcohol were illustrated in another study of 351 patients treated for tongue cancer.[17] Forty-three patients abstained from both tobacco and alcohol, and 308 were users of either or both. The abstainers had a mortality of 14% in five years; the users, 31%. A second primary occurred in 11% of the abstainers, as compared with 20% of the users.

PIPES, CIGARS, SNUFF, AND CHEWING TOBACCO

Carcinogenic agents have been isolated from pipe, cigar, and smokeless tobaccos. Although studies of these forms of tobacco use have not been as extensive as those of cigarettes, the data show a strong association between non-cigarette forms of tobacco and mouth cancer.[19] The Surgeon General's report of 1964 concluded that "the causal relationship of the smoking of pipes to the development of cancer of the lip appears to be established" (Fig. 2-1). Fortunately, the incidence of lip cancer has been declining slowly. Interestingly, the production and consumption of small and large cigars as well as pipe tobacco have decreased slightly since 1976.

The carcinogenic hazard of snuff dipping and tobacco chewing is of special concern because of the marked up-

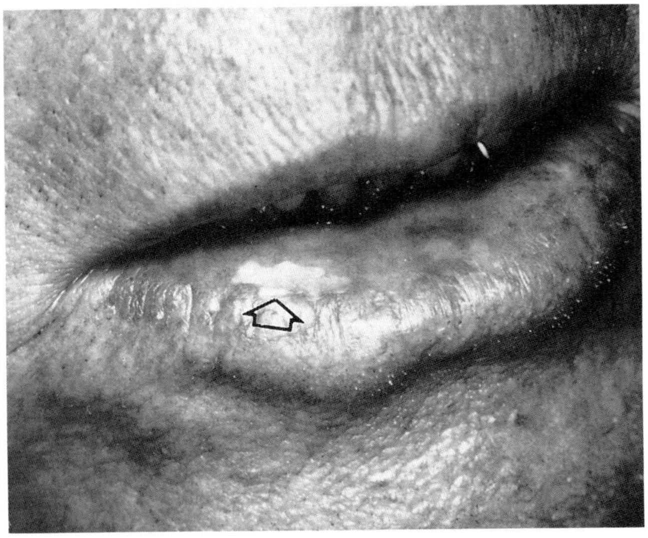

A

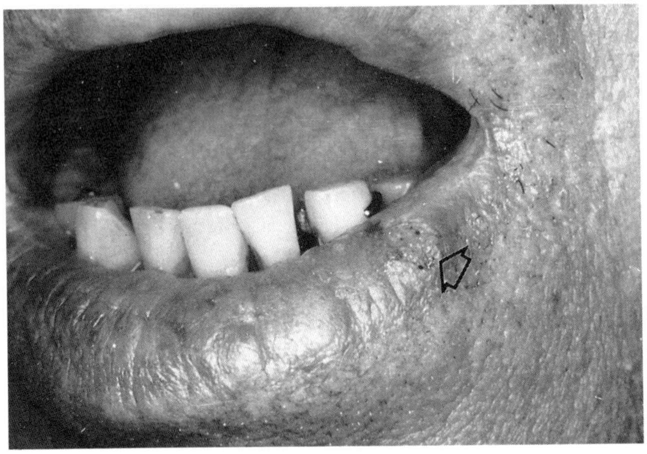

B

Fig. 2-1. Relationship between pipe smoking and lip cancer. **A**, Precancerous leukoplakic lesion (arrow) at site of chronic contact with pipe stem. **B**, Early squamous carcinoma (arrow) at site where pipe stem was habitually held for more than 10 years.

swing of smokeless tobacco consumption in the United States.[20–26] It has been estimated that over 12 million Americans (3 million under age 21) use smokeless tobacco. Its use among teenagers is increasing and poses a danger for increased oral cancer in the future (Fig. 2-2). In the southeastern United States, where women frequently use snuff or chewing tobacco, there is a higher-than-expected incidence of oral cancer in women together with a higher mortality.[27] A case-control study in North Carolina of 255 women with oral and oropharyngeal cancer showed an up to fiftyfold risk for cancers of the gingiva and buccal mucosa in long-term habitual snuff dippers.[28] A report on 201 oral cancer patients at M.D. Anderson Hospital in Texas showed that 46 (23%) used snuff or chewing tobacco. Twenty of these patients reported that, for an average of 44 years, they had consistently held the tobacco at the site where the cancer arose.

Nitrosamines (nitrosonornicotine being the most potent) have been identified as noncombustible products in snuff and chewing tobacco that possess carcinogenic activity. Other carcinogens are found in smaller quantities (hydrocarbons and polonium). Of interest, tobacco products are not regulated by the Food and Drug Administration and the nitrosamine levels far exceed those permitted in foods (as preservatives). Both sugar and fluoride contents are higher in chewing tobacco than in other forms of tobacco.[29] However, a relationship between different tobacco forms and dental caries has not been established. Nicotine levels are high and serve as a potent factor in habituation, addiction, and hypertension. Since smokeless tobaccos contain salt, this also contributes to high blood pressure. The most common conditions found are gingival recession, hyperkeratosis, and staining. In addition, the risk of oral epithelial dysplasia or carcinoma increases with long-term usage of smokeless tobacco products.

SMOKING AND SURVIVAL

The hazards of smoking can also be demonstrated by the survival time of oral cancer patients after diagnosis and treatment. In a University of California, San Francisco, study of 874 patients with intraoral squamous carcinoma, the five-year survival rate for nonsmokers was 43%, compared with 27% for smokers.[30] In the study of 203 oral and laryngopharyngeal cancer patients cited earlier,[16] 65% of the nonsmokers were alive at the end of 13 years, while only 30% of the smokers survived the same period.

SMOKING CESSATION

Since tobacco plays such an important role in oral carcinogenesis, stopping the habit is a fundamental part of treatment.[31,32] Following are some approaches.

Fear. While fear motivates some people to stop smoking, in others it may backfire and even increase tobacco use.

Drugs. Drugs have been used as tobacco substitutes or dissuaders, and the use of tranquilizers and sedative-hypnotic drugs has also been studied. None of these approaches has reproducibly or significantly helped. Studies have suggested the potential benefits of a nicotine-containing chewing gum (Nicorette) in helping people to stop smoking.[33–35] Each stick of this gum contains 2 mg nicotine, the habituating factor in tobacco, and it has no pathologic effect on oral mucosa, gingiva, or teeth. Many individuals find this gum unacceptable, and long-term effects are not clear.

Filters. Apparently, as filters become more effective in reducing "tar" and nicotine, their effectiveness in breaking the tobacco habit decreases.[36] This points out the importance of taste and habituation, which are related to tar and nicotine content.

Aversive conditioning. Methods to make tobacco smoking or taste objectionable, such as chemical additives, electric shock, and hypnosis, have not been reproducibly effective. Clinics, organized groups, self-help methods, and manuals have helped some persons and are promoted widely. Studies have not yet convincingly documented their long-term value.

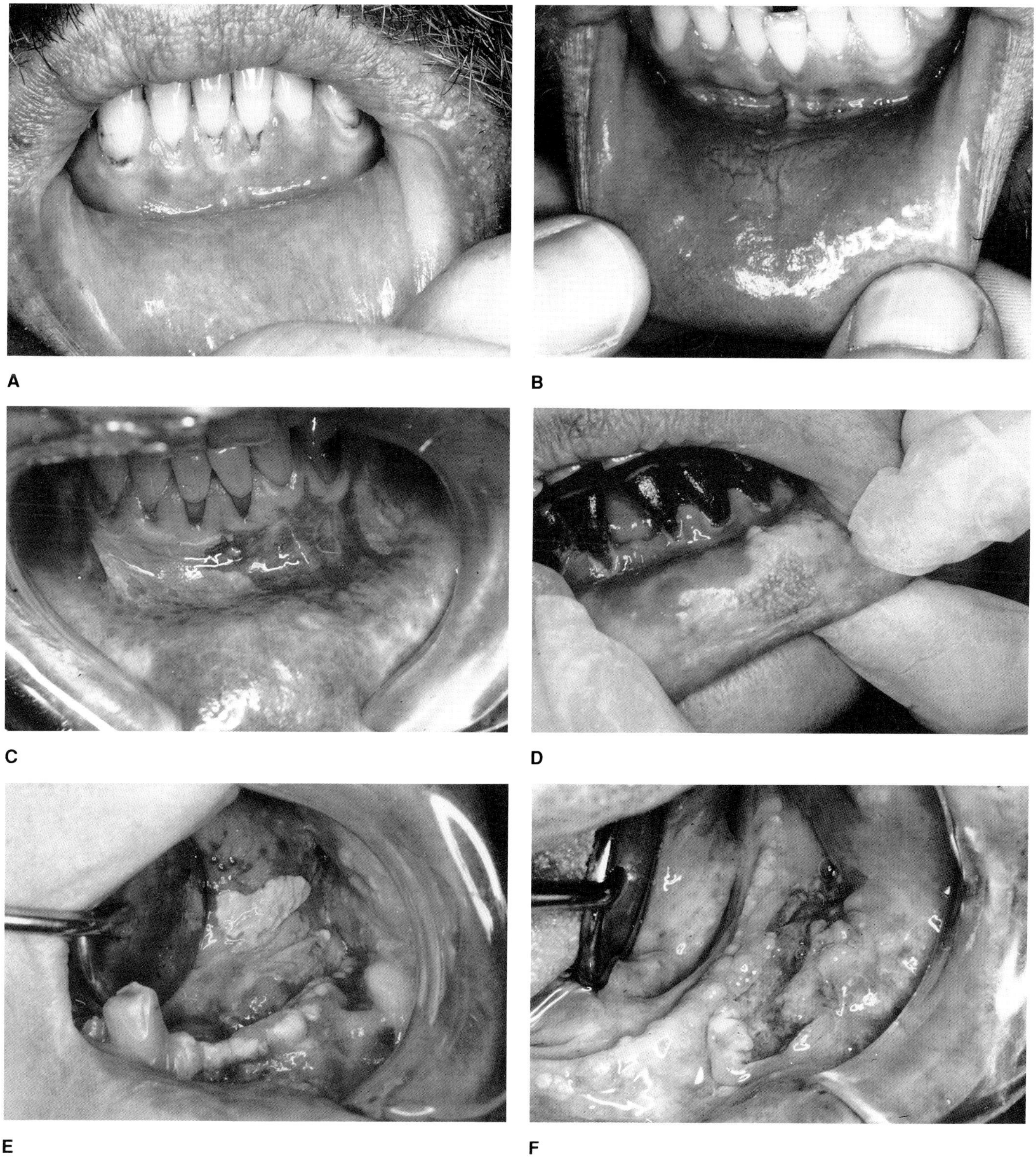

Fig. 2-2. Tissue changes caused by prolonged contact with tobacco. **A,** Gingival recession and loss of attachment are common early changes at sites where smokeless tobacco is held. **B,** Patient habitually held tobacco at this site for more than 5 years. **C,** Patient held tobacco between lower lip and gingiva for more than 5 years, inducing this erythroleukoplakic mucosal lesion. **D,** Leukoplakia of the lower labial mucosa at site where patient held tobacco during a 27-year habit. There was microscopic epithelial dysplasia and intense dental staining. **E,** Leukoplakia in a 60-year-old woman at the site where smokeless tobacco was used habitually for more than 30 years. A biopsy from the floor of mouth showed early invasive squamous carcinoma. **F,** Squamous carcinoma at site where tobacco was habitually held for more than 30 years.

"Cold Turkey." Stopping abruptly rather than gradually has been successful for some patients who are well motivated and can effectively assign priorities to their life-style and goals.

Advertising regulations and legislation. These approaches have been ineffective in stemming the increasing consumption of tobacco and habituation at an early age. However, taxation and the increased cost of smoking seem to have some influence.

OTHER CARCINOGENIC HABIT FORMS

Social customs that can lead to cancer are complex and far-reaching. Some customs, such as betel- and tobacco-dipping, are widespread and seem to satisfy important human desires. In the areas of the world where these habits are practiced, the incidence of oropharyngeal tumors is comparatively high. There are considerable variations in prevalence in different countries, depending upon the manner in which the ingredients are prepared for chewing.

Reports from India[37] reveal that oral carcinoma accounts for a high percentage of total cancers, ranging from 15% to 65%. A relationship appears to exist between this extremely high occurrence of oral malignancy and the use of various forms and combinations of tobacco, slaked lime, betel nuts, and spices (Fig. 2-3).

In many areas throughout the world, members of the low economic groups smoke rolled tobacco leaves or small cigars with the lit end placed in the mouth (Fig. 2-4). In some of these areas the incidence of palatal carcinoma is high.[38]

PRECANCEROUS LESIONS

It is well recognized that tobacco may induce benign clinical changes of the oral mucosa (Fig. 2-5). Mucosal changes in the form of red and white lesions are considered premalignant since they may unpredictably transform into malignancies (see below, **Leukoplakia and Erythroplasia**). However, it must be remembered that not all oral cancers are preceded by clinical precancerous lesions.

SUMMARY

In conclusion, the use of tobacco in all forms—cigarettes, cigars, pipes, chewing preparations, and snuff—increases the risk of eventually developing oral carcinoma which appears to be causally related. This is based on the following facts:

1. Carcinogenic agents have been isolated from tobacco condensates.
2. Tobacco can induce cellular change and tissue atypia (Fig. 2-6).
3. There is a greater use of tobacco among patients with oral carcinoma than among persons in control groups.
4. Tobacco used in various forms has been associated with an unusually high prevalence of carcinoma of specific oral sites.
5. Continued smoking is a factor in the development of multiple oral carcinomas.
6. There is an increased mortality ratio from oral carcinoma for smokers as compared with nonsmokers.

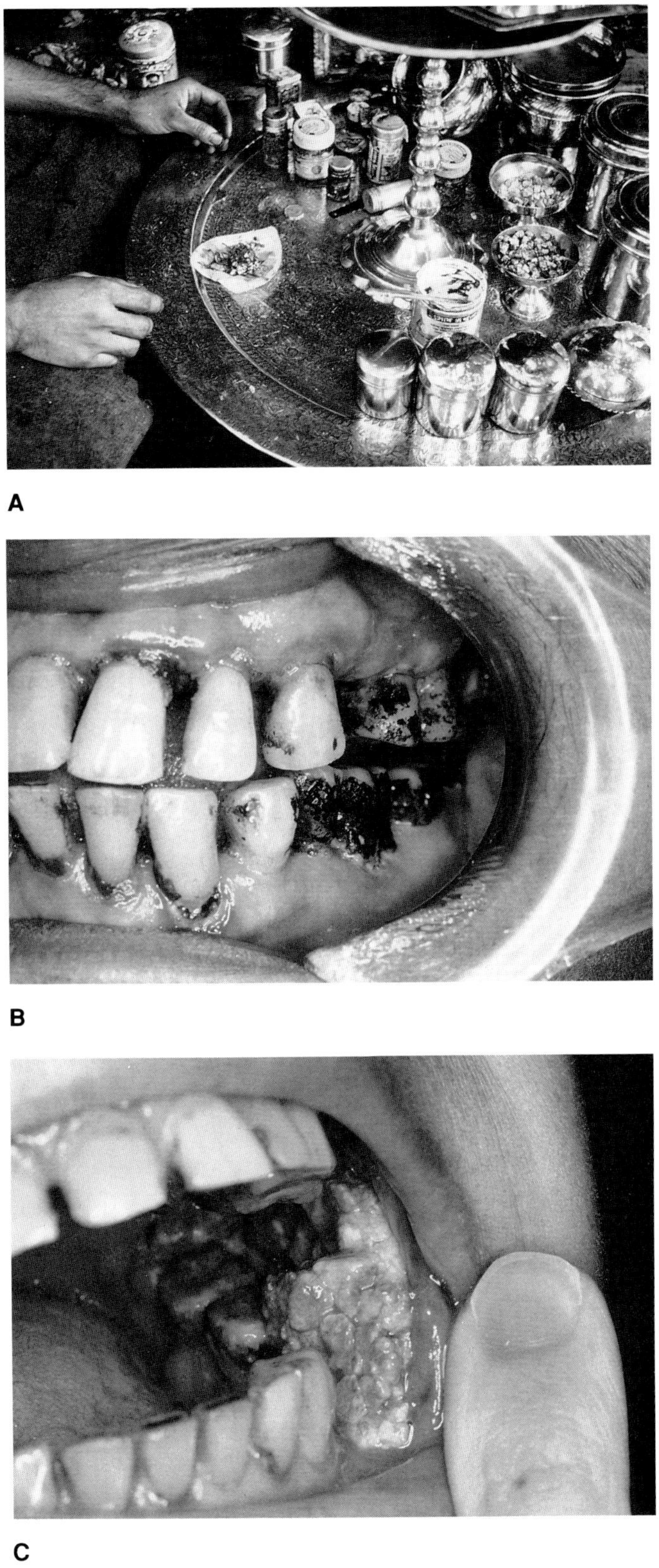

Fig. 2-3. Pan habit in India. **A,** Varying ingredients, including tobacco, areca (betel) nut, lime, and spices are placed in the betel leaf to be folded and held in the mouth for prolonged periods of time. **B,** Note usual tooth staining which is the result of the use of pan. **C,** After prolonged usage, the risk increases for squamous carcinoma to develop at the habit site.

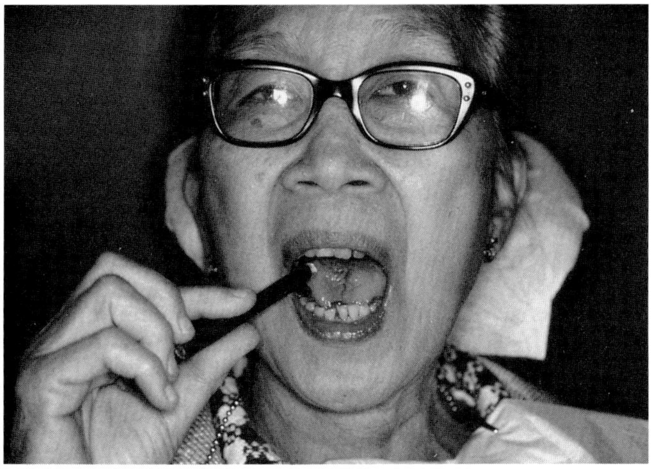

A

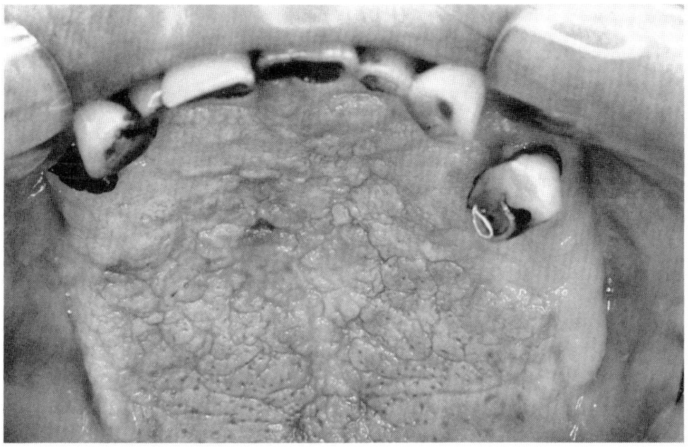

B

Fig. 2-4. Reverse smoking habit of many decades duration. **A,** Lit end of cigarillo is held inside the mouth. **B,** The palatal leukoplakia is mildly symptomatic. Risk for dysplastic and malignant changes are moderately high.

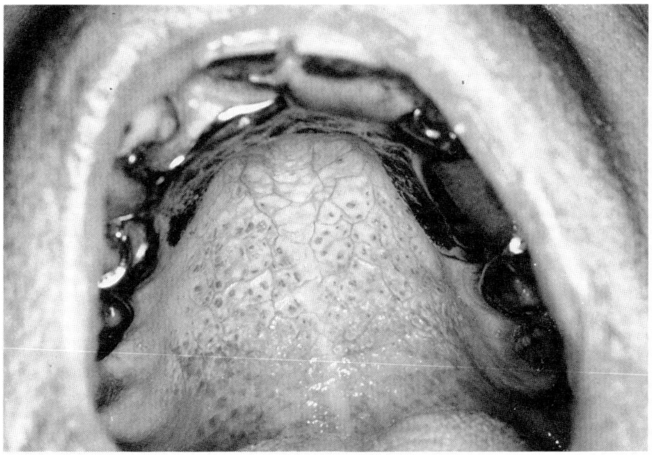

Fig. 2-5. Smoker's palate (nicotinic stomatitis), primarily seen in pipe smokers. Typical clinical picture includes hyperkeratosis and swollen minor salivary glands with dilated and reddened orifices (giving the speckled appearance). Malignant transformation is very rare.

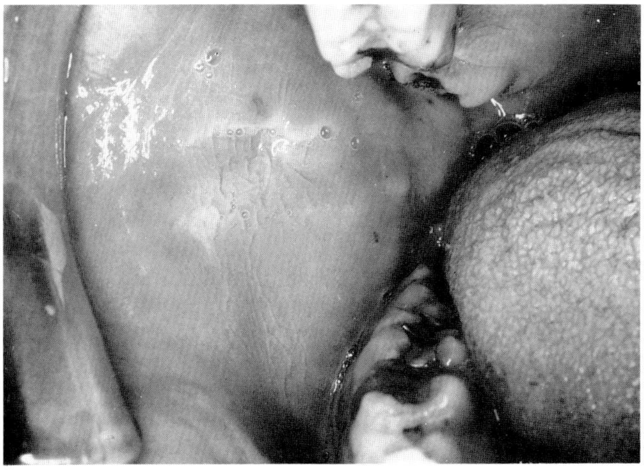

A

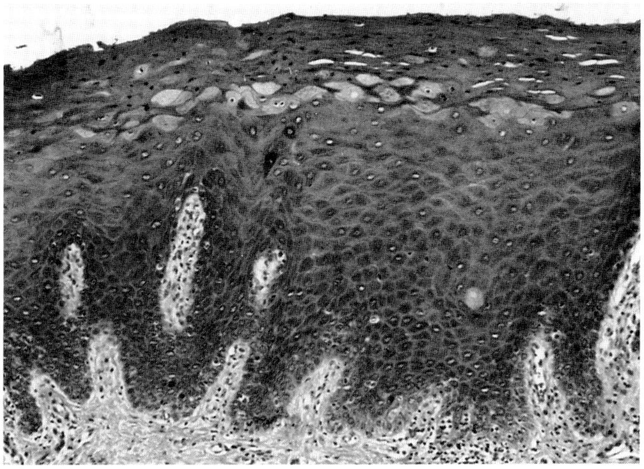

B

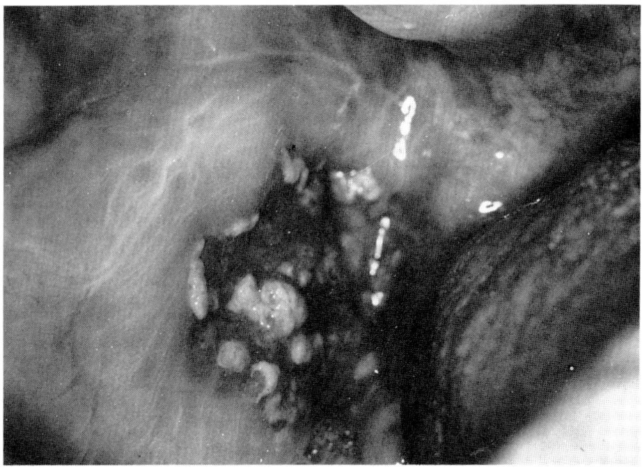

C

Fig. 2-6. Leukoedema, a tissue change usually seen on buccal mucosa in response to tobacco irritation. **A,** Mucosa appears boggy and coated with a thin, whitish film. **B,** Microscopic examination shows typical hyperparakeratosis, hyperplasia, and vacuolization. **C,** Leukoedema and associated squamous carcinoma. The precancerous nature of leukoedema has not been established.

ALCOHOL AND CIRRHOSIS

Death from cirrhosis (primarily due to alcohol intake) is the eighth leading cause of death in the United States. This high incidence of alcoholism is significant because alcohol intake has been related to an increased risk of developing oral cancer[12] and a higher-than-expected mortality.[39]

More than 30 years ago, a study determined heavy alcohol consumption to be a significant factor in the development of mouth cancer.[40] It was found that of 543 male oral cancer patients, one third drank more than 7 ounces of whiskey per day, as compared with 12% of a control group.

The association between alcoholism and oral and laryngeal cancer was further affirmed in a study showing a large excess mortality (observed-expected ratio more than 3:1) in a group of alcoholics with oropharyngeal carcinoma.[41] A report from Utah, a state whose population is approximately 72% Mormon (a religious group abstaining from alcohol and tobacco), indicated an incidence of oropharyngeal cancer less than that of the western United States or the nation as a whole.[42]

One group of investigators found that 44% of 108 patients with cancer of the tongue and 59% of 68 patients with cancer of the floor of the mouth, palate, or tonsillar fossa had unequivocal evidence of hepatic cirrhosis.[43] Approximately 75% drank alcohol excessively. Another investigator, studying 2,177 male oral cancer patients, found no relationship between liver cirrhosis and tongue cancer; however, he did find an association between cancer of the floor of the mouth and cirrhosis.[44] In an additional study of 408 oral cancer patients with age-matched controls, he confirmed the correlation of cirrhosis of the liver with cancer of the floor of the mouth in finding clinically diagnosed liver cirrhosis in 20% of the cases of floor-of-mouth carcinoma in contrast to 9% of controls.[45] He concluded that liver cirrhosis, heavy drinking, and smoking were associated with cancer of the floor of the mouth.

Of 213 patients studied at the University of California for whom the information was available, 41 (19%) had laboratory-diagnosed cirrhosis and an additional 26 (12%) demonstrated clinical cirrhotic changes.[30] In the 41 patients with diagnosed cirrhosis, 40% had carcinoma of the tongue (only slightly more than the distribution of tongue cancer in the entire group), but 46% had floor-of-mouth carcinoma (significantly higher than the rate in the entire group). In patients with cancer of the floor of the mouth (information available for 54 patients), 35% had cirrhosis.

The underlying mechanisms for this association are poorly understood.[46] The cause might be related to the dehydrating effects of alcohol (rendering the mucosa more susceptible to carcinogens), to carcinogens contained in alcoholic beverages (nitrosamines, hydrocarbons), or to liver-induced cellular changes in target tissues (e.g., increased acetaldehyde content). Experiments in animals have confirmed the clinical association between alcohol ingestion and tumorigenesis.[47]

Patients with liver cirrhosis often demonstrate what appear to be smooth, erythematous, glossy-appearing oral mucosae (atrophic mucous membranes). Interestingly, in the past, patients with Plummer-Vinson syndrome (atrophic-appearing oral mucous membranes, dysphagia, and iron deficiency anemia) had a high incidence of carcinoma of the tongue and pharynx.

It should be pointed out that most heavy drinkers are also smokers, and many of the predisposing factors may work in combination rather than independently. Several studies confirm an independent and synergistic relationship between oral cancer and consumption of tobacco and alcohol.[10,12,39,48–50] Another study has shown the risk of developing head and neck cancer for heavy consumers of alcohol is increased almost tenfold with the heavy use of tobacco.[18]

No oral cancer risk associations have been found in individuals who are regular users of mouth rinses containing alcohol.

LEUKOPLAKIA AND ERYTHROPLASIA

White and red lesions of the oral mucosa are the most common precancerous clinical lesions. Although not all oral cancers are preceded by premalignant mucosal changes, such changes give a warning of risk and present an opportunity for preventive measures. Early cancer can even appear as an innocuous white or red lesion. Although white changes (leukoplakia) are the most common premalignant lesion, red changes (erythroplasia) or white changes with a red component (speckled leukoplakia, erythroleukoplakia) carry a greater risk.

LEUKOPLAKIA

The term "leukoplakia" is used to designate a clinical white patch or plaque on the oral mucous membranes that cannot be removed by scraping and cannot be classified clinically or microscopically as another disease entity (Fig. 2-7). Most of these lesions, which can occur in all areas of the oral cavity, are reflections of benign hyperkeratosis (Fig. 2-8). Although tobacco or trauma may induce hyperkeratosis, causes for the occurrence of many leukoplakias are unknown (Fig. 2-9).

Epidemiology of Leukoplakia

The age range and the tobacco habits of patients with oral leukoplakia are similar to those of patients with oral carcinoma. These facts indicate possible biologic similarities and comparable risks. The relationship of tobacco to the causation of leukoplakia is not always clear since abstinence from tobacco may not lead to remission of the lesion and some patients with leukoplakia are nonsmokers.

The prevalence of oral leukoplakia in the general population is unknown. Prevalence studies have been attempted in certain parts of the world, but the results are variable and do not support any generalizations as to rates. In a Minnesota study of 27,443 adults, the occurrence of leukoplakia was found to be 0.1%[51], yet in a study of more than 180,000 army recruits, ranging in age from 17 to 26 years, 1.5% had oral leukoplakia.[52] A study of 51,000 villagers in India found that the prevalence rates in four states ranged from 0.2% to 5%.[53] A study from Ahmedabad, India indicated that in a selected population consisting of 57,518 textile mill workers (a low socioeconomic class) over 35 years of age, the occurrence of leukoplakia was close to 12%.[54]

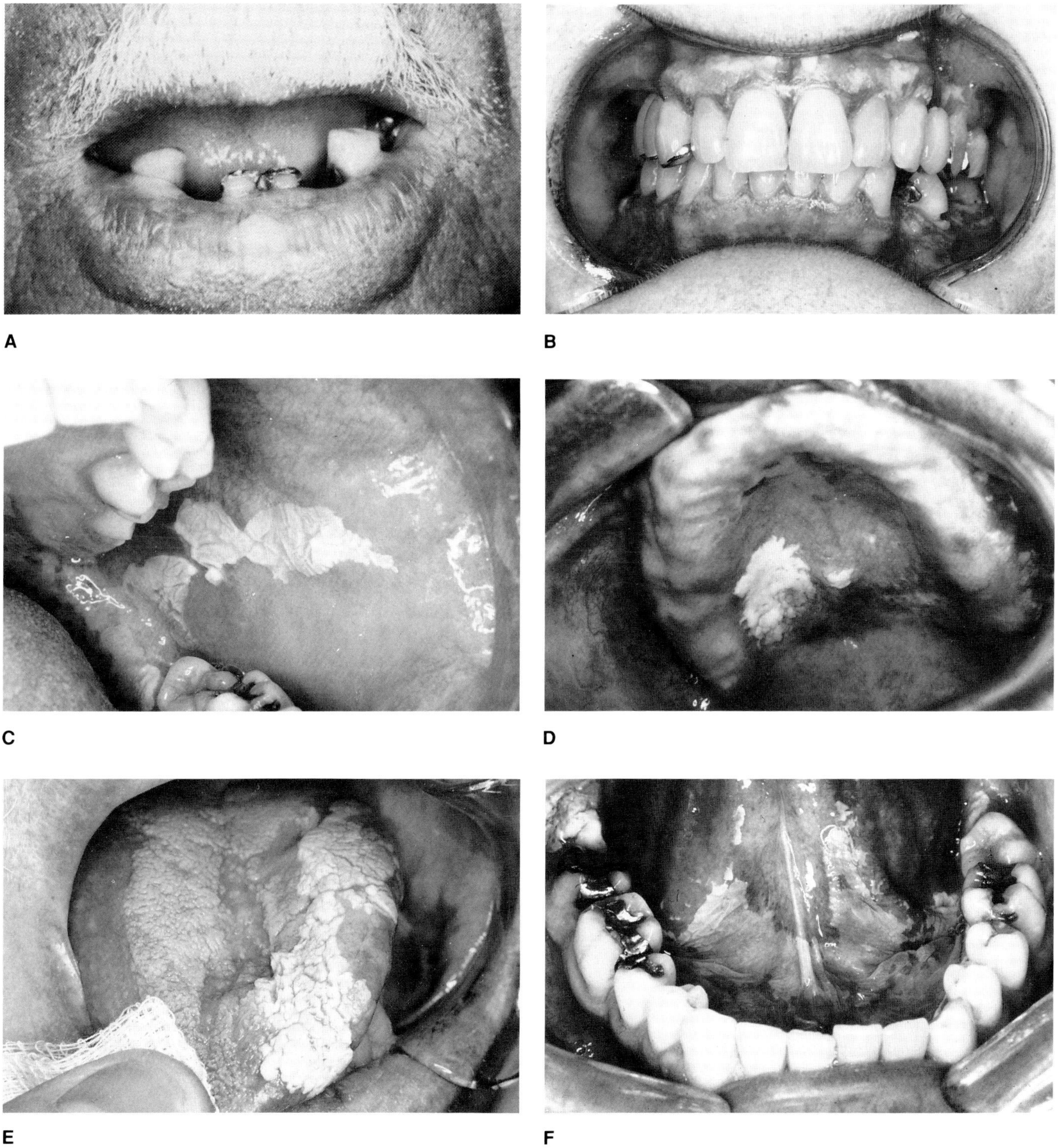

Fig. 2-7. Clinical appearance of leukoplakia in various oral sites. **A,** Lower lip. **B,** Gingiva. **C,** Buccal mucosa. **D,** Palate and alveolar mucosa. **E,** Tongue. **F,** Floor of mouth.

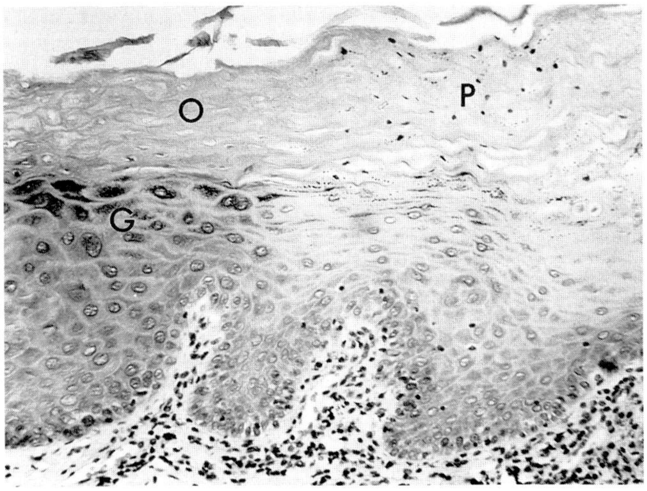

Fig. 2-8. Section from buccal leukoplakia revealing marked hyperkeratosis (O = orthokeratosis, P = parakeratosis). Note increased granular layer (G) associated with orthokeratosis.

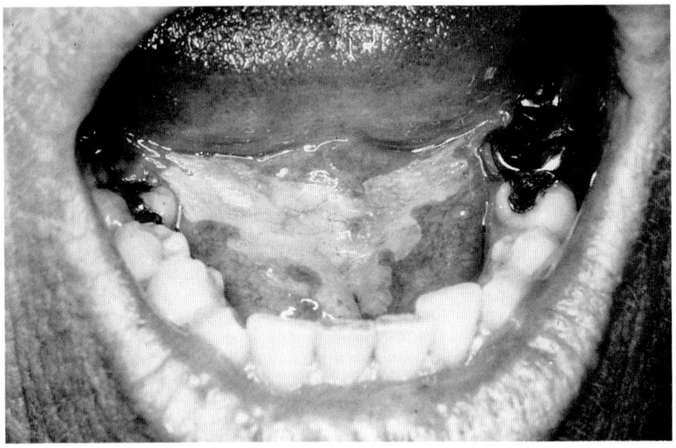

A

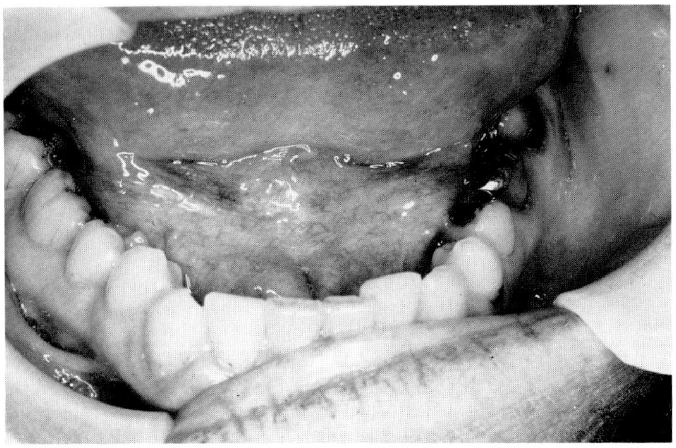

B

Fig. 2-9. Tobacco-induced leukoplakia. **A,** Leukoplakia followed for 20 years in a woman who smoked two packages of cigarettes daily. **B,** After 1 year of abstinence and without any other changes, the leukoplakia slowly attained complete remission.

Precancerous Classification

Oral leukoplakia is a premalignant lesion.[55–66] This conclusion is based on the findings that (1) a large number of oral carcinomas have been associated with leukoplakic changes (Tables 2-5 and 2-6), and (2) there has been a significant occurrence of malignant transformations in oral leukoplakias observed over a period of time (Table 2-7, Figs. 2-10, 2-11).

Table 2-5. LEUKOPLAKIA ASSOCIATED WITH CARCINOMA*

Site of Carcinoma	Total No. Patients	No. (%) Patients with Leukoplakia
Buccal mucosa	35	8 (23)
Gingiva, alveolar mucosa	43	9 (21)
Lip	24	38 (15)
Tongue	261	37 (14)
Floor of mouth	126	17 (13)
Oropharynx, palate	160	18 (11)
Total	874	127 (15)

*Data from Chierici, Silverman and Forsythe, 1968.[30]

Table 2-6. MALIGNANCIES AMD PREMALIGNANT CHANGES FOUND IN BIOPSY SPECIMENS CLINICALLY DIAGNOSED AS LEUKOPLAKIA

Source (Country) Year	No. Patients	Frequency of Malignancy or Premalignant Changes
Pindborg (Denmark) 196355	185	3% carcinoma 12% dysplasia
Silverman (USA) 1968[58]	117	10% carcinoma
Waldron (USA) 1975[73]	3,256	3% carcinoma 17% dysplasia
Banoczy (Hungary) 1976[70]	500	10% carcinoma 24% dysplasia

Tobacco, Leukoplakia, Carcinoma

Tobacco usage increases the risk for individuals to develop oral cancer. Paradoxically, in patients with oral leukoplakia, nonsmokers are at higher risk. This was shown in a study of patients from the UCSF Oral Medicine Clinic (Table 2-8) and in a previous report,[58] and has also been reported by others. Einhorn and Wersall[56] cited an eightfold risk and Roed-Petersen[67] a fivefold risk for nonsmoking leukoplakic patients to develop a carcinoma. Although an explanation for this finding is not clear, it might be speculated that in the absence of tobacco as a causative irritant, there may be a more lethal initiating or potentiating factor. Banoczy confirms this increased risk in nonsmokers in her long-term reports on leukoplakic patients.[62]

Table 2-7. MALIGNANT TRANSFORMATION IN ORAL LEUKOPLAKIAS OBSERVED OVER A PERIOD OF TIME*

Source (Country) Year	No. Patients	Malignant Transformation (%)	Observation Period Years	(mean)
Silverman (Gujarat, India) 1976[54]	4762	0.13	2	
Gupta (Bhavnagar, India) 1980[63]	360	0.3	1-10	(7)
Gupta (Ernakulan, India) 1980[63]	410	2.2	1-10	(7)
Roed-Petersen (Denmark) 1971[67]	331	3.6	>1	(4.3)
Einhorn (Sweden) 1967[56]	782	4.0	1-20	
Pindborg (Denmark) 1968[57]	248	4.4	1-9	
Kramer (England) 1969[59]	187	4.8	1-16	
Banoczy (Hungary) 1977[62]	670	5.9	1-30	(9.8)
Silverman (USA) 1968[58]	117	6.0	1-11	(3.5)
Silverman (USA) 1984[64]	257	17.5	1-39	(7.2)

*Number of transformations varied according to selection of patients and duration of observation. A larger number of patients with leukoplakic lesions, selected at random and followed up over a longer period of time, would be necessary to determine a transformation rate in a given population.

Table 2-8. ASSOCIATION BETWEEN TOBACCO HABITS AND FOLLOW-UP CHANGES IN LEUKOPLAKIA IN 257 UNTREATED PATIENTS*†

No. Patients	Tobacco Use‡ At Diagnosis	Tobacco Use‡ After Diagnosis	Leukoplakia Unchanged or Extended (%)	Leukoplakia Improved or Disappeared (%)	Leukoplakia Transformed to Carcinoma (%)
74	–	–	73	3	24
133	+	+	47	37	16
50	+	–	44	44	12

*Data from Silverman, Gorsky and Lozada, 1984.[64]
†Mean follow-up time 7.2 years.
‡+ = Current tobacco users.
– = Never smoked or stopped permanently at time of diagnosis.

Dynamic Nature of Oral Leukoplakia

The precancerous nature of oral leukoplakia was confirmed in a two-year follow-up study of 4,762 persons with oral leukoplakia residing in Gujarat, India.[54] Although essentially there was no change in habits in the persons with oral leukoplakia during the two-year interval, almost one third experienced complete regression of their lesions.

The prevalence rates for oral leukoplakia in the entire Gujarat study group at the beginning and end of the two-year period were similar, 11.7% and 12.0% respectively. This indicates that development and regression rates were comparable, so that the occurrence of oral leukoplakia in this population was relatively constant. The incidence was 2.6% per year. Since others have found incidences of complete regression in oral leukoplakia in different Indian population groups ranging from 26.4% to 45.3% in five-year intervals[60,68], this remission phenomenon appears to be real. Similarly, a Danish study found that 37.4% of 214 leukoplakic lesions were totally or partially reversed without any intervention during a follow-up period that ranged up to 15 years,[57] and a study of 520 Hungarian patients with oral leukoplakia observed from one to 25 years found regressive changes in 9%.[61]

Dysplasia and Oral Carcinoma

Some clinical leukoplakias demonstrate microscopic cellular changes that warrant a classification of dysplasia (Table 2-6). The diagnosis of dysplasia is an interpretation based upon abnormal tissue patterns and cell morphology combined with individual judgment (see Chapter 3, Fig. 3-3). The question arises: What is the significance of a histologic diagnosis of dysplasia? The significance derives from studies that document the increased risk for malignant transformation of dysplastic leukoplakic lesions on an unpredictable basis (Table 2-9).[64,69–71]

Diagnosis of Leukoplakia and Risk Factors

Patients with leukoplakia are usually asymptomatic. The lesion is often discovered upon routine examination or by patients feeling roughness in their mouths. There are no consistent or reliable clinical signs and symptoms associated with oral leukoplakia that allow differentiation or prediction of a premalignant or early malignant change. Since the clinical appearance of oral leukoplakia—thick or scant, large or small—does not reliably indicate its biologic potential, clinicians should be suspicious of all-white patches and should carefully evaluate and observe patients with such lesions.

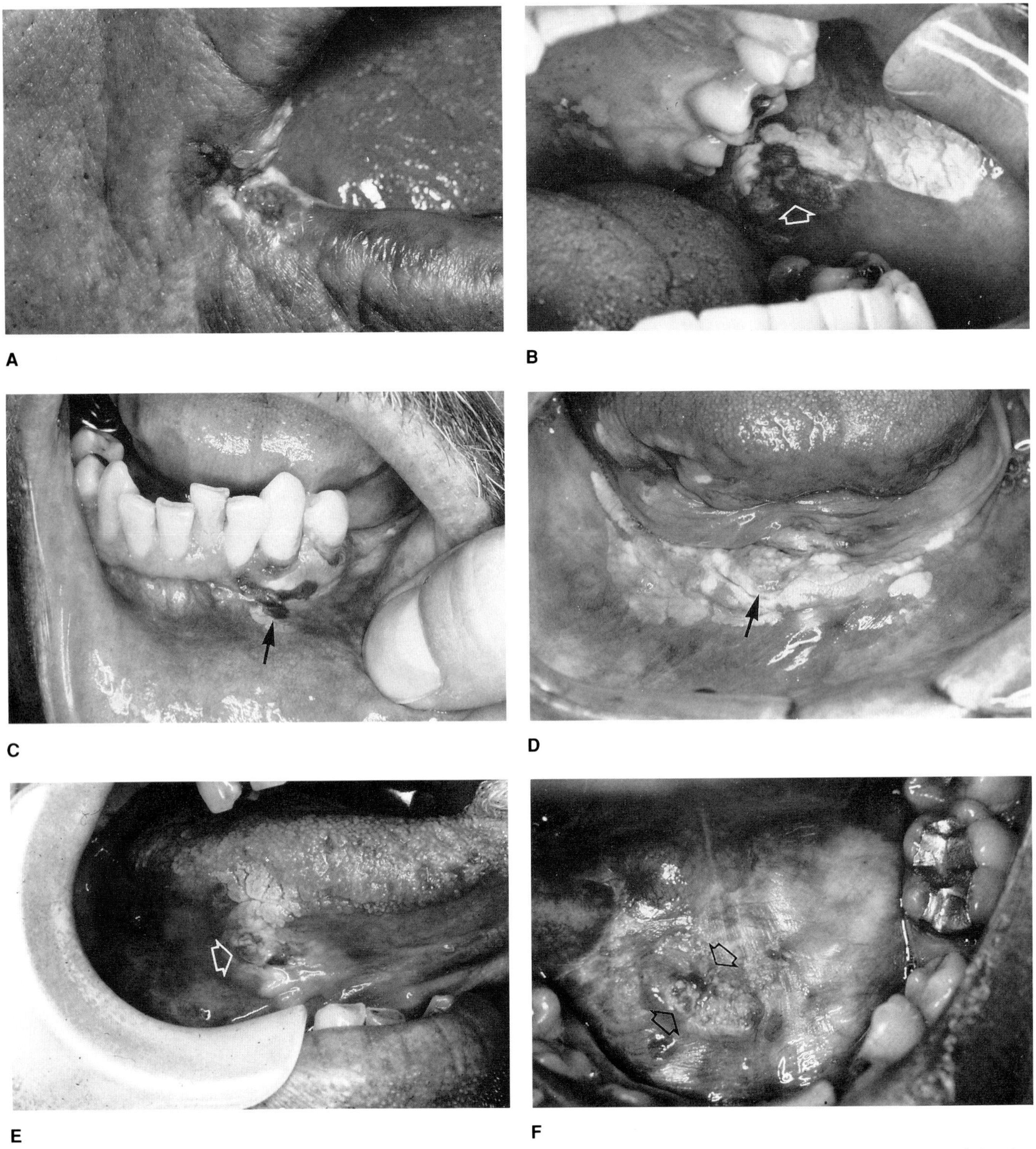

Fig. 2-10. Malignant transformation in oral leukoplakias. **A,** Carcinoma at the commissure associated with leukoplakia involving the buccal mucosa and lip. **B,** Carcinoma (arrow) developed in this buccal leukoplakia after 12 years. **C,** Carcinoma (arrow) appeared as a symptomatic red lesion in this gingival leukoplakia which had persisted for 8 years. **D,** Squamous carcinoma on alveolar mucosa (arrow), associated with widespread leukoplakia of 15 years' duration involving ventral tongue, floor of mouth, and alveolar mucosa. **E,** This leukoplakia, which had been noticed for 6 years, became symptomatic at the site of cancer formation (arrow). **F,** Carcinoma occurring in leukoplakia of the floor of the mouth (arrows), observed for more than 5 years.

Table 2-9. PROGRESSION OF DYSPLASIA IN CLINICAL LEUKOPLAKIA TO CARCINOMA

Source (Country) Year	No. Patients	No. (%) Malignancies	Time Span (years)
Mincer (USA) 1972[69]	45*	5 (11)	1-8
Banoczy (Hungary) 1976[70]	68†	9 (13)	1-20
Pindborg (India) 1977[71]	21‡	3 (14)	7
Silverman (USA) 1984[64]	22	8 (36)	1-39

*17 persisted, 3 disappeared spontaneously; and 20 were excised, of which 7 recurred.

†45 of the 68 lesions were excised; 8 of the 9 malignant changes were in the 23 lesions not subjected to surgery.

‡In a control group of 40 dysplasias not associated with leukoplakia, only 1 became malignant.

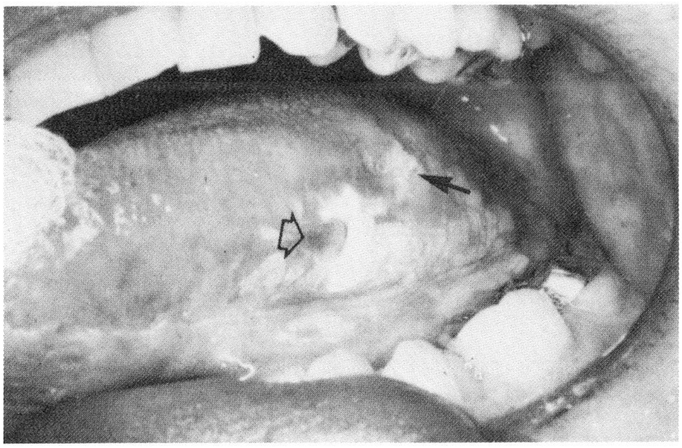

A

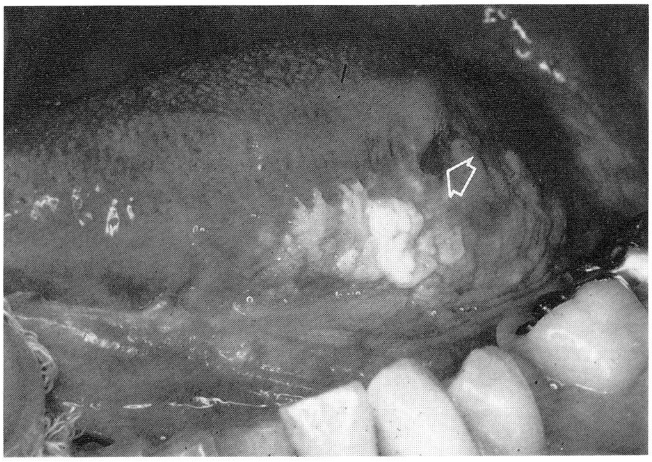

B

Fig. 2-11. Malignant transformation of an oral leukoplakic lesion. **A,** This asymptomatic leukoplakia was noticed for 1 year in a 40-year-old nonsmoking woman. Note biopsy site (open arrow) and site of subsequent transformation (closed arrow). **B,** One year later, examination revealed an erythematous, painful area (open arrow) which proved to be squamous carcinoma. Note complete healing of the original biopsy site which had shown only a benign hyperkeratosis.

ERYTHROLEUKOPLAKIA AND ERYTHROPLASIA

Leukoplakia that clinically has an erythematous or red component (erythroleukoplakia) is far more likely to undergo dysplastic or malignant epithelial changes than other forms of leukoplakia (Fig. 2-12). In the 1984 University of California study,[64] the risk of malignant transformation in the erythroleukoplakia group was seen to be almost fourfold that of the patients with homogeneous leukoplakia (Table 2-10). With this in mind, clinicians should take biopsy specimens from erythematous areas, particularly if the choice is between red- and white-appearing mucosa (Fig. 2-13). In the UCSF study group, 53% of the patients with leukoplakia had an associated erythematous area, whereas 82% of the patients who eventually developed a carcinoma demonstrated a red component. Other investigators have also found this increased risk associated with erythroleukoplakia. Roed-Petersen[67] reported a sevenfold risk for malignant transformation in individuals whose leukoplakia had an erythematous component. His patients showed a 1.3% transformation rate in homogeneous leukoplakia versus a 9.1% rate in red-and-white lesions. Kramer and coworkers,[72] in a study limited to leukoplakias of the tongue and mouth floor, reported a 15% transformation rate in an average period of 4.3 years. The risk for formation of carcinoma on the red-and-white lesions was five times that of the homogeneous leukoplakias. Banoczy[62] described an erosive form of leukoplakia lesions with an erythematous component which had a fivefold greater risk of malignant transformation than other leukoplakia.

The high risk of malignancy in erythroplasia was reaffirmed further in a microscopic review of 58 clinically red

Table 2-10. TRANSFORMATION RATES OF LEUKOPLAKIC FORMS*

Leukoplakia	No. Patients	Subsequent Carcinoma	Transformation Rate (%)
Homogeneous†	107	7	6.5
Erythroleukoplakia‡	128	30	23.4
Dysplasia§	22	8	36.4

*Data from Silverman, Gorsky and Lozada, 1984.[64]

†All-white appearance.

‡Red component.

§20/22 appeared clinically as erythroleukoplakia.

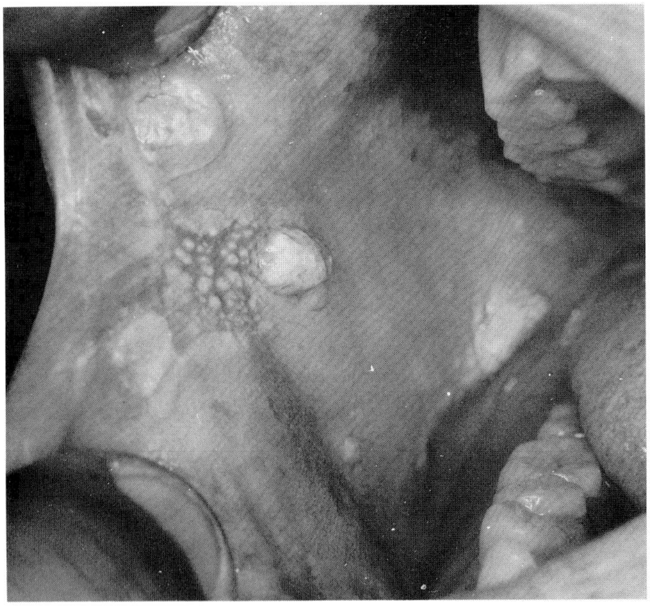

A

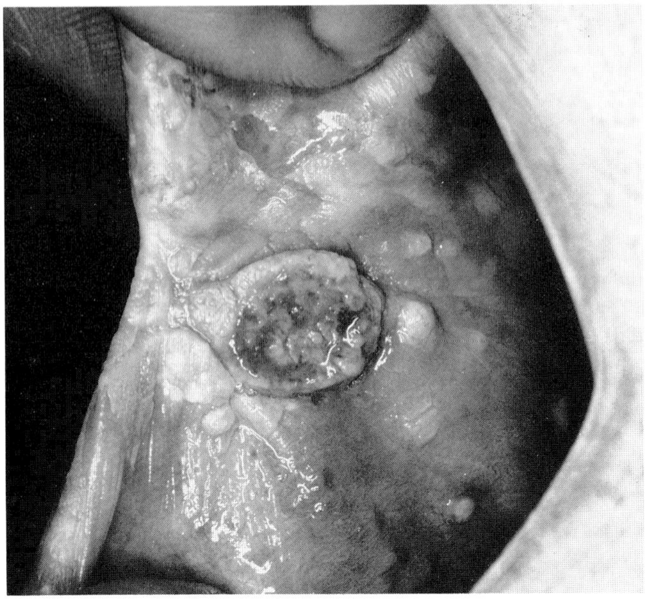

B

Fig. 2-12. Malignant transformation in erythroleukoplakia. **A,** Red-and-white leukoplakia of right commissure demonstrated mild epithelial dysplasia. Patient refused suggested excision. **B,** Two years later, lesion has transformed into carcinoma.

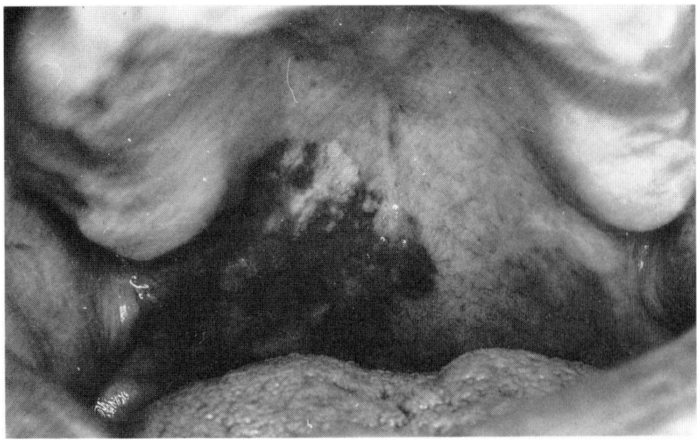

A

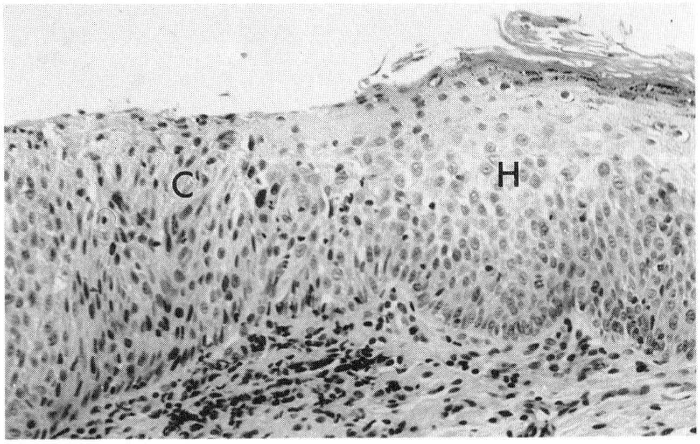

B

Fig. 2-13. Erythroplasia and malignant transformation. **A,** Mildly symptomatic, predominantly red (erythematous) lesion of right soft palate, noticed by patient for about 4 months. Biopsy specimen contained some hyperkeratotic tissue along with adjacent red-appearing tissue. **B,** Microscopic view reveals transition between clinically red area showing intraepithelial carcinoma (C) and clinically white area showing hyperkeratosis (H). This case illustrates the need to include erythematous tissue in biopsy material in order to assess the most dangerous areas.

lesions, of which 91% were found to be either invasive carcinoma, carcinoma in situ, or severe dysplasia.[73] Another series of studies showed that persistent erythroplasia rather than leukoplakia in high-risk sites is the earliest and predominant sign of oral carcinoma.[74–76] In a prospective study of 222 asymptomatic oral carcinomas, 28% were red only, 62% were red and white, 97% occurred in the mouth floor, oral tongue, and oropharynx, and 84% were less than 2 cm at their largest diameter.[75]

Proliferative Verrucous Leukoplakia (PVL)

This form of leukoplakia fortunately is rare because its course is invariably one of progression and it is often associated with dysplasia and malignant transformation.[77] It can usually be recognized clinically by the irregular exophytic wart-like and papillary features and its capacity to extend its margins (Fig. 2-14). A red component is sometimes present. Microscopically, at first there is no dysplasia, but there is an irregular, extensive epithelial hyperplasia (pseudoepitheliomatous hyperplasia) and often dyskeratosis. A heavy subepithelial lymphocytic infiltrate is frequently found (which sometimes causes PVL to be confused with lichen planus). Since the lesions are extensive, multiple microscopic changes, from simple hyperkeratosis to dysplasia to carcinoma, may be present simultaneously (Fig. 2-15). Therefore, adequate tissue sampling and careful follow-up are essential.

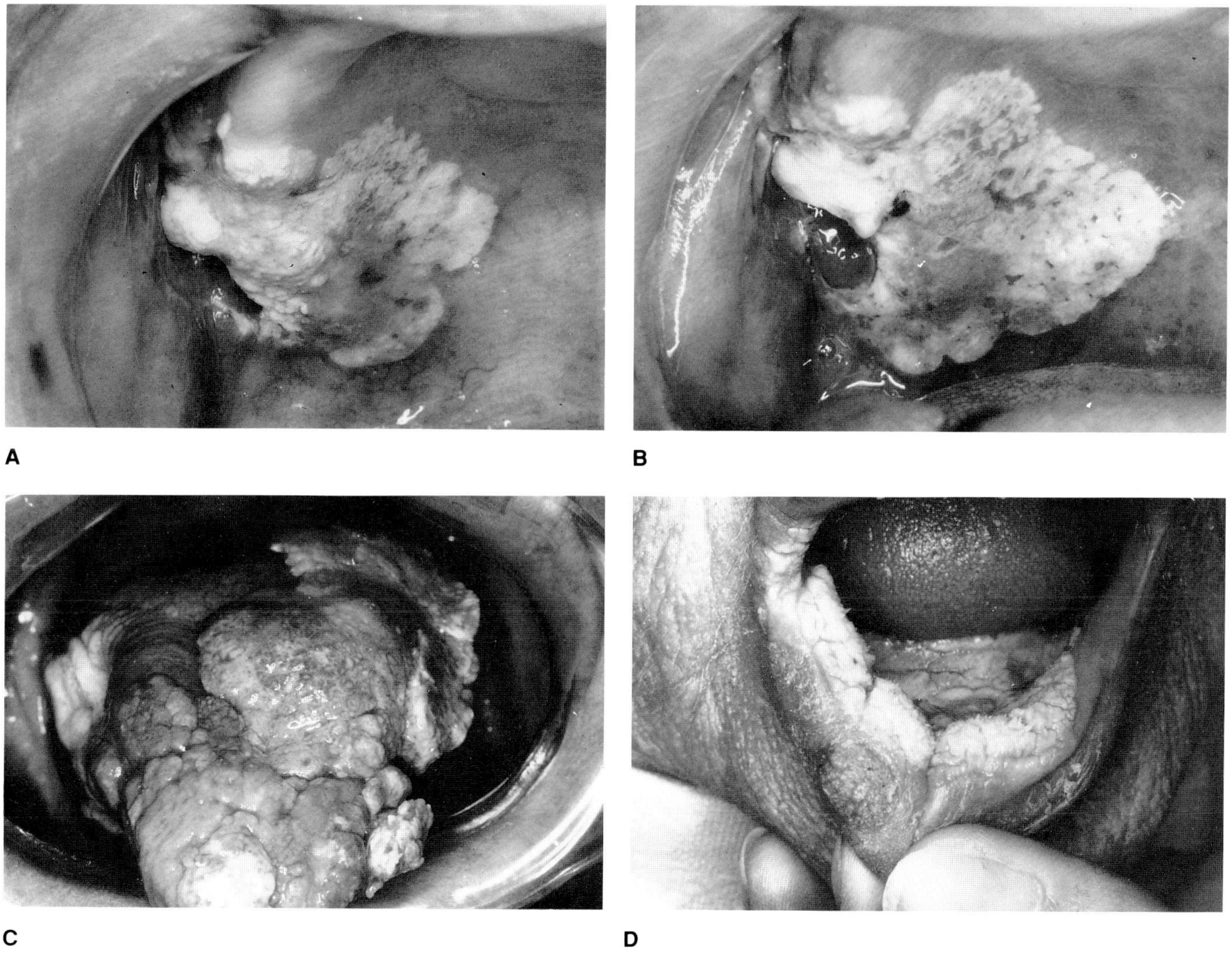

Fig. 2-14. Proliferating verrucous leukoplakia (PVL). **A,** Mildly symptomatic lesion on right palatal alveolar mucosa, noticed by patient for about 6 months. **B,** Three months later lesion has spread, illustrating the characteristic clinical progression and extension of this form of leukoplakia. Biopsy revealed transformation from apparently benign pseudoepitheliomatous hyperplasia to verrucous carcinoma. **C,** Another PVL, with more prominent papillary features. This lesion was present for 4 years and eventually transformed into carcinoma. **D,** PVL in a 75-year-old woman. The progressive changes had been noticed for 2 years and were mildly bothersome. Multiple biopsies revealed hyperkeratosis and hyperplasia with cellular atypia.

Candidal organisms are often associated with PVL, but antifungal treatment has not been beneficial. No cause, whether it is irritative, nutritional, viral, or genetic, has been identified. Interestingly, while leukoplakia seems to be more common in men, the female-male ratio for PVL is about 4 to 1.

The lesion tends to recur after excision. Irradiation has been helpful in extensive cases, but the best management is earliest possible recognition and aggressive excision if possible. Chemotherapy with methotrexate (see Chapter 5) has been a consideration in assisting control.

Candidiasis, Leukoplakia, and Erythroplasia

Candidiasis (thrush, moniliasis) is caused almost always by an overgrowth of the fungus *Candida albicans*. Although this fungus is found in more than one third of normal-appearing mouths, overgrowth does not occur unless the "balance" of the oral flora is disturbed, for example, by debilitating or acute illness, immune suppression, xerostomia, or antibiotic therapy. The diagnosis of candidiasis is suspected when there are creamy-white or erythematous mucosal changes (Fig. 2-16) and may be confirmed by smear, culture, and biopsy, or by response to antifungal therapy (Fig. 2-17).

Studies in the Oral Medicine Clinic at the University of California, San Francisco, indicate that candidiasis is a potential risk factor for, or at least a complication of, leukoplakia (Fig. 2-18). Although cultures showed that 31% of the clinic's leukoplakia patients fostered this fungal organism in their mouths,[64] a rate similar to the occurrence in normal populations,[78] 53% of the leukoplakia patients who developed carcinomas were *Candida*-positive prior to tumor formation. However, mutagenicity and carcinogenicity of *Candida albicans* has not been shown.

Fig. 2-15. **A,** Proliferating verrucous leukoplakia in a 55-year-old woman. The chief complaints were discomfort and inability to wear her denture. Biopsy tissue from different sites showed the histologic extremes of (**B**) benign hyperkeratosis and hyperplasia and (**C**) squamous carcinoma.

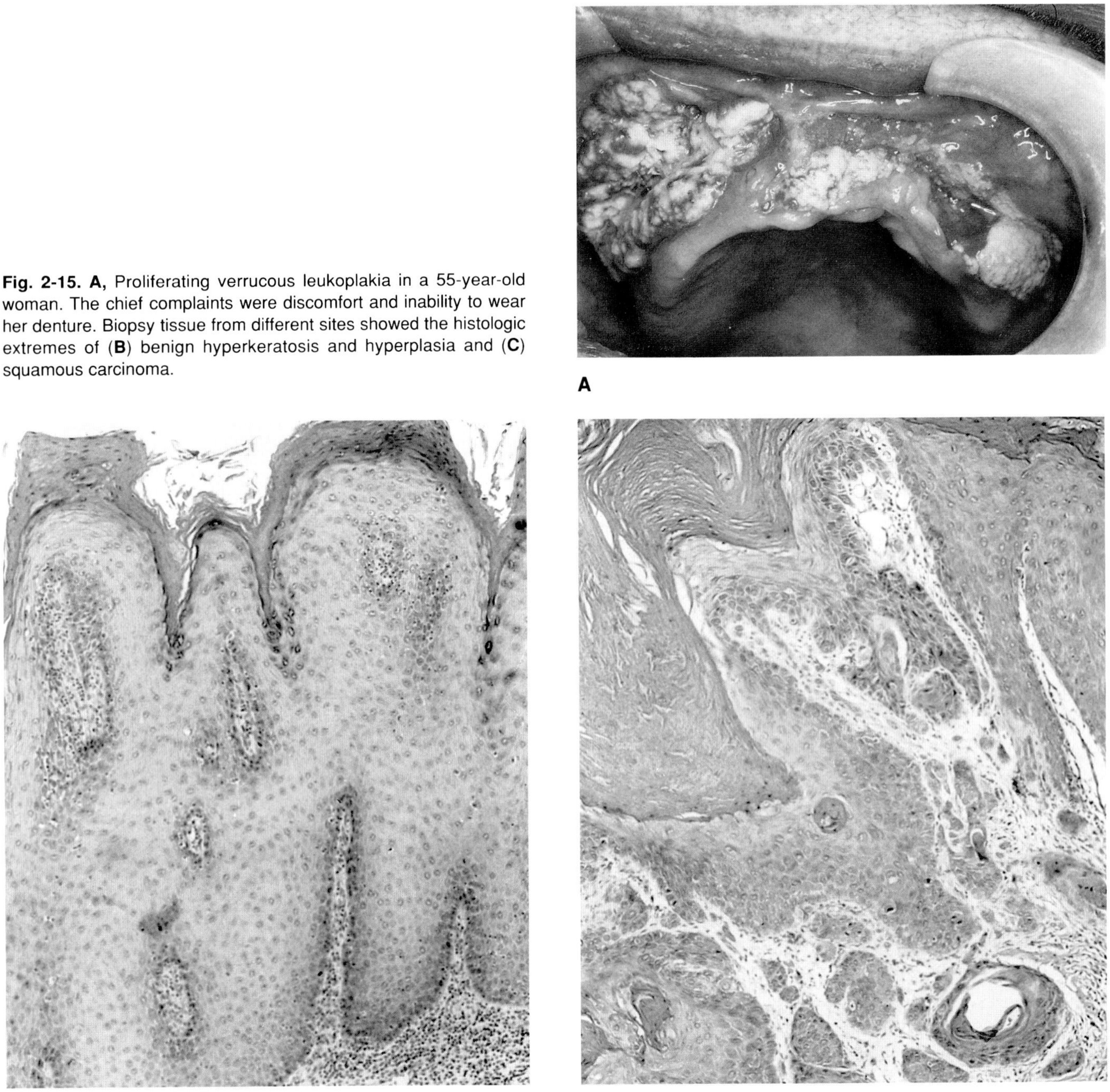

A

B

C

Other studies have reported similar incidences of *Candida* in leukoplakia.[79–81] These studies also demonstrated a higher prevalence of *Candida* in speckled leukoplakia than in homogeneous leukoplakia. Specifically, Renstrup[81] found that while 55 of 235 patients with leukoplakia (23.4%) were *Candida*-positive, further analysis showed that in the homogeneous group four of 152 (2.6%) were positive, but in the speckled leukoplakia group 51 of 83 (61.4%) were positive. The UCSF Oral Medicine Clinic experience confirms the greater risk of fungal infection in the red-and-white lesion. It seems that the candidal organisms in these situations are secondary transients since treatment will most often only convert erythroleukoplakia into the homogeneous form. It is possible but infrequent that candidal organisms stimulate hyperkeratosis (hyperplastic candidiasis), since adequate treatment of the candidal infection rarely leads to disappearance of the clinical lesion.

These reports show that candidiasis may complicate the observation and management of oral leukoplakia, but there has been no study documenting a cause-and-effect relationship between candidal-associated leukoplakia and malignant transformation.

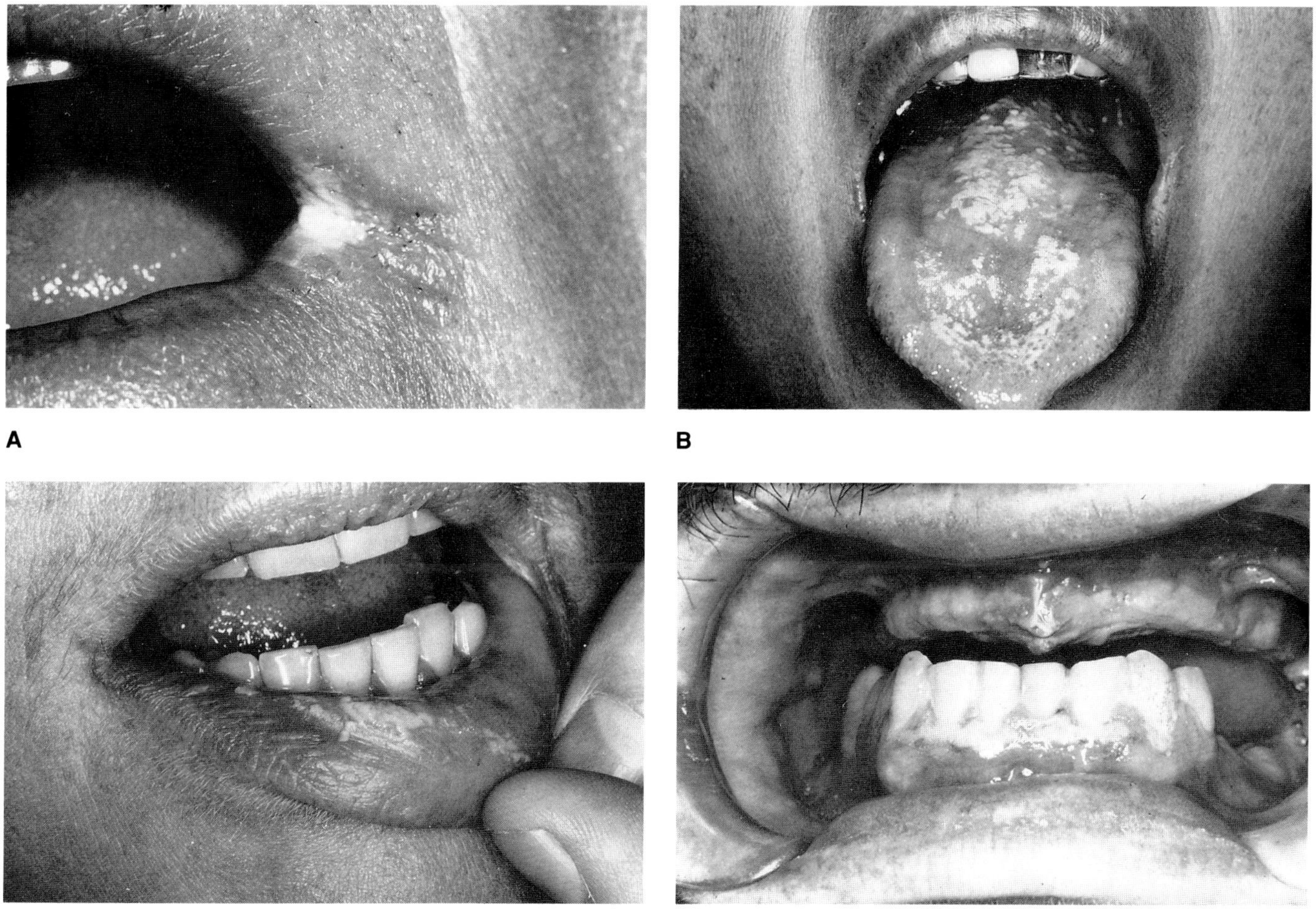

Fig. 2-16. Candidiasis. These infections often resemble leukoplakia in clinical appearance. The following four cases were clinically misdiagnosed as leukoplakia. Cultures for *Candida* were positive, and all lesions disappeared after antifungal therapy. **A,** White patch at angle of mouth, present for 1 month. **B,** Chronic, mildly symptomatic white changes of the dorsal tongue. **C,** Asymptomatic white changes of lower lip, thought to be hyperkeratotic change caused by chronic lip chewing. **D,** Mildly symptomatic keratotic changes of lower gingiva.

Hairy Leukoplakia

Oral "hairy leukoplakia" (HL) describes white-appearing lesions that almost always occur unilaterally or bilaterally on the borders of the tongue.[82] HL frequently appears as hair-like projections and/or corrugations, but HL may also have a plaque-like appearance (Fig. 2-19). HL will appear occasionally on other oral sites such as the buccal mucosa, oropharynx, and mouth floor. There is no evidence that HL is biologically similar to hyperkeratotic leukoplakia that has premalignant connotations.

Microscopically HL appears as an epithelial hyperplasia with a parakeratotic surface and vacuolated cells often referred to as koliocytes (cells suggestive of viral infection). The presence of EBV in these vacuolated cells have been confirmed by electron microscopy and DNA probes. Since sometimes non-HL lesions can have similar clinical, even microscopic appearances to EBV, ultimate confirmation is the demonstration of EBV. Connective tissue inflammation may vary from moderate white cell infiltrates to the appearance of a noninflammatory lesion. In about half the cases, candidal organisms can be demonstrated in the epithelial surface; however, antifungal treatment does not appreciably alter HL.

The cause of HL is unknown. Whether EBV is a cause or result is as yet not clear. HL can occur in all HIV-infected groups, although it is by far more common in both homosexual and bisexual men than in women. Of utmost significance is that HL indicates HIV infection and is highly predictive for the development of AIDS, probably within 3 years.

Treatment is elective. These lesions are usually asymptomatic, but chronic. They are treated only if they are bothersome in some way to the patient, or by coincidence when another disease is the target of treatment. HL may disappear following high doses of antiviral drugs (acyclovir, azidothymidine) which interrupt viral replication, topical Retin-A solution, and sulfa-type antibiotics given for controlling pneumocystis pneumonia. HL usually recurs when treatment is modified or discontinued. In any event, HL augers a poor prognosis and is most definitely a sign of AIDS-related complex (ARC).

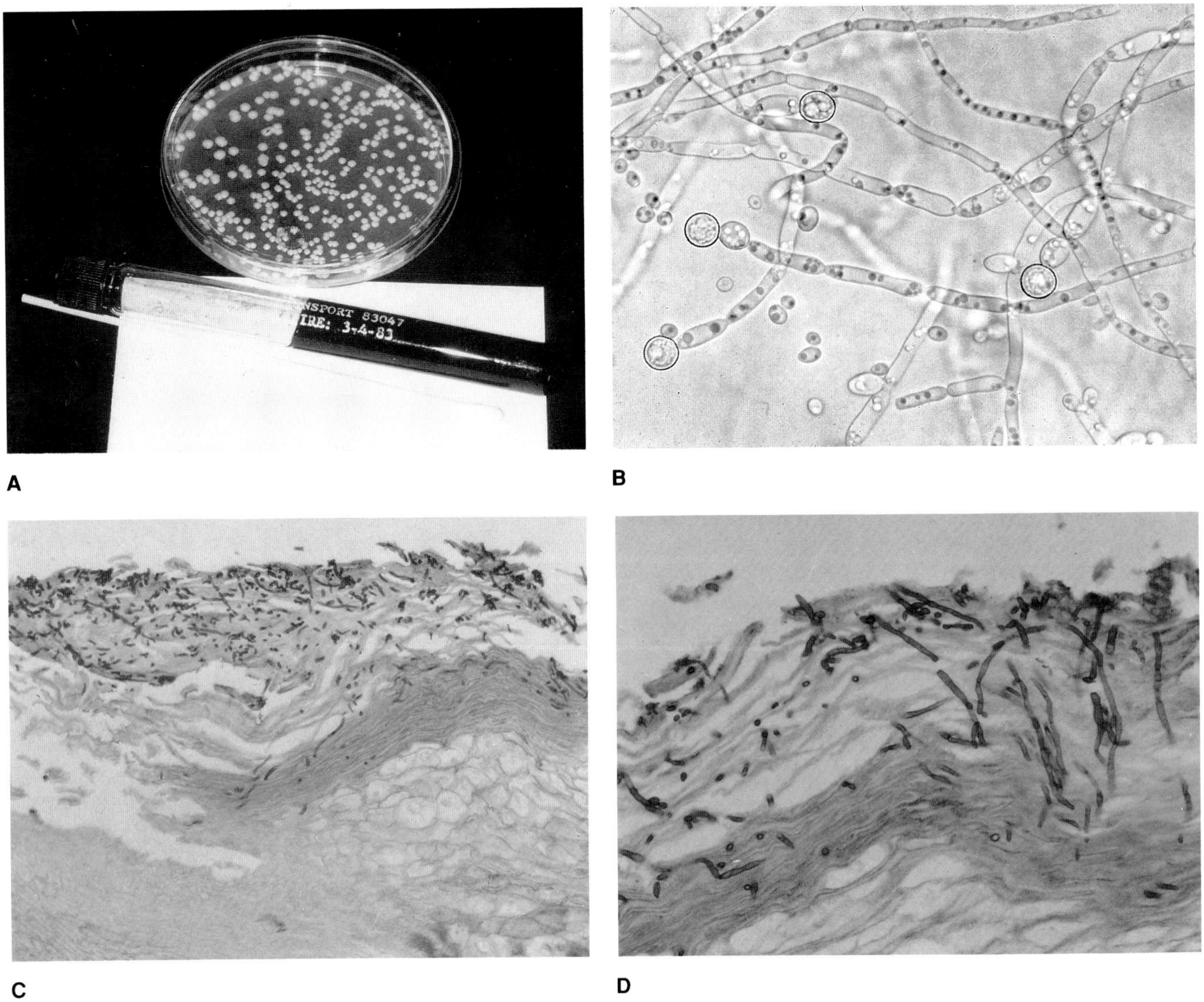

Fig. 2-17. Oral candidiasis. **A,** Colonies of *Candida albicans* growing on culture medium (Sabaroud's). **B,** Scraping from these colonies reveals the typical pseudomycelia and spores of the fungus. **C,** Biopsy of fungally infected oral mucosa shows the candidal organisms growing in the surface cells of the epithelium (PAS stain). **D,** Higher-power view of the fungal organisms.

Erythroplasia with Ulceration

Another rare, but high-risk premalignant lesion is the chronic erythematous change associated with constantly recurring erosive changes. These lesions are often mistaken for "recurrent aphthous stomatitis of the herpetiform variety" or a "nonspecific inflammatory vesiculoerosive disease" (Fig. 20). A biopsy of the early lesion may show only hyperkeratosis and inflammation not suggestive of any specific disease. Clinical responses to empirical corticosteroid therapy may help rule out a premalignant status by indicating a benign inflammatory response associated with a vesiculo-erosive disease. In the lesion that has been present for some time, an initial biopsy might reveal a carcinoma or dysplasia, thereby mandating treatment. However, even a nondysplastic pattern in this type of lesion that cannot be classified deserves close follow-up or attempted removal because clinical experience indicates that a definite risk exists that it will eventually develop into a carcinoma.

MANAGEMENT

The first step in management of leukoplakia is the removal of all irritants. If the leukoplakia is not reversible, excision is the most effective treatment. However, since these lesions may spread over a large area, they cannot always be surgically excised. In addition, recurrence after excision is common, due possibly to continuation of an irritant or the biologic potential in adjacent tissue that morphologically appears normal. The use of the carbon dioxide laser (Figs. 2-21 and 2-22) has proved extremely useful and effective (see Chapter 5).[83] Electrodesiccation and cryosurgery (Fig. 2-23) have not been uniformly effective in permanently removing

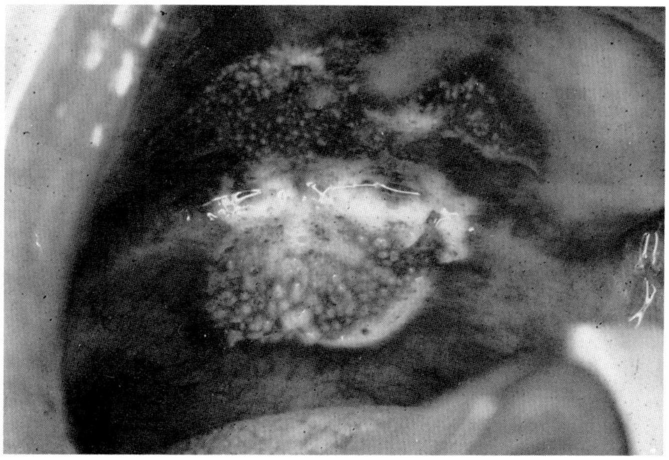

A

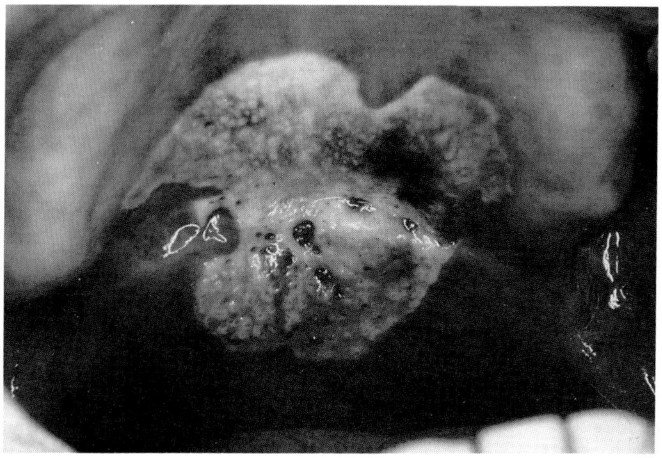

B

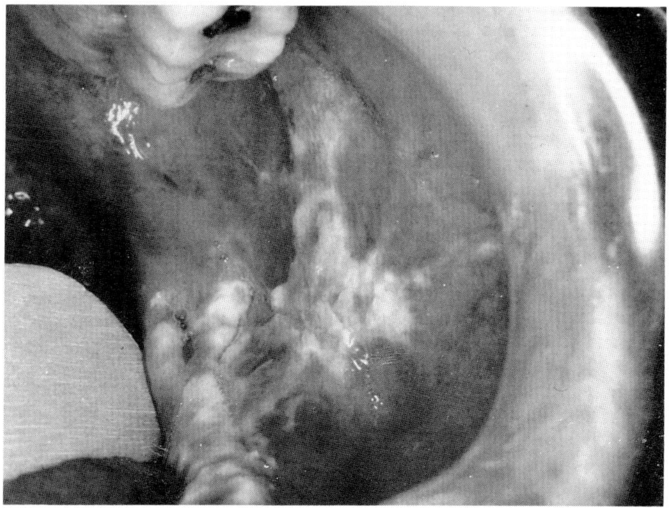

C

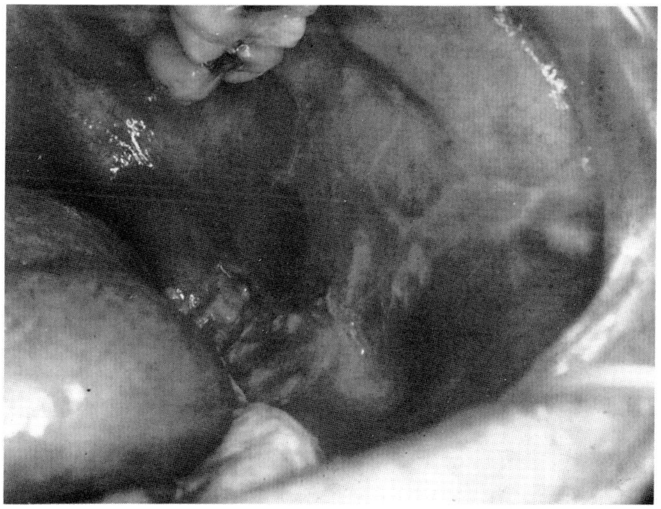

D

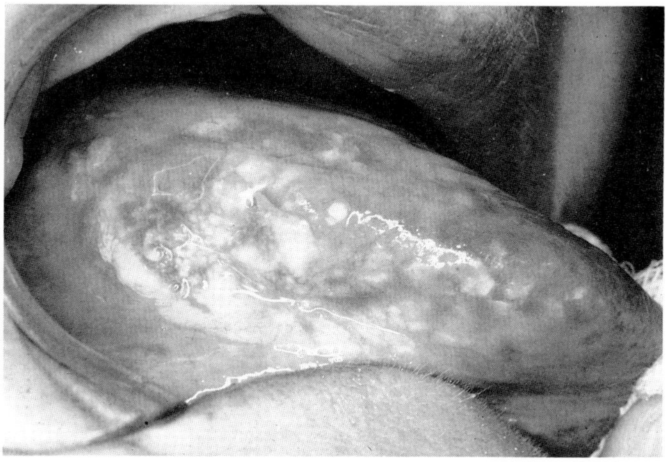

E

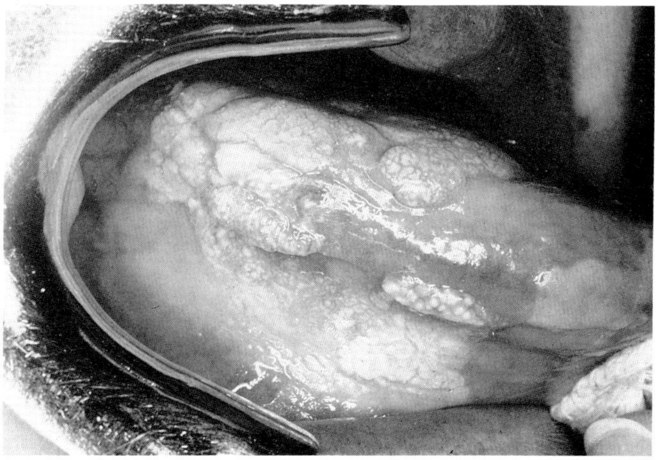

F

Fig. 2-18. Candidiasis and leukoplakia. **A,** Mildly symptomatic candidal erythroleukoplakia of the palate. **B,** After treatment with antifungal medications, the leukoplakia became more homogeneous and asymptomatic. **C,** Moderately painful candidal leukoplakia of the buccal and alveolar mucosae. **D,** Forty-eight hours after antifungal medicine, the signs and symptoms greatly regressed. **E,** Erythroleukoplakia of the tongue associated with a positive candidal culture and pain. **F,** Years later the lesion transformed into a squamous carcinoma.

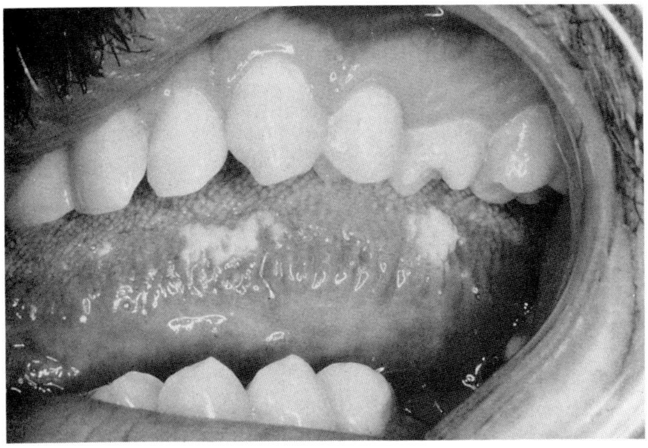

A

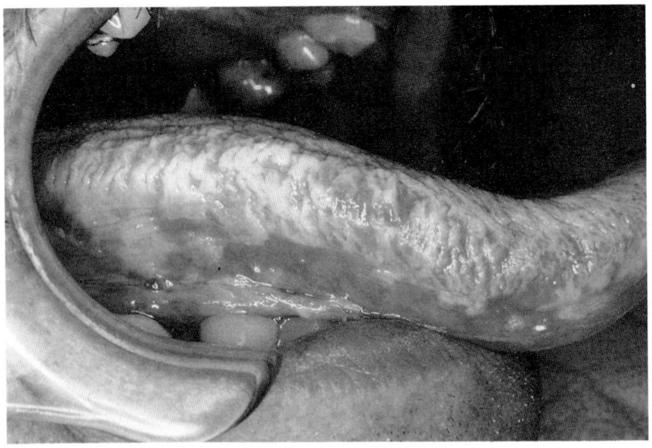

B

Fig. 2-19. A, Minimal oral hairy leukoplakia in an HIV-infected homosexual male. B, Extensive oral hairy leukoplakia in an AIDS patient.

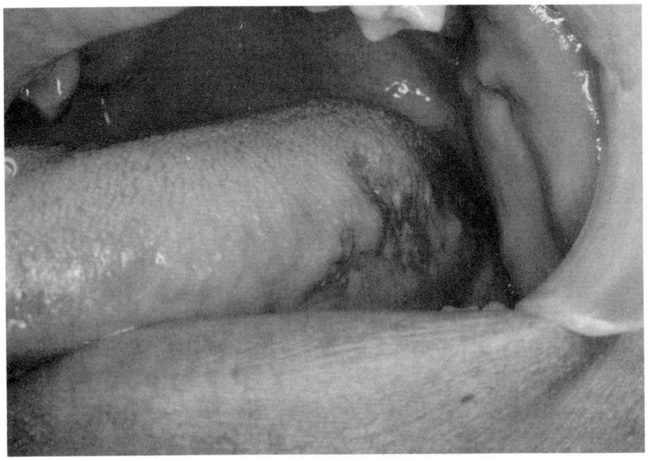

Fig. 2-20. This 45-year-old man had a persistently sore tongue for two years which was thought to be an "aphthous or herpetiform" lesion. A biopsy showed this erosive and erythematous tongue lesion to be a squamous carcinoma.

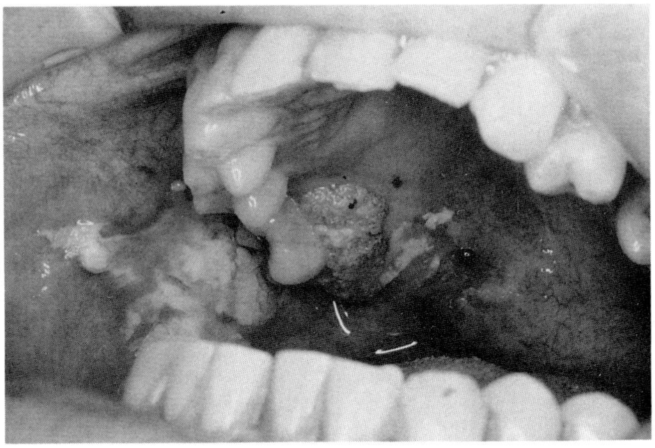

A

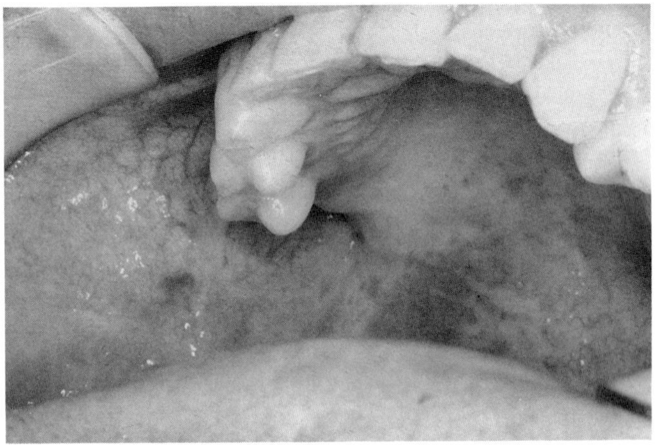

B

Fig. 2-21. Proliferative verrucous leukoplakia. A, Mildly symptomatic, widespread growth of lesion. Microscopy showed tissue variations from hyperkeratosis to severe dysplasia. B, Seven weeks after CO_2 laser excision-evaporation, plus extraction of the upper right molar, the patient was asymptomatic, completely functional, and without evidence of leukoplakia. Follow-up at 3 years remained negative.

keratotic lesions. Proteolytic enzymes have been of no value since keratin is resistant to them.

Vitamin A in high dosages (more than 300,000 units per day in troche form) has been effective in some patients in reversing hyperkeratosis.[84] The mechanism of action is unknown, and upon withdrawal of vitamin A the hyperkeratosis returns. Vitamin A tolerance is short lived with the required high dosages because of limited liver storage and detoxification. Common side effects are dry skin, rash, and pruritus. In a few instances, oral squamous carcinomas have developed. The role of vitamin A and its analogues in carcinogenesis is not known, and studies are inconclusive. Most animal studies have shown protective effects.[85] A human study indicated some beneficial effects of vitamin A analogues (beta-carotene and 13-cis-retinoic acid) on oral leukoplakia in short-term observations.[86] Retinoic acid solution has been approved for use in acne. In our experience,

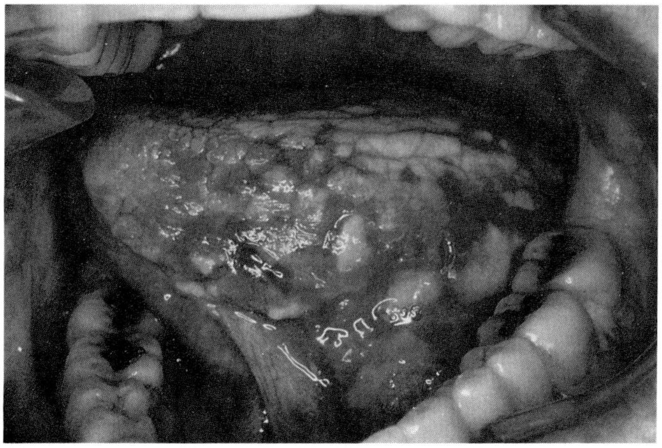

A

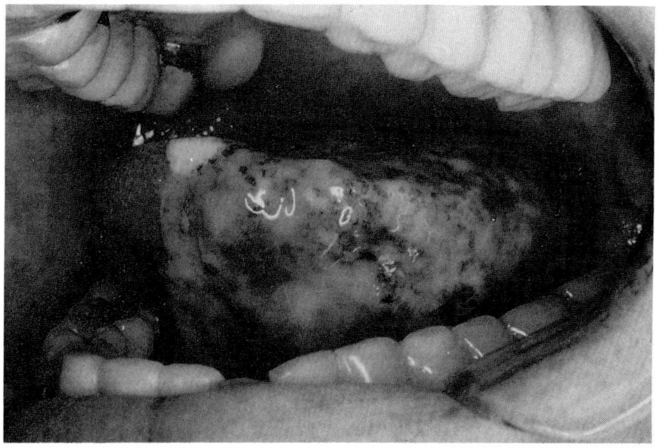

B

Fig. 2-22. Erythroplakia of the tongue. **A,** Erythroleukoplakia of the left tongue in a non-smoking 72-year-old man. The lesion was painful and had been present for more than 3 years. Biopsies revealed severe epithelial dysplasia. **B,** Immediately following CO_2 laser excision-evaporation. Tylenol and codeine controlled the pain, and the patient was able to manage a liquid-soft diet. **C,** Eight weeks following treatment the patient was asymptomatic and had no difficulties with speech or swallowing.

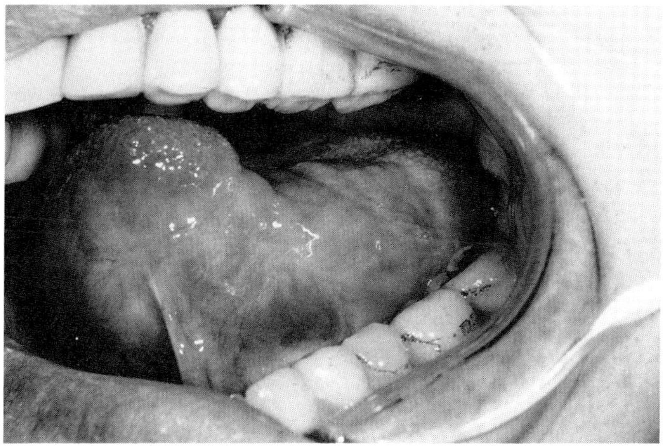

C

daily topical applications of 0.05% retinoic acid solution to oral leukoplakia has achieved partial remissions without untoward side effects (Fig. 2-24). Long-term implications are unknown.

Since many methods of managing leukoplakia are not always feasible or effective, these patients must be observed periodically. The follow-up examination includes careful clinical observation and an occasional biopsy. Exfoliative cytology and vital staining with toluidine blue are helpful to supplement clinical judgment and to serve as an adjunct to biopsy (see Chapter 3). A negative cytologic report must be balanced with clinical judgment. Therefore, if clinical suspicion persists despite a negative cytologic smear, a biopsy must be considered.

Follow-up

The risk for malignant transformation in oral leukoplakia is always present. The UCSF long-term follow-up study[64] confirmed the persistent, somewhat constant, and unpredictable danger of malignant transformation (Table 2-11). Table 2-12 describes the 45 patients (17.5%) in this study who developed carcinomas in associated leukoplakic lesions. Interestingly, the follow-up times and patient ages were similar to those of all the patients in the study group as a whole.

SUMMARY

Because leukoplakia and carcinoma can occur simultaneously and an established prognostic clinical guide is lacking, all white lesions characterized as leukoplakia must be microscopically diagnosed and either removed or monitored with care. Biopsy is the only definitive way to establish the exact nature of oral leukoplakias.

When seeking dysplastic or malignant areas in leukoplakic lesions, it is important to remember that erythematous and speckled regions are more likely to be cancerous than thick and homogeneous white regions. It must also be remembered that the diagnosis of a previously biopsied benign white patch must be periodically reaffirmed, since a leukoplakia may unpredictably transform into a malignancy. Moreover, although a leukoplakic lesion may regress and disappear when an irritant is reduced or removed, it can recur and may subsequently become cancerous.

In determining the aggressiveness of treatment, consideration of risk factors is essential. These factors are: (1) an erythematous component, (2) microscopic dysplasia, (3) a clinical appearance of proliferative verrucous leukoplakia, (4) associated candidiasis, (5) a nonsmoking patient, and (6) pain.

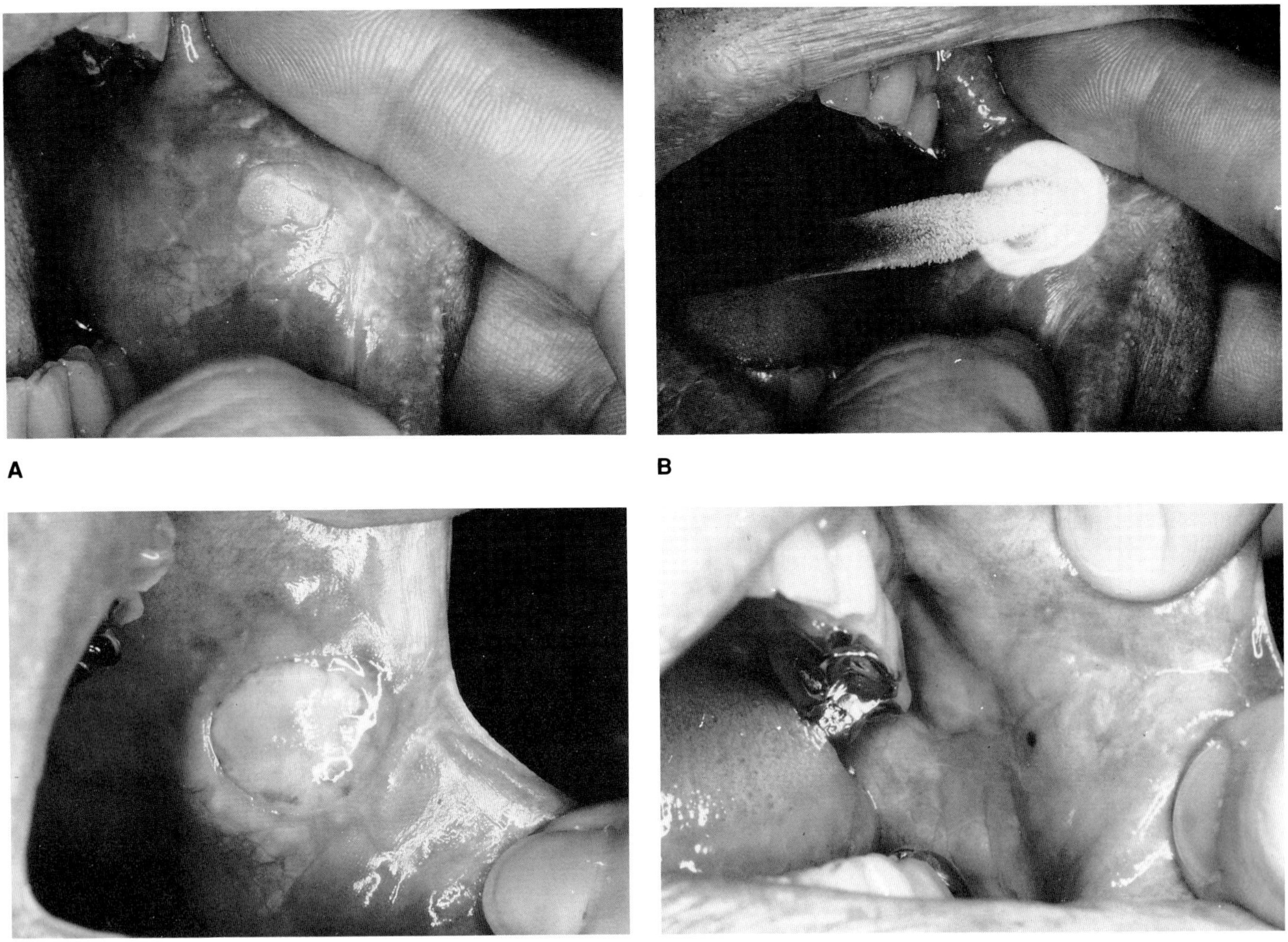

A B C D

Fig. 2-23. Cryosurgery in management of leukoplakia. **A,** Longstanding asymptomatic leukoplakia of left buccal mucosa. **B,** A cryoprobe is used to administer two 2-minute freezes, two minutes apart, at temperature of about $-140°$ C. **C,** One week later, ulcer has been produced due to cell death by freezing. **D,** One month later, leukoplakia has been temporarily controlled and patient is asymptomatic.

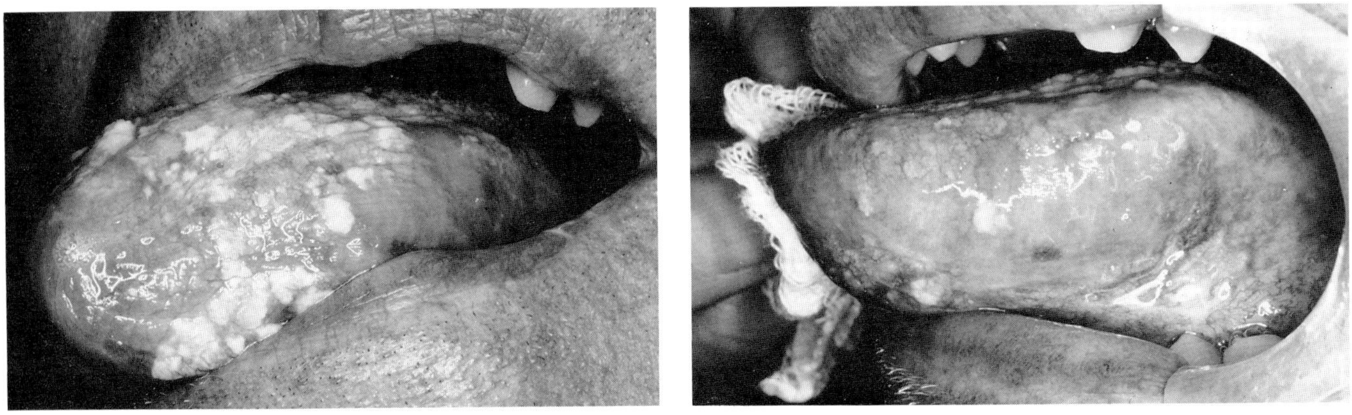

A B

Fig. 2-24. Retinoic acid (tretinoin) in treatment of leukoplakia. **A,** Patient with leukoplakia of the tongue of 10 years' duration applied 0.05% retinoic acid solution once a day. **B,** One month later, tongue is asymptomatic and most of the hyperkeratosis has been reversed.

Table 2-11. OCCURRENCES OF CARCINOMAS RELATED TO FOLLOW-UP PERIODS IN 257 PATIENTS WITH LEUKOPLAKIA*

Follow-up (yrs)	Occurrences of Carcinoma in 45 Patients (%)	Patients Followed for Each Period (%)	Rate of Carcinoma in Patients Followed (%)	Rate of Carcinoma Per Year (%)
0.5-1	9	100	2	4
1-2	24	84	5	5
2-5	20	70	5	1.6
5-10	22	46	8	1.6
10-20	16	27	10	1
20-39	9	8	19	1

*Data from Silverman, Gorsky and Lozada, 1984.[64]

Table 2-12. PROFILE OF 45 PATIENTS WITH TRANSFORMATION OF LEUKOPLAKIA TO CARCINOMA*

				Age at Onset of Leukoplakia (yr)		Transformation Time (yr)			Tobacco Usage†			
Transformation Site	F	M	% of Total Lesions	Range	Mean	Range	Mean	Pre-Existing Dysplasia	Cigarette	Pipe	Cigar	Snuff
Tongue	9	4	28.9	37-79	55	1-18	6.4	1	2		1	
Gingiva	6	5	24.4	46-84	66	1-21	8.6	3	2	1		
Floor	2	5	15.6	30-69	50	0.5-30	10.2	2	6	1		
Buccal	3	2	11.1	48-71	60	1-16	8.8	1	1	1		
Palate	4	1	11.1	38-76	54	2-39	9.3	1	2			1
Lip	2	2	8.9	45-65	54	3-11	6.6	0	3			
Total	26	19	100	30-84	57.3	0.5-39	8.1	8	16	3	1	1

*Data from Silverman, Gorsky and Lozada, 1984.[64]
†Of the 24 nonsmokers, 18 had never smoked and 6 stopped smoking when diagnosed.

ORAL LICHEN PLANUS

Lichen planus is a complex chronic inflammatory disease: mucosa and skin both may be affected, microscopic features vary, and the oral lesions appear in different forms (Figs. 2-25 and 2-26). The prevalence of lichen planus is unknown, but it may be present in as much as 1% of the adult population.

The etiology of this inflammatory (probably autoimmune) mucocutaneous disease is unknown, and there is no definitive curative treatment, although corticosteroids are beneficial for control. The oral lesions are frequently symptomatic and chronic, persisting indefinitely in most patients. Our experience has shown spontaneous remission in less than 3% of patients. Lichen planus is primarily a disease of adults with the average age of onset being about 50 years. It is rarely found in persons less than 30 years old. Women predominate, about 2 to 1. Lichen planus can be found in all ethnic groups, and there is little evidence of familial clustering.

DIAGNOSIS

Oral lichen planus can usually be recognized by the unique clinical features of reticular, annular, or punctate keratotic (white) patterns on the mucosal surface. The diagnosis, however, can be confusing since these keratotic changes may be associated with pseudomembrane-covered ulcerations and marked erythema. Because many lichen planus patients are asymptomatic, signs are sometimes recognized unexpectedly during routine oral examination or by chance observation. Although lichen planus can occur in any oral site, the buccal mucosa is by far the most common location. The majority of oral lichen planus patients do not have skin involvement. Diagnosis is confirmed by biopsy.

MALIGNANT ASSOCIATION

There is inadequate evidence relating to malignant transformation to substantiate that lichen planus is a precancerous lesion. Initially five oral carcinomas (2.5%) were found in a follow-up study of 200 patients with oral lichen planus at the UCSF Oral Medicine Clinic.[87] In a later prospective study in the clinic of 570 oral lichen planus patients, malignant transformation occurred in seven patients(1.2%).[88] Considering a mean age of 52 and a mean duration of lichen planus of 5.5 years, this prevalence was in excess of that expected in a comparable sample of the general population (see Chapter 1). There was no association with gender, smoking, or site of oral lichen planus. Other investigators also have reported

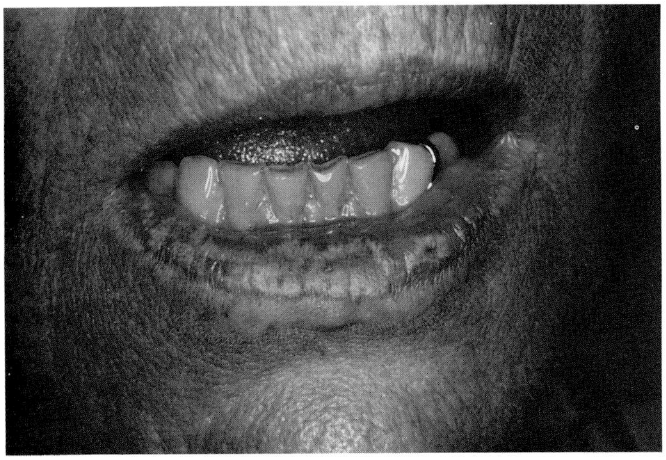

A

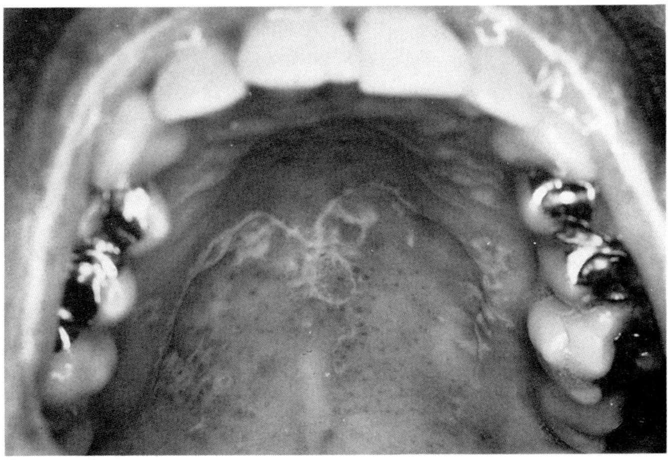

B

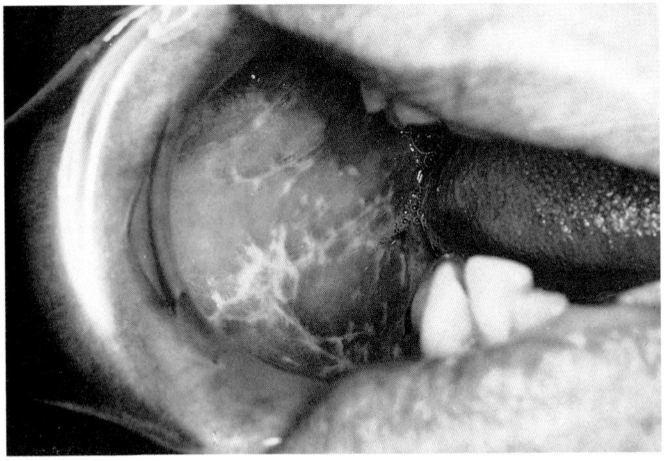

C

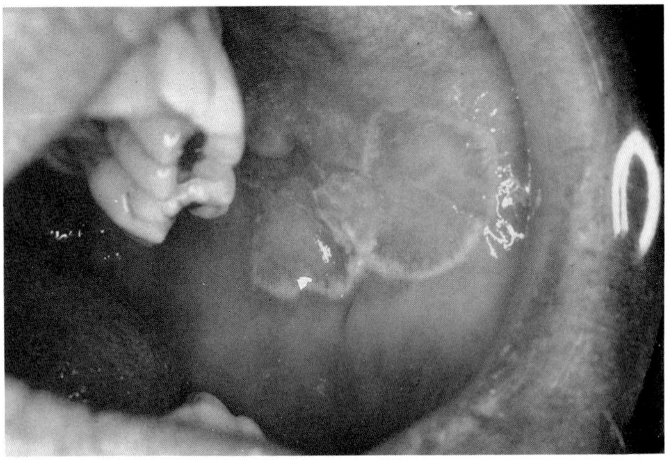

D

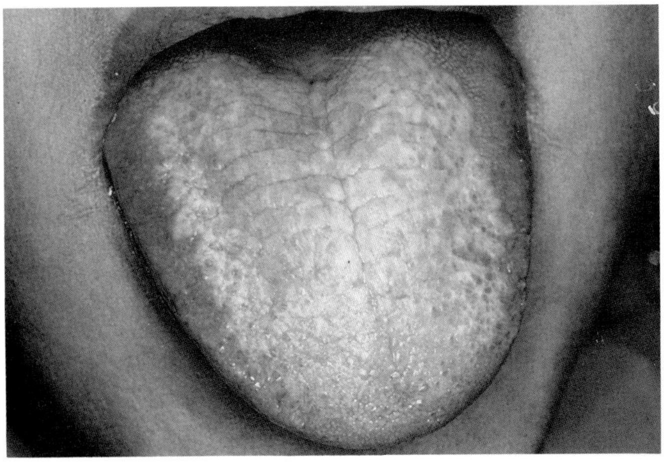

E

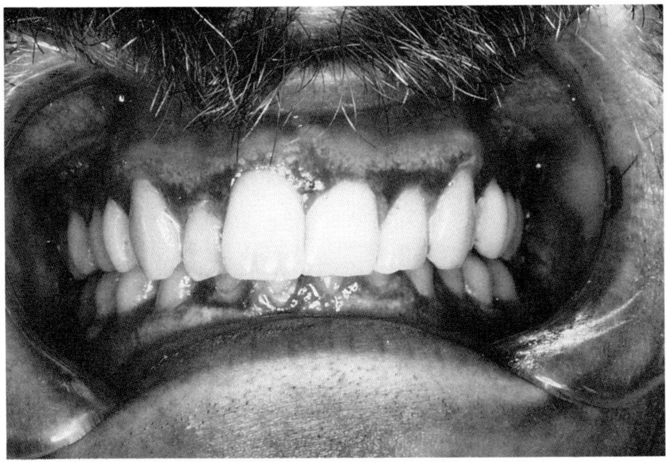

F

Fig. 2-25. Clinical forms of oral lichen planus. **A,** Reticular form, lip. **B,** Reticular form, palate. **C,** Reticular and punctate forms, buccal mucosa. **D,** Annular form, buccal mucosa. **E,** Reticular and plaque forms, tongue. **F,** Atrophic form, gingiva.

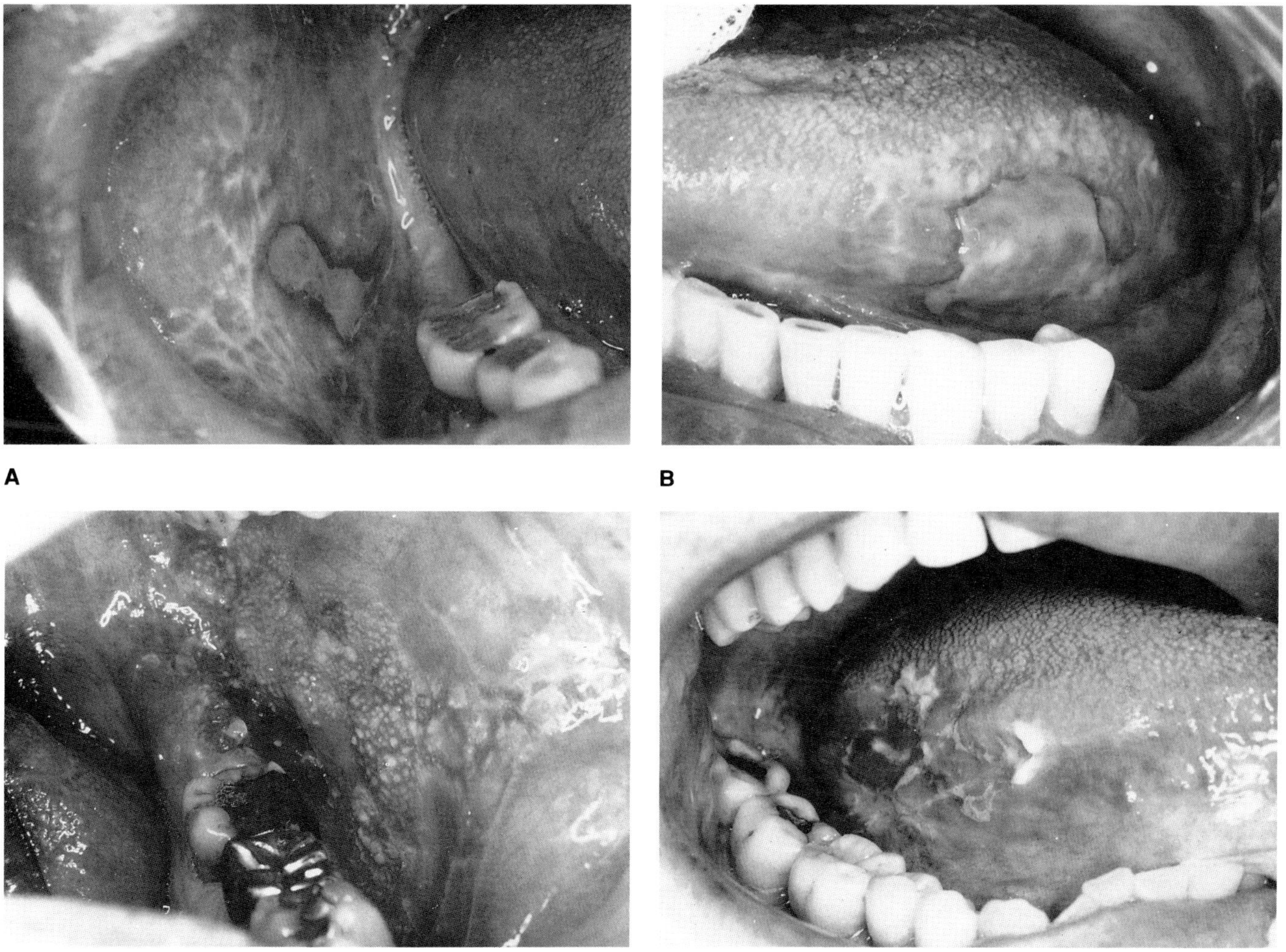

A B C D

Fig. 2-26. Oral lichen planus. **A,** Erosive form, buccal mucosa. **B,** Erosive form, tongue. **C,** Lichen planus and associated squamous carcinoma, buccal mucosa (transformation after 12 years.) **D,** Lichen planus and associated squamous carcinoma, tongue (transformation after 3 years).

finding oral carcinoma in patients with lichen planus, suggesting an association, particularly in erythematous (erythroplastic) portions.[89,90]

It is of interest to compare lichen planus with leukoplakia. The similarities between patients with lichen planus and those with leukoplakia are comparable age of onset and hyperkeratotic propensity of the epithelium. Red areas seem to increase the risk for dysplasia and carcinoma in both lesions. The two diseases differ in that lichen planus seems to be more common in women, is primarily inflammatory, and bears no relationship to tobacco use.

In summary, the findings indicate a risk of associated malignancy in patients with oral lichen planus, particularly in the erosive form and in erythematous areas (Fig. 2-26). However, a "formal" classification as a precancerous lesion is reserved until transformation rates can be more confidently confirmed. Therefore, all patients with oral lichen planus should be carefully evaluated and observed periodically since a continued benign disease state cannot be indefinitely assured.

SYPHILIS

A positive syphilitic history in the general American population has been estimated at 5% to 8%. Currently, according to the U.S. Center for Disease Control's weekly morbidity and mortality report, almost 800 cases of syphilis are being reported each week in the United States, a 6% increase over 1988. This is probably related to sexual promiscuity, prostitution, and drug abuse.

The evidence for a relationship between oral carcinoma in general and a positive luetic history or active lues is equivocal. A 1958 study found that 18.5% of 108 patients with carcinoma of the tongue had a positive serology or a history of syphilis; histories and serologic tests were positive in 9% of 68 patients with cancer of the floor of mouth, palate, or tonsillar fossa.[91] Another study reported that of 243 patients with primary carcinoma of the tongue, 6% had positive evidence of syphilis.[92] However, a study of 2,177 patients with oral cancer showed that an association with syphilis could not be established.[44] In a 1968 University of California study of oral cancer patients, 8% of 520 patients for whom the information was available had a luetic history.[30] In 412 of these patients whose serology was recorded, 36 (9%) also had positive serologic tests. Half the patients with positive serology had cancer of the tongue. In summary, there is little current evidence supporting an association between syphilis and oral cancer.

The syphilitic lesion (chancre and gumma) may clinically resemble carcinoma. When there is doubt in these cases, appropriate serologic and microscopic examinations must be performed.

VIRUSES

Many factors can cause cells to become malignant, but the role of viruses is being increasingly examined. The phenomenon of viral carcinogenesis is well established in experimental animal systems, but, although there is little doubt that several viruses would cause cancer in human beings if given the opportunity, viral carcinogenesis in humans remains unproven.

HERPES VIRUSES

Any enveloped virus containing double-stranded DNA within an icosahedral capsid about 100 to 150 nm in diameter is known as a herpes virus. The characteristic morphology which is easily recognized under the electron microscope is illustrated in Fig. 2-27. Most animal species are infected by particular herpes viruses, and there are six that cause human disease: *Herpes simplex* virus type-1 (HSV-1), *Herpes simplex* virus type-2 (HSV-2), Epstein-Barr virus (EBV), cytomegalovirus (CMV), *Varicella zoster* virus (VZV), and human herpesvirus 6. Each of these viruses causes an acute human infection, and HSV, EBV, and CMV have been implicated in certain malignant diseases as well.

EBV is almost certainly a cause of Burkitt's lymphoma and nasopharyngeal carcinoma since the virus is epidemiologically associated with those diseases and can transform the target cell type. More recently it has been found that EBV can infect oral epithelial cells[93] and is present in hairy leukoplakias.[94] However, EBV has not been reported in association with oral squamous cell carcinomas.

CMV can transform human cells to a malignant phenotype. It may seem paradoxical that a virus could either lyse cells or convert them to malignancy, but, in fact, many oncogenic animal viruses are capable of performing either function, depending on the conditions that prevail.

Herpes Simplex Virus

HSV can cause acute and recurrent infections at two principal sites: the genital and the oral epithelia. In 1967 it was proposed that the virus isolated from oral lesions be termed HSV-1, and the virus from genital lesions be termed HSV-2. This proposal has been generally adopted, although the two types are remarkably similar. Genital infections with type-1 are often seen, although oral infections with type-2 are rare.[95]

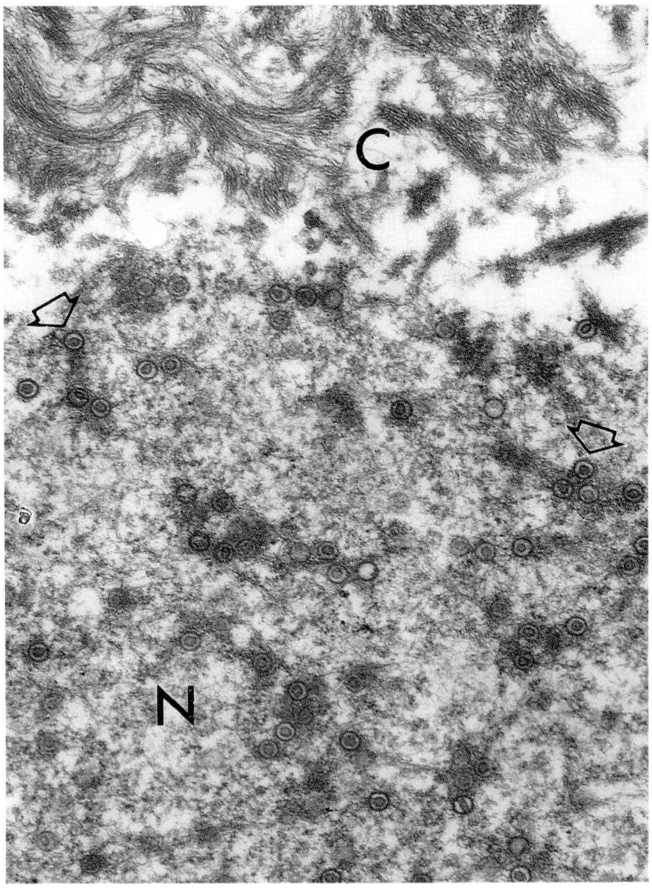

A

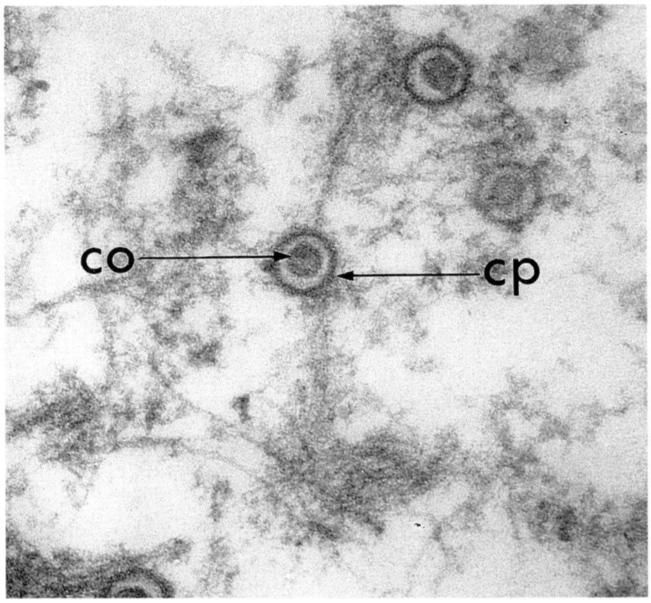

B

Fig. 2-27. Appearance of herpes viruses in the nucleus of a squamous cell. **A,** Low-power electron micrograph showing nucleus (N), fibrillar cytoplasm (C), and herpes viruses (arrows). **B,** High-power view revealing virus core (co) and capsid (cp). This patient had a primary herpetic gingivostomatitis. (From Shillitoe and Silverman, 1979).[96]

The natural history of HSV infections is now well known. During a primary infection with HSV-1 or HSV-2 in mature persons, the lesions are localized to mucous membranes, but the virus travels back along sensory nerves toward the regional sensory ganglion. In the case of primary herpetic gingivostomatitis, this will be the trigeminal ganglion. In a very small proportion of cases the virus passes into the central nervous system and causes encephalitis, but usually the virus remains latent in the ganglion for the lifetime of the individual. The nature of the virus during this time and the factors that maintain latency are not understood, although recent evidence suggests that an 'anti-sense' RNA transcript could be responsible.

Recurrent herpetic infections are not due to exogenous reinfection with HSV but are due to release of virus from latency, followed by its passage along the sensory nerves to the skin. An important finding is that reactivation of the virus is not always accompanied by epithelial lesions. Therefore oral epithelial cells are repeatedly exposed to HSV without being killed, and the long-term effects of this are not known.

The earliest reports of an association between HSV and human cancer concerned a total of eight patients in whom carcinoma of the lip had developed at a site of previous frequent recurrent herpetic infection. These reports were entirely anecdotal, and the cases were selected from a patient population of unknown size. No confirmatory reports have been published since, and in our clinical experience there is no association between recurrent herpes labialis and cancer of the lip or mouth. In 51 consecutive patients with oral cancer, only one had a history of herpes labialis, and that patient's tumor was not associated with the lip.[96] Attempts to culture HSV from swabs taken from the tumor surfaces of oral carcinomas are usually not successful and clinically there is no evidence of a herpetic infection. A comprehensive electron microscopic examination of oral carcinomas in this study showed cytoplasmic disorganization, but no virus particles.

Seroepidemiology

Serologic studies of patients with oral cancer made in the University of California Oral Medicine Clinic over several years have confirmed an association between HSV-1 and oral cancer. In one study researchers first compared the complement-fixing HSV antibody levels in 24 patients with oral cancer with the levels in control subjects, but no significant difference was found. The patients were reexamined two weeks later since a rise in virus antibody titers is diagnostically more significant than any single value. No change in titer was found in 23 of the 24 cases; the remaining patient showed a rise from 1:8 to 1:64.[96]

When neutralizing antibodies were measured, it was seen that patients who were smokers had higher levels of antibody to HSV-1 than non-smokers.[97] This raised the interesting possibility that the irritant effect of cigarette smoke might reactivate latent virus, thereby boosting the level of antibodies. A cocarcinogenic effect of HSV and cigarette smoke is entirely consistent with the experimental evidence discussed below. When antibody of different classes was measured, it was seen that patients with oral cancers had higher levels of IgM and IgA antibodies than the control subjects. These antibodies were directed at two different antigens of the virus, although the nature of those antigens is still unknown.[98,99]

Since these serological studies indicated an association between oral cancer and HSV, a long-term follow-up study was initiated. The levels of IgG, IgA, and IgM antibody to HSV-1, and as a control to CMV, were measured, and the patients were observed for the following five years. It was found that those patients with the highest level of IgM antibody had five-year survivals about half those of patients with the lowest levels of IgM antibody. The inverse was seen with IgG antibodies, as would be expected given the known associations between these antibody classes, and no association was found with antibody to CMV.[100]

Carcinogenicity of HSV

When the earliest clinical studies began to reveal an association between HSV and human carcinomas, experimental work was begun by various researchers to find out if the virus can be carcinogenic under any particular conditions. It was seen that if the cytolytic properties of the virus were inhibited by exposure to ultraviolet light, the virus became capable of transforming hamster cells in a culture. These cells grew as carcinomas if they were reintroduced into the original host. Cells from a variety of species, including human, have now been transformed, both by HSV-1 and HSV-2. The virus was also shown to be oncogenic if exposed first to neutral red and then to visible light. This sequence was recommended at one time as a treatment for recurrent herpetic infections, but it should now be discontinued, or at least used with extreme caution, since some patients developed carcinoma in situ.

Experiments in animals have not yet demonstrated a direct carcinogenic effect of HSV in vivo, but a cocarcinogenic effect has been shown. When the skin of mice was painted with a low concentration of the carcinogen 3-methylcholanthrene, a low incidence of skin tumors was found. The simultaneous application of HSV significantly increased the yield of tumors and also increased the proportion of tumors that became malignant. It may be relevant that in cattle, "spontaneous" oral carcinomas are the result of simultaneous exposure to a papilloma virus and a dietary agent, each of which is noncarcinogenic by itself. An interesting series of experiments carried out in Sweden has shown that if rats are infected in the mouth with HSV-1 and are also given chewing tobacco, many of them develop oral cancer or precancerous lesions.[101] The rats given only HSV-1, or given only chewing tobacco, did not develop any tumors.

HSV cannot be detected in animal tumors established from cells that were transformed by the virus, and no tumor antigens nor DNA fragments are retained by these cells. For these reasons it is now accepted that HSV transforms cells by a 'hit and run' mechanism, leaving behind no traces of its former presence.[102,103] This, of course, makes it extremely difficult to establish the role of HSV in oral cancer. Even if the tumor is induced by the virus, how could this be shown beyond all doubt?

PAPILLOMA VIRUSES

Papilloma viruses are the cause of warts.[104] Unfortunately, human papilloma viruses do not grow in cell cultures or in laboratory animals which has limited the pace of research, but the availability of powerful new techniques of molecular biology has resulted in many important findings regarding these viruses. It has been suspected for a long time that some oral cancers or leukoplakias (such as verrucous carcinoma and atypical verrucous hyperplasia) might be caused by papilloma viruses because of their clinical appearance and slow growth.

The number of human papilloma viruses is very large. More than 50 types were recognized by the end of 1988 with new ones being reported every few months. Some of these types are found mainly in benign lesions, while others are more prevalent in malignant skin tumors and in cervical carcinomas.[105]

Many oral carcinomas contain papilloma viruses. In verrucous carcinomas about one third of the tumors contain HPV 2, which is commonly found in warts,[106] while about half of squamous cell carcinomas contain types 16 or 18 which are also associated with cervical cancer.[107,108] A long-term follow-up study has been initiated to find if there are significant clinical differences between those patients whose tumors contain HPV and those whose do not.

Under experimental conditions papilloma viruses can transform cells to benign or malignant phenotypes. It is, therefore, quite possible that these viruses, like HSV, could be involved in the etiology of oral cancer. Indeed, it is possible that the two viruses could interact with each other to produce tumors.

SUMMARY AND FUTURE RESEARCH

The etiology of oral cancer is complex, but viruses offer a variety of approaches that should clarify the biologic mechanisms involved. The interactions of different virus genes with each other and with other agents such as cigarette smoke are all likely to be important in the etiology of the disease, and they are all accessible for study by modern research techniques. If oral tumors are shown to be under the control of virus gene products, then new targets for rational therapy will have been identified.

DENTURES

Although many carcinomas appear to develop in areas covered by a prosthetic appliance (Fig. 2-28), adequate studies have not been designed to conclusively demonstrate whether this is a coincidental or a cause-and-effect relationship. Careful histories in some oral carcinoma cases indicate that the initial changes resemble traumatic denture ulcers, beginning in the areas where an appliance was chafing or injuring the mucous membrane.

Denture irritation, at most, must only be a cocarcinogenic factor in specifically predisposed individuals. This supposition is based on the fact that more than 35 million Americans over 30 years of age wear one or two full dentures, yet carci-

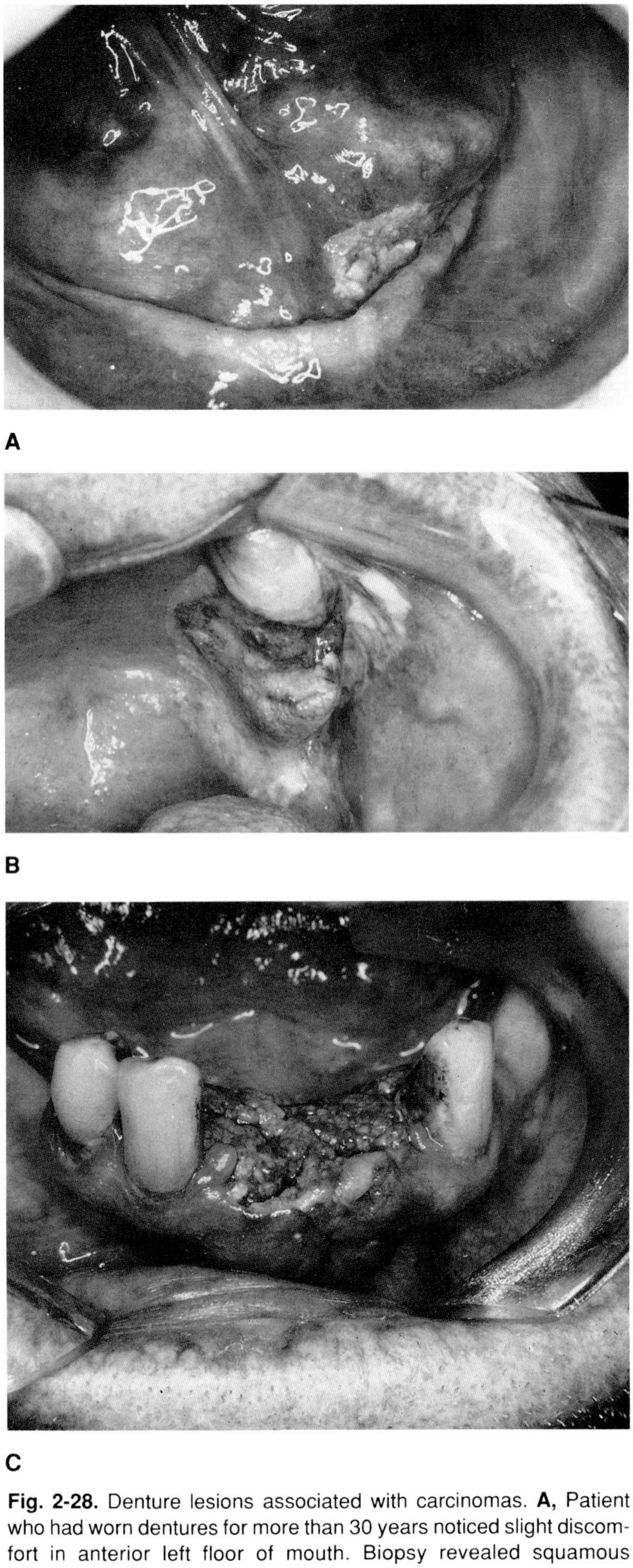

A

B

C

Fig. 2-28. Denture lesions associated with carcinomas. **A,** Patient who had worn dentures for more than 30 years noticed slight discomfort in anterior left floor of mouth. Biopsy revealed squamous carcinoma. **B,** Painful ulcer noticed by patient for 3 months. Biopsy revealed squamous carcinoma. **C,** Mildly symptomatic granular, exophytic lesion, present under partial denture for at least 6 months. Biopsy revealed verrucous carcinoma.

Table 2-13. COMPARISON OF CANCER SITE AND USE OF DENTURES IN 400 CANCER PATIENTS*

			Type of Denture		
Cancer Site	% of Total Lesions	Denture Wearers (%)	Complete Upper and Lower (%)	Complete Upper or Lower (%)	Other Combinations (%)
Tongue	34	42	60	30	10
Floor of mouth	23	49	56	27‡	17
Oropharynx	20	35	54	36	10
Gingiva†	10	43	61	28	11
Buccal mucosa	6	54	62	23	15
Palate	3	43	0	67	33
Lip	4	29	75	0	25
Total	100	43	56	30	14

*Data from Gorsky and Silverman, 1984.[109]
†Seven in maxilla.
‡All upper dentures.

nomas of the palate and alveolar mucosa account for only about 10% of all oral cancers (less than 0.3% of all cancers). Occasionally carcinomas are directly associated with a denture-bearing area. This raises concern that in some patients, even though the risk is low, irritation in addition to other unidentified factors may serve to promote neoplastic activity.

In the University of California Oral Medicine Clinic, 400 patients with oral cancer were studied to determine if there appeared to be a risk related to denture wearing.[109] Forty-three percent of the group wore dentures, and there seemed to be no correlation between the wearing of dentures and any specific cancer site (Table 2-13). Furthermore, there was no difference between denture wearers and other patients relative to age, sex, time from first signs or symptoms to diagnosis, tumor stage, or tobacco use. Other studies[110,111] have also shown no difference between denture wearers and control groups in the occurrence of oral cancer. Therefore, at this time it does not seem plausible to consider denture irritation as a significant carcinogenic aggravating factor. However, since chronic denture irritation and oral cancer have been associated, care should be taken by patient, as well as the dentist, to minimize local irritation and to examine any changes with utmost care.

The same principle might be thought to apply to patients who have poor oral hygiene or jagged teeth or fillings that may act as irritants. There is, however, little controlled evidence to support this supposition, although it is frequently mentioned in almost all articles dealing with etiologic factors of oral cancer. In animal experiments testing various carcinogenic agents, oral tumor induction has been facilitated by trauma.[112] Denture material per se has not been shown to be carcinogenic.

Placement of jaw-bone implants is increasing at a rapid pace, however, there has been no indication of a carcinogenic factor. But since these patients are generally in the higher risk age group, careful examinations and follow-up are indicated.

PALATAL PAPILLARY HYPERPLASIA

This lesion, which is moderately common among denture wearers, is manifested by grape-like clusters of erythematous tissue on palatal mucosa that is covered by either a plastic or a metal prosthetic appliance (Fig. 2-29). It is found mainly in patients who do not have good adaptation. Paradoxically, poor adaptation does not necessarily indicate that a subsequent tissue hyperplasia will develop.

The microscopic picture may sometimes be confusing, since the chronic tissue irritation can cause a reactive-type hyperplasia with resultant nuclear pleomorphism and hyperchromatism. Therefore, lack of familiarity with this lesion may lead to an erroneous interpretation of carcinoma.

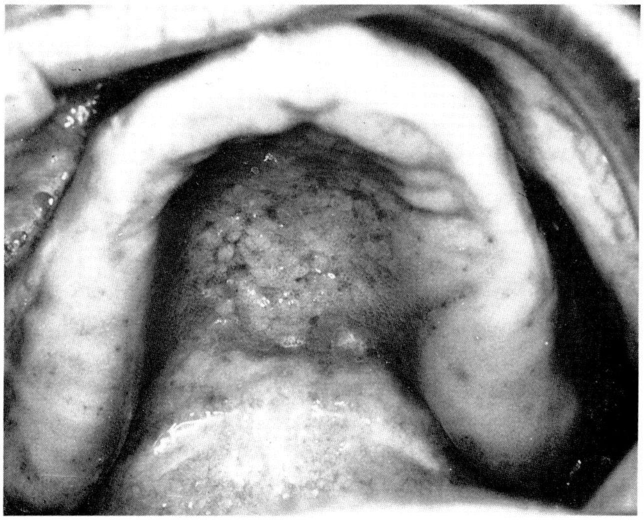

Fig. 2-29. Palatal papillary hyperplasia. This usually asymptomatic lesion is due to a nonspecific tissue reaction to dentures and is not considered precancerous.

Numerous years of observing patients, plus the lack of reports in the literature correlating this lesion with carcinoma, lead to the conclusion that palatal papillary hyperplasia is not a premalignant change.[113,114]

Management demands careful follow-up and elimination of irritation. In case of doubt, periodic cytology and occasional biopsy is advised. Removal of the lesion is elective. However, when indicated for denture adaptation, hygienic purposes, or discomfort, many surgical techniques and prosthodontic approaches have been useful in modifying the hyperplastic tissue. Candidiasis can complicate the diagnosis by producing palatal erythema and symptoms of burning or pain.

NUTRITION

High dietary fat intake may be a factor in colon cancer, indicating that food selection may play a role in carcinogenesis in some sites.[115] Other dietary factors, such as fiber content, have been inconsistently related.[116,117] However, no dietary characteristics have been recognized that distinguish patients with cancer of the oral cavity.[11] In addition, there has been no body of evidence linking oral cancer with deficiencies or excesses in dietary proteins, fats, and carbohydrates. While there have been suggestions that poor dental health and denture status might be related to oral cancer risk by causing chewing difficulties that could adversely affect nutrition, studies have not confirmed this indirect relationship.

Deficiencies of vitamins A or C have been postulated as cocarcinogenic factors. There have been reports of an inverse relationship between ingestion of carotenoids (carotene-rich vegetables) and cancer risk.[118] More specifically, cancers of the mouth, larynx, and esophagus have been negatively related to the intake of fruits and vegetables. Low dietary or serum levels of vitamin A have been associated with oral precancerous lesions and subsequent cancer (see discussion of **Leukoplakia** earlier in this chapter). This association has been based upon the correlation between vitamin A deficiencies and hyperkeratosis, as well as upon demographic studies showing high rates of oral cancer in countries where vitamin A intake is low. Animal studies of oral carcinogenesis using vitamin A in various forms have resulted in inconsistent findings. As for vitamin C, it appears to participate in blocking the conversion of nitrites to nitrosamines (potent carcinogens).[119] However, there are no data to indicate vitamin C deficiencies occur in oral cancer patients.

Minerals have been studied also. Iron deficiency anemia is part of the Plummer-Vinson syndrome, which has been associated with an increased risk for developing carcinoma of the tongue. Iron deficiency has not been shown to be a common finding in patients presenting with oral cancer, although high iron storage has been indicated as a possible marker or factor in cancer.[120] Zinc and copper also have been implicated in head and neck cancer, but a recent study of zinc and copper in oropharyngeal cancer patients found that serum levels of these elements were not different from those of control subjects and were not useful as markers.[121] While hypercalcemia indicates a poor prognosis in patients with head and neck cancer, alterations in calcium metabolism have no cause-effect relationship.

Nutrition is an important factor in the management of patients during treatment and in rehabilitation (see Chapters 6 and 10). Poor nutrition and abnormal weight loss is usually associated with cachexia, intercurrent infections, and a poor prognosis.[122] On the other hand, obesity appears to be equally associated with poor survival.[123,124] Obviously then, factors that encourage adequate food intake and a nutritious diet are important to survival in conjunction with tumor control.

DENTAL RADIATION

There is no evidence at the present time to indicate that exposure to radiation from periodic routine diagnostic dental x-ray examination is mutagenic or carcinogenic.[125–127] However, to minimize any potential risk to patients, it is advisable that all procedures that will reduce radiation exposure consistent with patients' diagnostic requirements be used. Some dentists have carelessly exposed themselves to radiation over a period of years, leading to carcinomas of their fingers.

FLUORIDATED WATER

In September 1977, Dr. Arthur Upton, then Director of the National Cancer Institute, made the following statement to the House Committee on Government Operations of the U.S. Congress: "No trends in cancer rates can be ascribed to the consumption of water that is artificially or naturally fluoridated." Numerous studies and comprehensive reviews that compare mortality data between communities with fluoridated and nonfluoridated water document this statement. No study has suggested that fluoridation poses any hazard to health or increased the risk for cancer.[128,129]

REFERENCES

1. Farber E: Cancer development and its natural history. *Cancer* 62:1676, 1988.
2. Scully C: The immunology of cancer of the head and neck with particular reference to oral cancer. *Oral Surg Oral Med Oral Pathol* 53:157, 1982.
3. Eskinazi DP, Perna JJ, Mihail R: Mononuclear cell subsets in patients with oral cancer. *Cancer* 60:376, 1987.
4. Friend SH, Dryja TP, Weinberg RA: Oncogenes and tumor-suppressing genes. *N Engl J Med* 318:618, 1988.
5. Benowitz NL: Drug Therapy. Pharmacologic aspects of cigarette smoking and nicotine addiction. *N Engl J Med* 319:1318, 1988.
6. Fielding JE: Smoking: Health effects and control. *N Engl J Med* 313:555, 1985.
7. Newell GR, Vogel VG: Personal risk factors. What do they mean? *Cancer* 62:1695, 1988.
8. Ernster VL: Trends in smoking, cancer risk, and cigarette promotion. Current priorities for reducing tobacco exposure. *Cancer* 62:1702, 1988.
9. Hammond EC, Horn D: Smoking and death rates—report on forty-four months of follow-up of 187,783 men. *CA* 38:28, 1988.
10. Enstrom JE: Cancer mortality among Mormons. *Cancer* 36:825, 1975.
11. Graham S, Dayal H, Rohrer T et al: Dentition, diet, tobacco and alcohol in the epidemiology of oral cancer. *J Natl Cancer Inst* 59:1611, 1977.

12. Mashberg A, Garfinkel L, Harris S: Alcohol as a primary risk factor in oral squamous carcinoma. *CA* 31:146, 1981.
13. Silverman S Jr, Gorsky M, Greenspan D: Tobacco usage in patients with head and neck carcinomas: A follow-up study on habit changes and second primary oral/oropharyngeal cancers. *J Am Dent Assoc* 106:33, 1983.
14. McKenzie M, McLemore T, Rankin P et al: A human plasma component that binds benzo(a)pyrene. *Cancer* 42:2733, 1978.
15. McLemore TL, Martin RR, Wray NP et al: Reassessment of the relationshp between aryl hydrocarbon hydroxylase and lung cancer. *Cancer* 48:1438, 1981.
16. Moore C: Cigarette smoking and cancer of the mouth, pharynx and larynx. A continuing study. *JAMA* 218:533, 1971.
17. Johnston WD, Ballantyne AJ: Prognostic effect of tobacco and alcohol use in patients with oral tongue cancer. *Am J Surg* 134:444, 1977.
18. Wynder EL, Hoffman D: Tobacco and health. *N Engl J Med* 300:894, 1979.
19. Spitz MR, Fueger JJ, Goepfert H et al: Squamous cell carcinoma of the upper aerodigestive tract. A case comparison analysis. *Cancer* 61:203, 1988.
20. Christen AG, Swanson BZ, Glover ED: Smokeless tobacco: The folklore and social history of snuffing, sneezing, dipping, and chewing. *J Am Dent Assoc* 105:821, 1982.
21. Greer RO Jr, Poulson TC: Oral tissue alterations associated with the use of smokeless tobacco by teenagers. Part I. Clinical findings. *Oral Surg Oral Med Oral Pathol* 56:275, 1983.
22. Creath CJ, Shelton WO, Wright JT et al: The prevalence of smokeless tobacco use among adolescent male athletes. *J Amer Dent Assoc* 116:43, 1988.
23. Squier CA: The nature of smokeless tobacco and patterns of use. *CA* 38:226, 1988.
24. Connolly GN, Winn DM, Hecht SS et al: The reemergence of smokeless tobacco. *N Engl J Med* 314:1020, 1986.
25. Holmstrup P, Pindborg JJ: Oral mucosal lesions in smokeless tobacco users. *CA* 38:230, 1988.
26. Winn DM: Smokeless tobacco and cancer: The epidemiologic evidence. *CA* 38:236, 1988.
27. Alston R, Jacoway J: Verrucous carcinoma of the oral mucosa in North Carolina (Abstract 158). *J Dent Res* 59 (Special Issue A): 307, 1980.
28. Winn DM, Blot WJ, Shy CM et al: Snuff dipping and oral cancer among women in the Southern United States. *N Engl J Med* 304:745, 1981.
29. Going RE, Hsu SC, Pollack RL et al: Sugar and fluoride content of various forms of tobacco. *J Am Dent Assoc* 100:27, 1980.
30. Chierici G, Silverman S Jr, Forsythe B: A tumor registry study of oral squamous carcinoma. *J Oral Med* 23:91, 1968.
31. Gritz ER: Cigarette smoking: The need for action by health professionals. *CA* 38:194, 1988.
32. Schroeder KL, Soller HA, Chen MS et al: Screening for smokeless tobacco-associated lesions: Recommendations for the dental practitioner. *J Am Dent Assoc* 116:37, 1988.
33. Christen AG, McDonald JL Jr, Olson BL et al: Efficacy of nicotine chewing gum in facilitating smoking cessation. *J Am Dent Assoc* 108:594, 1984.
34. Tonnesen P, Fryd V, Hansen M et al: Effect of nicotine chewing gum in combination with group counseling on the cessation of smoking. *N Engl J Med* 318:15, 1988.
35. Cooper TM, Clayton RR: Stop-smoking program using nicotine reduction therapy and behavior modification for heavy smokers. *J Am Dent Assoc* 118:47, 1989.
36. Benowitz NL: Health and public policy implications of the "low yield" cigarette (editorial). *N Engl J Med* 320:1619, 1989.
37. Malaowalla AM, Silverman S Jr, Mani NJ et al: Oral cancer in 57,518 industrial workers of Gujarat, India. A prevalence and follow-up study. *Cancer* 37:1882, 1976.
38. Ramulu C, Raju MVS, Venkatarathnam G et al: Nicotine stomatitis and its relation to carcinoma of the hard palate in reverse smokers of chuttas. *J Dent Res* 52:711, 1973.
39. Schmidt W, Popham RE: The role of drinking and smoking in mortality from cancer and other causes in male alcoholics. *Cancer* 47:1031, 1981.
40. Wynder L, Bross IJ, Feldman RM: A study of the etiological factors in cancer of the mouth. *Cancer* 10:1300, 1957.
41. Monson RR, Lyon JL: Proportional mortality among alcoholics. *Cancer* 36:1077, 1975.
42. Smart CR, Lyon JL, Skolnick M et al: Cancer of the head and neck in Utah. *Am J Surg* 128:463, 1974.
43. Trieger N, Taylor GW, Weisberger D: The significance of liver dysfunction in mouth cancer. *Surg Gynecol Obstet* 108:230, 1959.
44. Keller A: The epidemiology of lip, oral, and pharyngeal cancers, and the association with selected systemic diseases. *Am J Public Health* 53:1214, 1963.
45. Keller A: Cirrhosis of the liver, alcoholism and heavy smoking associated with cancer of the mouth and pharynx. *Cancer* 20:1015, 1967.
46. McCoy GD, Wynder EL: Etiological and preventive implications in alcohol carcinogenesis. *Cancer Res* 39:2844, 1979.
47. Freedman A, Shklar G: Alcohol and hamster buccal pouch carcinogenesis. *Oral Surg Oral Med Oral Pathol* 46:794, 1978.
48. Rothman K, Keller A: The effect of joint exposure to alcohol and tobacco on risk of cancer of the mouth and pharynx. *J Chronic Dis* 25:711, 1972.
49. Kissin B, Kaley M, Su WH et al: Head and neck cancer in alcoholics: The relationship to drinking, smoking, and dietary patterns. *JAMA* 224:1174, 1973.
50. Keller AZ: Alcohol, tobacco and age factors in the relative frequency of cancer among males with and without liver cirrhosis. *Am J Epidemiol* 106:194, 1977.
51. Vickers RA, Shapiro BL: The incidence of oral malignant neoplasia in an adult population of Minnesota. A report of results in oral cancer detection (Abstract 486). 45th Gen Meeting, Int Assoc Dent Res, *Program and Abstracts of Papers*, 1967.
52. Knapp MJ: Oral disease in 181,338 consecutive oral examinations. *J Am Dent Assoc* 83:1288, 1971.
53. Pindborg JJ, Mehta FS, Gupta PC et al: Prevalence of oral submucous fibrosis among 50,915 Indian villagers. *Br J Cancer* 22:646, 1968.
54. Silverman S Jr, Bhargava K, Mani NJ et al: Malignant transformation and natural history of oral leukoplakia in 57,518 industrial workers of Gujarat, India. *Cancer* 38:1790, 1976.
55. Pindborg JJ, Renstrup G, Poulsen HE et al: Studies in oral leukoplakias. V. Clinical and histologic signs of malignancy. *Acta Odontol Scand* 20:407, 1963.
56. Einhorn J, Wersall J: Incidence of oral carcinoma in patients with leukoplakia of the oral mucosa. *Cancer* 20:2189, 1967.
57. Pindborg JJ, Renstrup G, Joist O et al: Studies in oral leukoplakia: A preliminary report on the period prevalence of malignant transformation in leukoplakia based on a follow-up study of 248 patients. *J Am Dent Assoc* 76:767, 1968.
58. Silverman S Jr, Rozen RD: Observations on the clinical characteristics and natural history of oral leukoplakia. *J Am Dent Assoc* 76:772, 1968.
59. Kramer IRH: Precancerous conditions of the oral mucosa. A computer-aided study. *Ann R Coll Surg Engl* 45:340, 1969.

60. Mehta FS, Shroff BC, Gupta PC et al: Oral leukoplakia in relation to tobacco habits: A 10-year follow-up of Bombay policemen. *Oral Surg Oral Med Oral Pathol* 34:426, 1972.
61. Banoczy J, Csiba A: Comparative study of the clinical picture and histopathologic structure of oral leukoplakia. *Cancer* 29:1230, 1972.
62. Banoczy J: Follow-up studies in oral leukoplakia. *J Maxillofac Surg* 5:69, 1977.
63. Gupta PC, Mehta FS, Daftary DK et al: Incidence rates of oral cancer and natural history of oral precancerous lesions in a 10-year follow-up study of Indian villagers. *Community Dent Oral Epidemiol* 8:287, 1980.
64. Silverman S Jr, Gorsky M, Lozada F: Oral leukoplakia and malignant transformation. A follow-up study of 257 patients. *Cancer* 53:563, 1984.
65. Shibuya H, Amagasa T, Seto K et al: Leukoplakia-associated multiple carcinomas in patients with tongue carcinoma. *Cancer* 57:843, 1986.
66. Bouquot JE, Weiland LH, Kurland LT: Leukoplakia and carcinoma in situ synchronously associated with invasive oral/oropharyngeal carcinoma in Rochester, Minn., 1935–1984. *Oral Med Oral Surg Oral Pathol* 65:199, 1988.
67. Roed-Petersen B: Cancer development in oral leukoplakia: Follow-up of 331 patients (Abstract 20). *J Dent Res* 50:711, 1971.
68. Mehta FS, Pindborg JJ: Spontaneous regression of oral leukoplakia among Indian villagers in a 5-year follow-up study. *Community Dent Oral Epidemiol* 2:80, 1974.
69. Mincer HH, Coleman SA, Hopkins KP: Observations on the clinical characteristics of oral lesions showing histologic epithelial dysplasia. *Oral Surg Oral Med Oral Pathol* 33:389, 1972.
70. Banoczy J, Csiba A: Occurrence of epithelial dysplasia in oral leukoplakia. Analysis and follow-up study of 12 cases. *Oral Surg Oral Med Oral Pathol* 42:766, 1976.
71. Pindborg JJ, Daftary DK, Mehta FS: A follow-up study of sixty-one oral dysplastic precancerous lesions in Indian villagers. *Oral Surg Oral Med Oral Pathol* 43:383, 1977.
72. Kramer, IRH, El-Labban N, Lee KW: The clinical features and risk of malignant transformation in sublingual keratosis. *Br Dent J* 144:171, 1978.
73. Waldron CA, Shafer WG: Leukoplakia revisited. A clinicopathologic study of 3,256 oral leukoplakias. *Cancer* 36:1386, 1975.
74. Mashberg A, Morissey JB, Garfinkle L: A study of the appearance of early asymptomatic oral squamous carcinomas. *Cancer* 32:1436, 1973.
75. Mashberg A: Anatomical site and size of 222 early asymptomatic oral squamous carcinomas. *Cancer* 37:2149, 1976.
76. Mashberg A: Erythroplasia: the earliest sign of asymptomatic oral cancer. *J Am Dent Assoc* 96:615, 1978.
77. Hansen LS, Olson JA, Silverman S Jr: Proliferative verrucous leukoplakia. A long-term study of 30 patients. *Oral Surg Oral Med Oral Pathol* 60:3, 1985.
78. Arendorf TM, Walker DM: The prevalence and intra-oral distribution of *Candida albicans* in man. *Arch Oral Biol* 25:1, 1980.
79. Samaranayake LP: Oral candidosis: predisposing factors and pathogenesis. *In* D.D. Derrick (ed) *The 1989 Dental Annual.* London: Wright, 1989, pp. 219–35.
80. Roed-Petersen B, Renstrup G, Pindborg JJ: *Candida* in oral leukoplakias. A histologic and exfoliative cytologic study. *Scand J Dent Res* 78:323, 1970.
81. Renstrup G: Occurrence of *Candida* in oral leukoplakias. *Acta Pathol Microbiol Scand* (Sect B) 78:421, 1970.
82. Greenspan JS, Greenspan D: Oral hairy leukoplakia: Diagnosis and management. *Oral Surg Oral Med Oral Pathol* 67:396, 1989.
83. Chu FW, Silverman S Jr, Dedo HH: CO;i2 laser treatment of oral leukoplakia. *Laryngoscope* 98:125, 1988.
84. Silverman S Jr, Eisenberg E, Renstrup G: A study of the effects of high doses of vitamin A on oral leukoplakia (hyperkeratosis), including toxicity, liver function and skeletal metabolism. *J Oral Ther Pharmacol* 2:9, 1965.
85. Shklar G: Oral leukoplakia. *N Engl J Med* 315:1544, 1986.
86. Hong WK, Endicott J, Itri LM et al: 13-*cis*-retinoic acid in the treatment of oral leukoplakia. *N Engl J Med* 315:1501, 1986.
87. Silverman S Jr, Griffith M: Studies on oral lichen planus. II. Follow-up on 200 patients, clinical characteristics, and associated malignancy. *Oral Surg Oral Med Oral Pathol* 37:705, 1974.
88. Silverman S Jr, Gorsky M, Lozada-Nur F: A prospective follow-up study of 570 patients with oral lichen planus: Persistence, remission, and malignant association. *Oral Surg Oral Med Oral Pathol* 60:30, 1985.
89. Holmstrup P, Pindborg JJ: Erythroplakic lesions in relation to oral lichen planus. *Acta Derm Venereol* 59 (suppl 85):77, 1979.
90. Fulling HJ: Cancer development in oral lichen planus. A follow-up study of 327 patients. *Arch Dermatol* 108:667, 1973.
91. Trieger N, Ship II, Taylor GW et al: Cirrhosis and other predisposing factors in carcinoma of the tongue. *Cancer* 11:357, 1958.
92. Meyer I, Abbey LM: The relationship of syphilis to primary carcinoma of the tongue. *Oral Surg Oral Med Oral Pathol* 30:678, 1970.
93. Sixbey JW, Nedrud JG, Raab-Traub N et al: Epstein-Barr virus replication in oropharyngeal epithelial cells. *N Engl J Med* 310:1225, 1984.
94. Greenspan JS, Greenspan D, Lennette ET et al: Replication of Epstein-Barr virus within the epithelial cells of oral "hairy" leukoplakia, an AIDS-associated lesion. *N Engl J Med* 313:1564, 1985.
95. Docherty JJ, Trimble JJ, Roman SR et al: Lack of oral HSV-2 in a college student population. *J Med Virol* 16:283, 1985.
96. Shillitoe EJ, Silverman S Jr: Oral cancer and herpes simplex virus: A review. *Oral Surg Oral Med Oral Pathol* 48:216, 1979.
97. Shillitoe EJ, Greenspan D, Greenspan JS et al: Neutralizing antibody to herpes simplex virus type I in patients with oral cancer. *Cancer* 49:2315, 1982.
98. Shillitoe EJ, Greenspan D, Greenspan JS et al: Immunoglobulin class of antibody to herpes simplex virus type I in patients with oral cancer. *Cancer* 51:65, 1983.
99. Shillitoe EJ, Greenspan D, Greenspan JS et al: Antibody to early and late antigens of herpes simplex virus type I in patients with oral cancer. *Cancer* 54:266, 1984.
100. Shillitoe EJ, Hwang CBC, Silverman S Jr et al: Examination of oral cancer tissue for the presence of the proteins ICP4 ICP5 ICP6 ICP8 and gB of herpes simplex virus type I. *J Natl Cancer Inst* 76:371, 1986.
101. Hirsch JM, Johansson SL, Vahlne A: Effect of snuff and herpes simplex virus I on rat oral mucosa. Possible association with development of squamous cell carcinoma. *J Oral Path* 13:52, 1984.
102. Galloway DA, McDougall JK: The oncogenic potential of herpes simplex viruses: Evidence for a 'hit-and-run' mechanism. *Nature* 302:21, 1983.

103. Macnab JCM. Herpes simplex virus and human cytomegalovirus: Their role in morphological transformation and genital cancers. *J Gen Virol* 68:2525, 1987.
104. Gross G, Pfister H, Hagedorn M et al: Correlation between human papillomavirus (HPV) type and histology of warts. *J Invest Dermatol* 78:160, 1982.
105. Lorinez AT, Temple GF, Kurman RJ et al: Oncogenic association of specific human papillomavirus types with cervial neoplasia. *J Natl Cancer Inst* 79:671, 1987.
106. Adler-Storthz K, Newland JR, Tessin BA et al: Human papillomavirus type 2 DNA in oral verrucous carcinoma. *J Oral Path* 15:472, 1986.
107. Milde K, Loning T: Detection of papillomavirus DNA in oral papillomas and carcinomas: Application of in situ hybridization with biotinylated HPV 16 probes. *J Oral Pathol* 15:292, 1986.
108. Maitland NJ, Cox MF, Lynas C et al: Detection of human papillomavirus DNA in biopsies of human oral tissue. *Br J Cancer* 56:245, 1987.
109. Gorsky M, Silverman S Jr: Denture wearing and oral cancer. *J Prosthet Dent* 52:164, 1984.
110. Wynder EL, Bross IJ, Feldman RM: A study of the etiological factors in cancer of the mouth. *Cancer* 10:1300, 1957.
111. Browne RM, Camsey MC, Waterhouse JAH et al: Etiological factors in oral squamous cell carcinoma. *Community Dent Oral Epidemiol* 5:301, 1977.
112. Fujita K, Kaku T, Sasaki M et al: Experimental production of lingual carcinomas in hamsters by local application of 9, 10-dimethyl-1,2 benzanthracene. *J Dent Res* 52:327, 1973.
113. Guernsey LH: Reactive inflammatory papillary hyperplasia of the palate. *Oral Surg Oral Med Oral Pathol* 20:814, 1965.
114. Bhaskar SN, Beasley JD III, Cutright DE: Inflammatory papillary hyperplasia of the oral mucosa: Report of 341 cases. *J Am Dent Assoc* 81:949, 1970.
115. Byers T: Diet and cancer. *Cancer* 62:1713, 1988.
116. Miller EC, Miller JA: Carcinogens and mutagens that may occur in foods. *Cancer* 58:1795, 1986.
117. Kritchevsky D: Diet and nutrition research. *Cancer* 62(8 suppl):1839, 1988.
118. Hennekens CH, Mayrent SL, Willett W: Vitamin A, carotenoids and retinoids. *Cancer* 58:1837, 1986.
119. Mivrish SS: Effects of vitamins C and E on N-nitroso compound formation, carcinogenesis and cancer. *Cancer* 58:1842, 1986.
120. Stevens RG, Jones DY, Micozzi MS et al: Body iron stores and the risk of cancer. *N Engl J Med* 319:1047, 1988.
121. Silverman S Jr, Thompson JS: Serum zinc and copper in oral/oropharyngeal carcinoma. A study of seventy-five patients. *Oral Surg Oral Med Oral Pathol* 57:34, 1984.
122. Grosvenor M, Bulcavage L, Chlebowski RT: Symptoms potentially influencing weight loss in a cancer population. Correlations with primary site, nutritional status, and chemotherapy administration. *Cancer* 63:330, 1989.
123. Heber D, Byerly LO, Chi J et al: Pathophysiology of malnutrition in the adult cancer patient. *Cancer* 58:1867, 1986.
124. Gross L: Inhibition of the development of tumors or leukemia in mice and rats after reduction in food intake. Possible implications for humans. *Cancer* 62:1463, 1988.
125. White SC, Frey NW: An estimation of somatic hazards to the United States population from dental radiology. *Oral Surg Oral Med Oral Pathol* 43:152, 1977.
126. Campbell JA: Where does dentistry stand on radiation? *J Calif Dent Assoc* 14(9):17, 1986.
127. Underhill TE, Kimura K, Chilvarguer I et al: Radiobiologic risk estimation from dental radiology. Part II. Cancer incidence and fatality. *Oral Surg Oral Med Oral Pathol* 66:261, 1988.
128. Newbrun E: Water fluoridation and fluoride supplements in caries prevention. *CDA Journal* 8:38, 1980.
129. Clemmesen J: The alleged association between artificial fluoridation of water supplies and cancer: A review. *Bull WHO* 61:871, 1983.

3

Diagnosis

SOL SILVERMAN, JR.
WILLIAM P. DILLON • Imaging

A clinician's dilemma in oral diagnosis stems from the multitude of ill-defined, variable-appearing, controversial, and poorly understood lesions that manifest themselves in the oral cavity. Most of these lesions are benign, and many present changes that may easily be confused with malignancy. Conversely, early malignancy may be mistaken for a benign change (Figs. 3-1, 3-2). Some lesions are considered premalignant because they are statistically correlated with subsequent associated cancerous changes. Inescapably, then, much clinical uncertainty is involved in the early detection of malignancy as well as in the understanding and management of other lesions that may not always remain benign.

DELAY IN DIAGNOSIS

Both public and professional awareness of oral cancer are fundamental for minimizing the time from onset of signs or symptoms to diagnosis. In most instances delay is due to patients' not seeking consultation. However, in a considerable number of cases diagnosis has been delayed because a clinician did not suspect the malignant nature of the lesion and treated it by empirical procedures inadequate for cancer control. Most patients will delay seeking professional advice for more than three months after becoming aware of an oral sign or symptom. Such delays in diagnosis can only lead to local extension of a lesion and increase the risk of metastatic spread (see Chapter 7).

SIGNS AND SYMPTOMS

Although some patients finally seek consultation only after developing severe and persistent pain, the most frequent chief complaint is that of a "sore" or "irritation" in the mouth. Early carcinoma of the oral cavity may be painless. Pain usually occurs when the lesion becomes ulcerated. Sometimes a patient seeks consultation because of a "lump in the neck" that represents a metastasis from an oral lesion of which the patient may be completely unaware.

The following are the most common presenting signs of oral carcinoma:

Ulceration or erosion—Destruction of epithelial integrity owing to discrepancy in cell maturation, loss of intercellular attachments, and disruption of basal lamina (basement membrane).

Erythema—Redness reflecting inflammation, thinness and irregularity of epithelium, and lack of keratinization.

Induration—Hardness due primarily to an increase in number of epithelial cells, and secondarily to an inflammatory infiltrate.

Fixation—Abnormally dividing cells invading to deeper areas and onto muscle and bone.

Chronicity—Failure to heal. Cancer is not a spontaneously reversible disease. Therefore, a malignant lesion normally will not disappear in the absence of definitive antitumor therapy. However, in the world literature 176 cases of spontaneous remission have been reported[1]; two involved the head and neck region (tongue and laryngeal carcinomas).

Lymphadenopathy—Hardening and/or enlargement of regional nodes due to engorgement with neoplastic cells that spread by lymphatic vessels (see Chapter 4). Nodes are usually painless and soon become fixed because of capsular erosion and local infiltration.

Leukoplakia—A white patch on the muscosal surface, reflecting excess keratin production. Hyperkeratosis is often associated with carcinomatous lesions (see Chapter 2).

Marked induration, fixation, and lymphadenopathy are signs of advanced lesions. Early carcinomas may appear as small, apparently harmless areas of induration or local changes (erosion, erythema, keratosis), frequently lulling the unsuspecting clinician into a false sense of security. In the premalignant and early cancerous stages, cellular proliferation may be slow, which in some cases may clinically obscure clinical recognition of growth or tumor activity. All lesions of the oral cavity that persist or do not respond to the usual therapeutic measures must therefore be considered malignant until proven otherwise.

An insight into the histopathogenesis of carcinoma may give the clinician a better understanding of presenting signs. Fig. 3-3 depicts the transformation from normal epithelium to dysplasia and finally to malignancy.

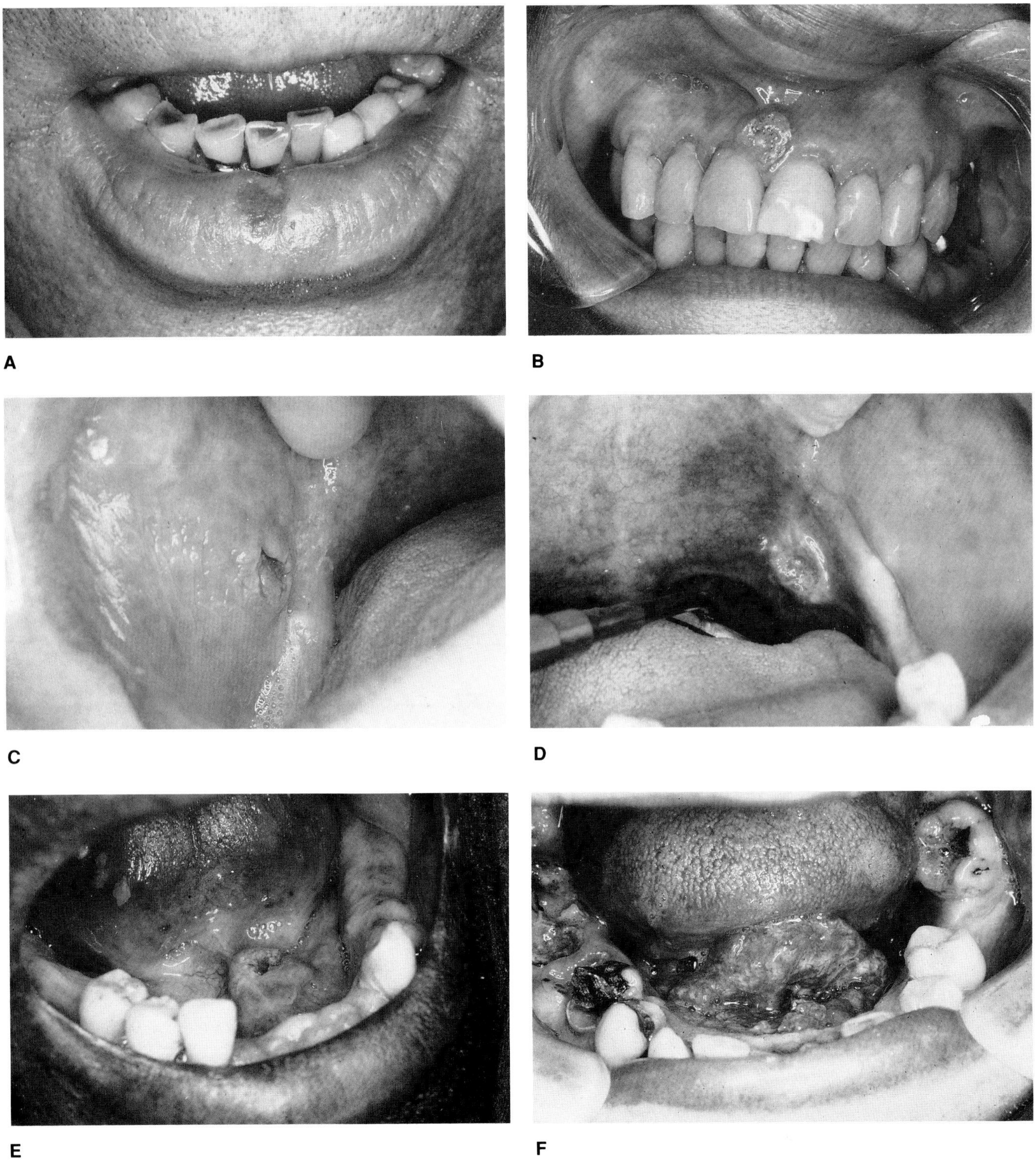

Fig. 3-1. Varied appearances of oral squamous cancers. **A,** Early carcinoma of lower lip, thought to be a "chronic cold sore" of 2 months' duration. **B,** Early carcinoma of the gingiva, thought to be a parulis. **C,** Early carcinoma of right buccal mucosa, thought to be a response to denture irritation. **D,** Early carcinoma resembling an aphthous ulcer, noticed on left soft palate, thought to be a traumatic or an aphthous ulcer. **E,** Early carcinoma of mouth floor first noticed because of mild pain of 3 weeks' duration. **F,** Advanced carcinoma of mouth floor. Signs and symptoms were ignored by patient for 6 months.

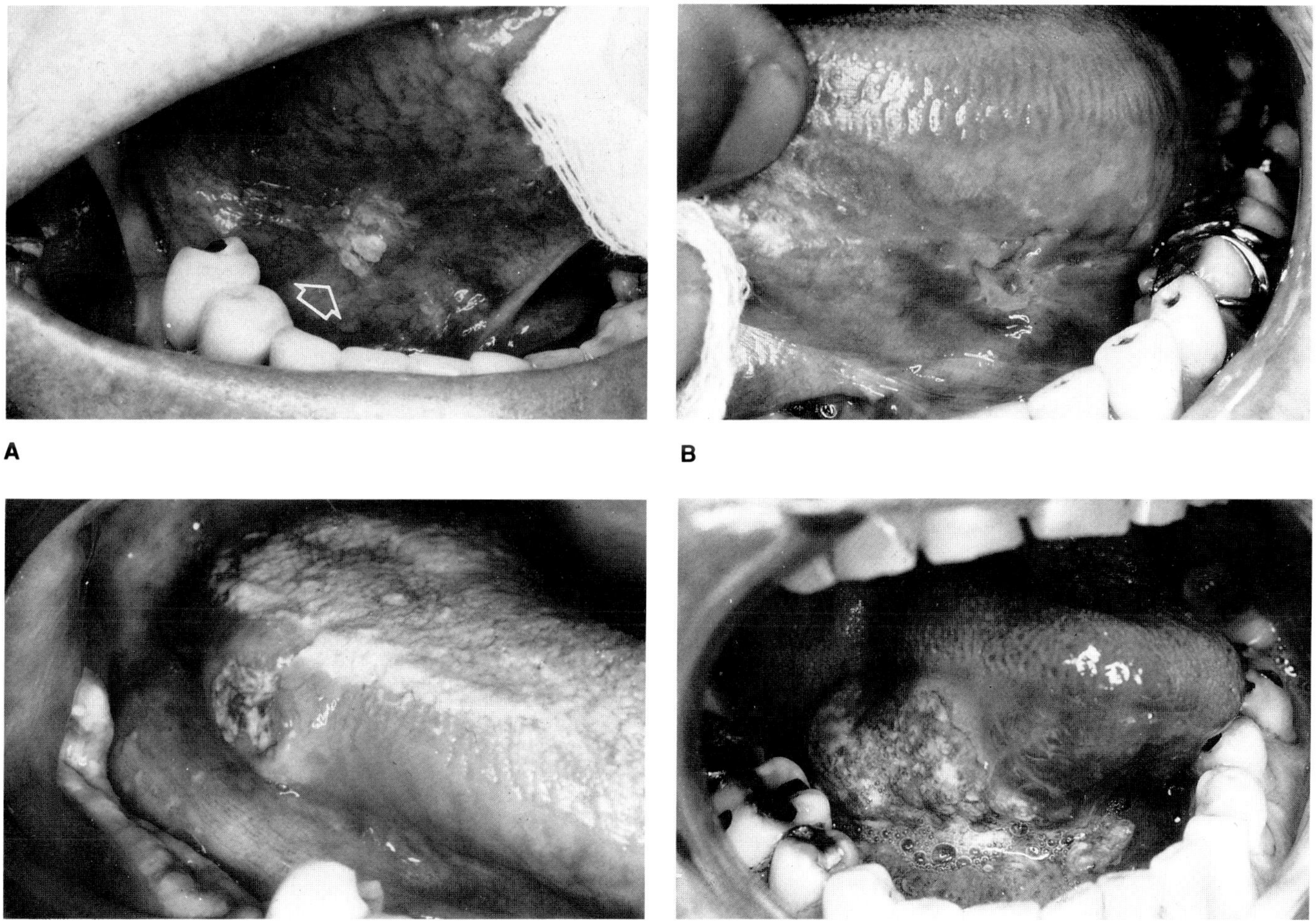

Fig. 3-2. Cancer of the tongue, the most common intraoral site. **A,** Squamous carcinoma of ventral lateral tongue, mimicking leukoplakia. **B,** Moderately painful carcinoma, noticed by patient for 2 weeks, thought to be an aphthous or traumatic lesion. **C,** Painful carcinoma of lateral tongue, thought to be an infectious process. **D,** Large carcinoma of right tongue, extending onto floor of mouth, noticed by patient for more than 6 months.

Once dysplasia becomes visible microscopically, there is no way of knowing whether it will reverse itself, because there are no clear-cut criteria for determining which dysplasias will transform into carcinoma and which will not. Therefore, the terms "carcinoma in situ" or "intraepithelial carcinoma" refer to severely dysplastic epithelium that most probably will proceed into malignancy. Once the disorderly activity of cells involves disruption of the basal lamina and invasion of the adjacent connective tissue, the diagnosis of malignancy can be made unequivocally.

BIOPSY AND EXFOLIATIVE CYTOLOGY

Because of the variability of signs and symptoms, even good clinical judgment and experience will not preclude diagnostic errors. Since oral cancer has such a poor prognosis, early detection and early adequate treatment are essential to the improvement of cure rates. Biopsy is the only method of definitively diagnosing a cancer.

Immediate biopsy of every ill-defined or innocuous-appearing lesion is impractical and not indicated. It is obvious, then, that a simple, reliable, and acceptable technique to support clinical judgment in differentiating benign from early malignant neoplasia is highly desirable. Exfoliative cytology is one technique that serves this purpose, but it must be remembered that cytology is an adjunct to, not a substitute for, biopsy.

EXFOLIATIVE CYTOLOGY

Exfoliative cytology is a technique used for observing the microscopic morphology of individual cells after they have been obtained from a tissue, spread on a slide, fixed, and stained (Table 3-1, Fig. 3-4). Because the oral epithelium renews itself fairly rapidly (probably within two weeks) and most superficial cells of the mouth contain nuclei, surface scrapings may be reliable indicators of dysplastic or neoplastic changes. The usefulness of cytology is augmented in oral

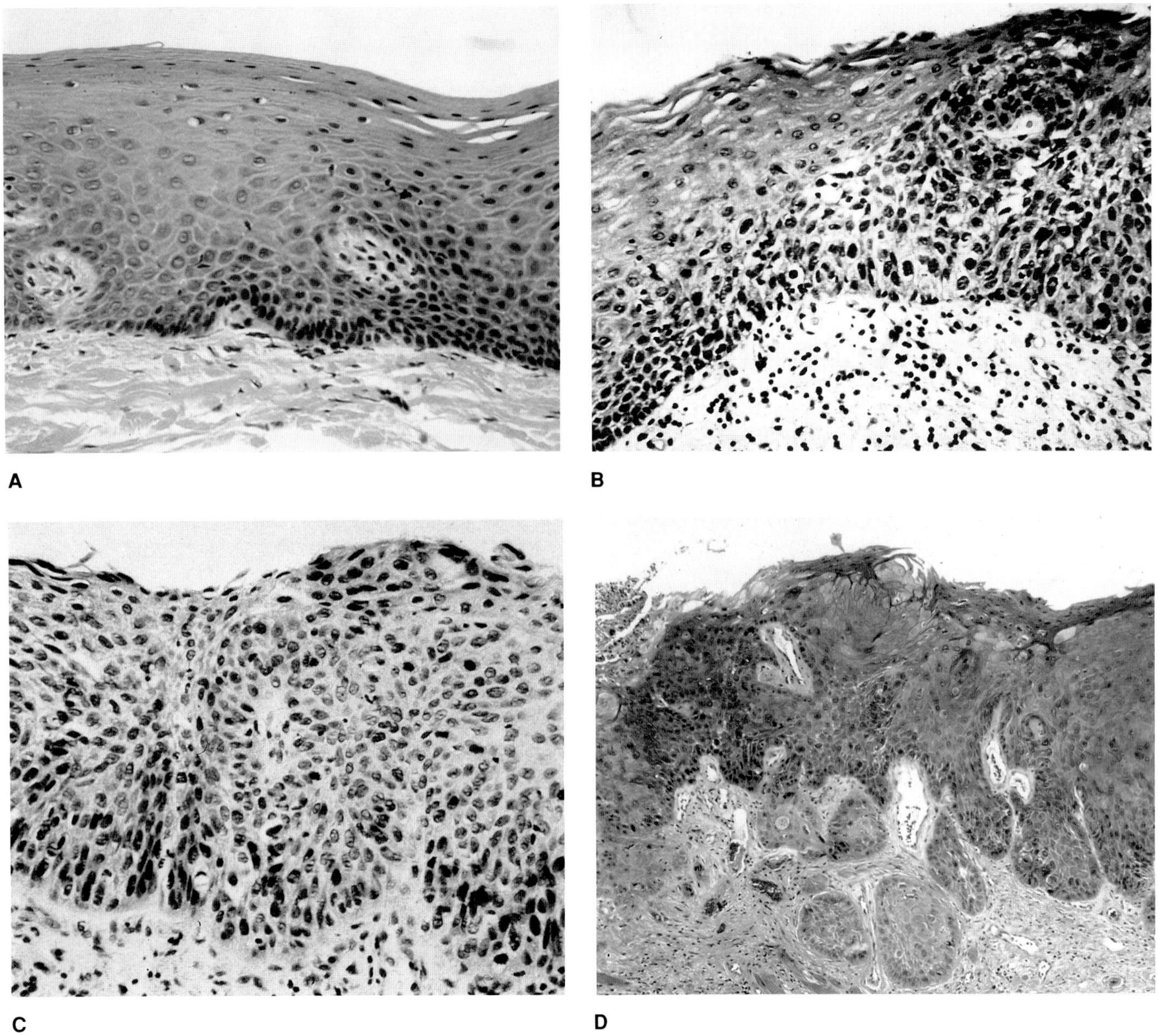

Fig. 3-3. Transformation of epithelium from normal to malignant. **A,** Normal buccal epithelium. **B,** Transition zone between normal buccal epithelium (left) and severe dysplasia or carcinoma in situ (right). **C,** Intraepithelial carcinoma. Note apparently intact basal lamina (basement membrane), which is confining all of the abnormal cells to the epithelial layer. **D,** Squamous cell carcinoma. Malignant cells, both individually and in groups, have penetrated the basal lamina and invaded the connective tissue.

cancer detection by the fact that over 95% of oral cancers are epithelial in origin. Direct smears allow for accurate sampling of a lesion and aid complete screening.[2] Numerous reports substantiate the fact that use of oral cytology has accelerated clinicians' use of biopsy of lesions that did not clinically appear to be oral cancers, thus leading to the early diagnosis of malignancies that would otherwise have remained unsuspected for longer periods of time.[3-6]

Screening of smears. It should be recalled that the entire oral cavity is lined with stratified squamous epithelium which varies in thickness and keratinization according to anatomic and functional sites (Fig. 3-5). A thorough examination of cellular scrapings must be made by a competent cytologist.

General features of *normal* intraoral squamous cells are as follows (Table 3-2, Fig. 3-6):

1. Keratinized surface cells (mature or cornified cells): more flattened and irregular in appearance; small pyknotic nucleus or anucleate; cytoplasm stains pink, yellow, or orange (acidophilic).

2. Unkeratinized surface cells (intermediate maturity): may be slightly flattened, with somewhat irregular cytoplas-

Table 3-1. EXFOLIATIVE CYTOLOGY TECHNIQUE

Collection of Smear: Label one end of a glass microscope slide with patient's name, date, and area from which material is to be obtained. Use a clean cotton-tipped applicator or wood spatula for collection of specimen. If the area to be scraped is dry, the applicator or spatula should be moistened. Usually saliva or tissue excretions are sufficient to prevent dehydration. Collect the material from the lesion by using slight rolling and scraping motions. Remember, smears may be inadequate if there is a pseudomembrane covering a lesion, saliva that is too thick, excess bleeding, or no moisture. The scrapings should be immediately smeared on the center area of the slide (approximately 2.5 cm).

Fixation of Smear: Alcohol (70%) is adequate for fixation. Commercial spray fixatives or hair sprays are satisfactory and also make it easier to handle the specimen. Do not allow the smear to dry before fixation.

Staining of Smear: The smear is stained by a modified Papanicolaou-Traut technique using Mayer's hematoxylin, orange G, eosin, and light green. The slide can be made ready for screening in less than one hour.

mic morphology; some degree of nuclear contraction; cytoplasm is usually basophilic, but may be acidophilic and stain pink or red.

3. Parabasal and immature prickle cells: spherical or cuboidal; centrally placed nucleus with even distribution of chromatin; cytoplasm stains green or blue-green (basophilic).

The following are criteria upon which cytologic interpretations of *malignant* cells are based (all criteria are not necessarily found in each specimen) (Fig. 3-7):

1. Enlarged nuclei.
2. Variation in nuclear size and shape (pleomorphism).
3. Prominent and irregular nuclear borders.
4. Increased nuclear-cytoplasmic ratio (decreased cytoplasm).
5. Multiple prominent and irregular nucleoli.
6. Hyperchromatism (increased nucleoproteins).
7. Abnormal chromatin pattern and distribution.
8. Discrepancy in maturation (extreme variations).

Cells from benign lesions may have atypical appearances, but they seldom display enough criteria to cause them to be misinterpreted as malignant (Table 3-3).[7-11] Classification of benign diseases from exfoliative cytologic studies has not been forthcoming.

False-positive and false-negative reports have been few. These errors, though undesirable, are not critical because of the manner in which cytologic reports are used and interpreted: (1) If clinical suspicion remains in the face of a negative or atypical report, further smears or biopsy should be performed. (2) A suspicious report indicates a definite need to establish a diagnosis immediately. (3) When smears contain cells consistent with malignancy, biopsy is mandatory.

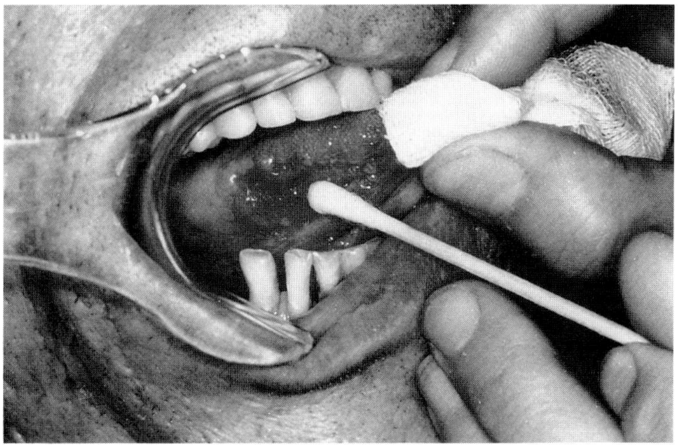

A

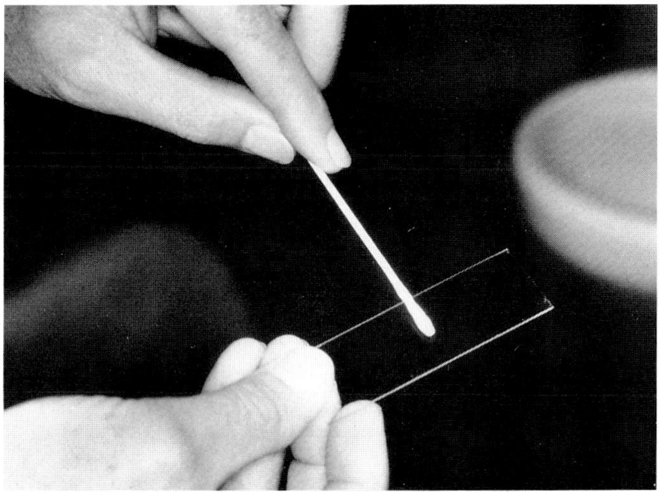

B

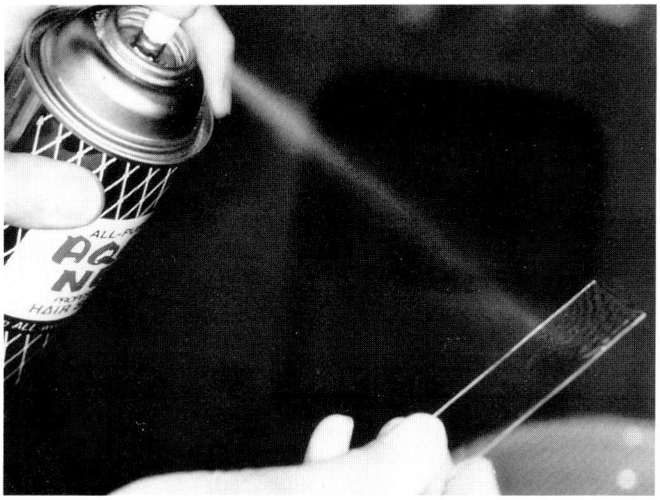

C

Fig. 3-4. Exfoliative cytology technique. **A,** Smear is obtained from a tongue ulcer with a cotton-tipped applicator used with a firm, rolling motion. **B,** Cells are transferred, using a streaking, rolling movement, to the central portion of a clean microscope slide. **C,** A short burst of spray adequately fixes the cells to the slide and preserves them for staining.

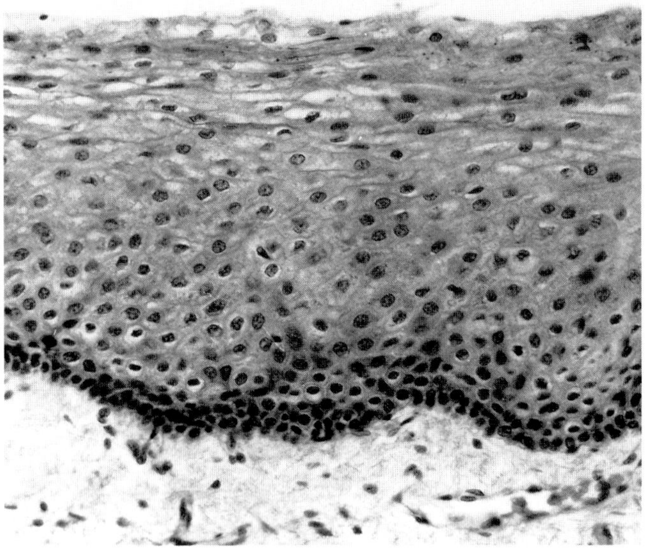

A

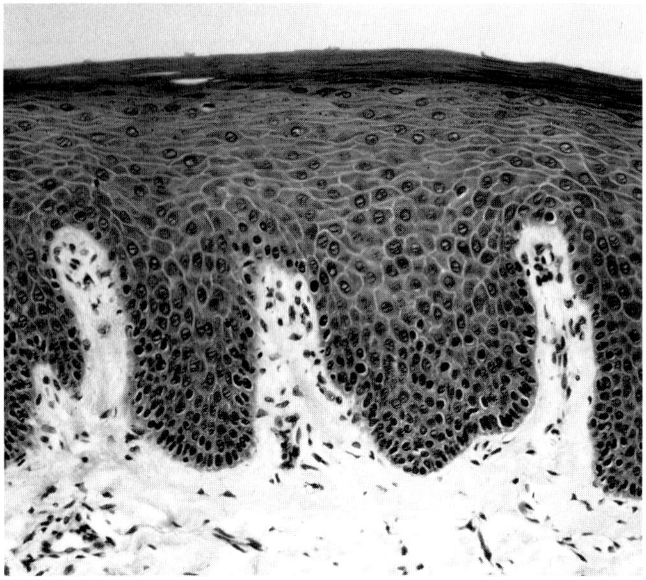

B

Fig. 3-5. Variations in maturation of normal oral epithelium. **A,** Unkeratinized soft palate. **B,** Keratinized hard palate.

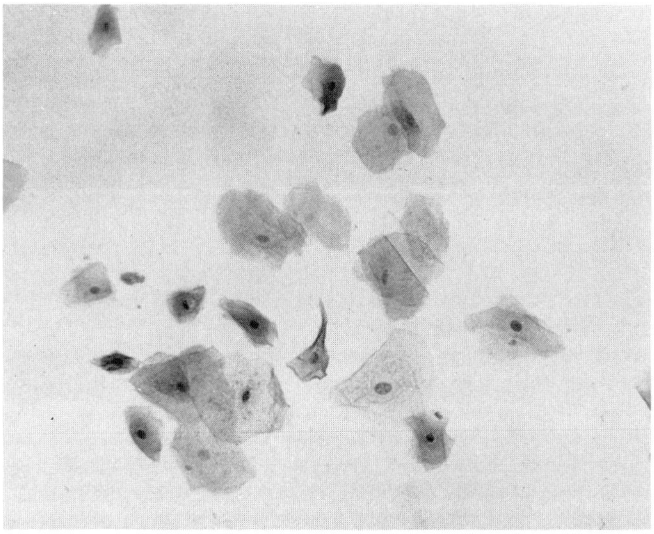

A

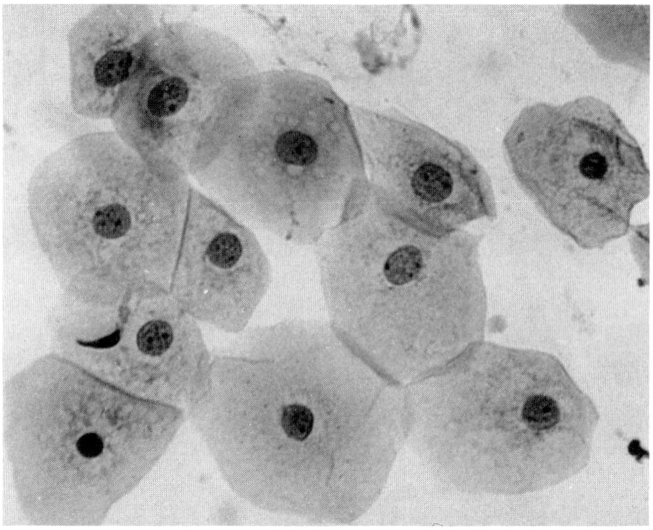

B

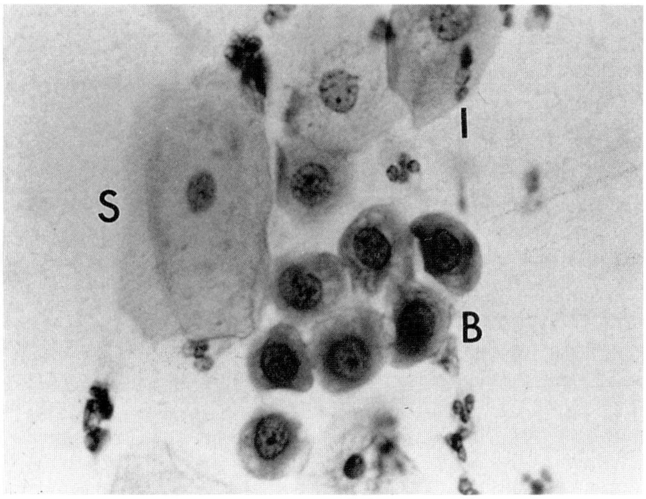

C

Fig. 3-6. Surface cells from normal epithelium. **A,** Mature epithelial cells from surface of keratinized epithelium. Note that some cells are anucleate and in others the nucleus is disappearing by proteolytic action. **B,** Squamous cells from unkeratinized epithelium. Note uniform size, shape, and position of nuclei with adequate surrounding cytoplasm. **C,** Cells from a newly healed ulcer. Note clump of basal cells (B), characterized by large nuclei and small amount of surrounding cytoplasm; compare these intermediate cells (I) and mature squamous cells (S).

Table 3-2. APPEARANCE OF SURFACE CELLS IN RELATION TO LOCATION

Hard palate, gingiva, dorsal tongue	**Mature cells:** High degree of cornification and some cells anucleated.
Buccal and labial mucosae	**Intermediate maturity:** Nucleated basophilic- and acidophilic-staining cells.
Floor of mouth, ventral tongue, soft palate, oropharynx	**Least maturity:** Preponderantly basophilic cells with large nuclei.

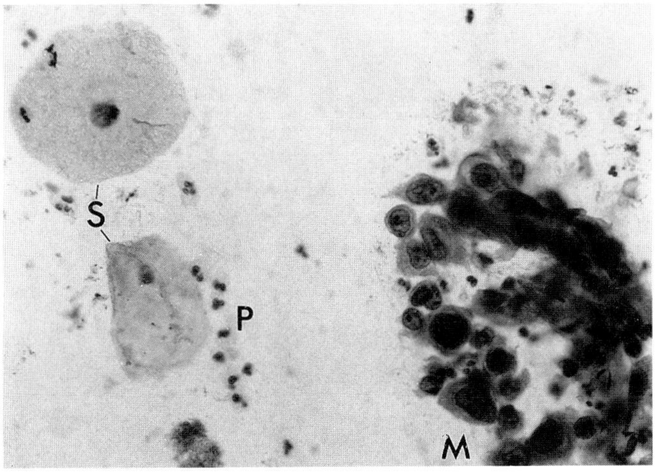

A

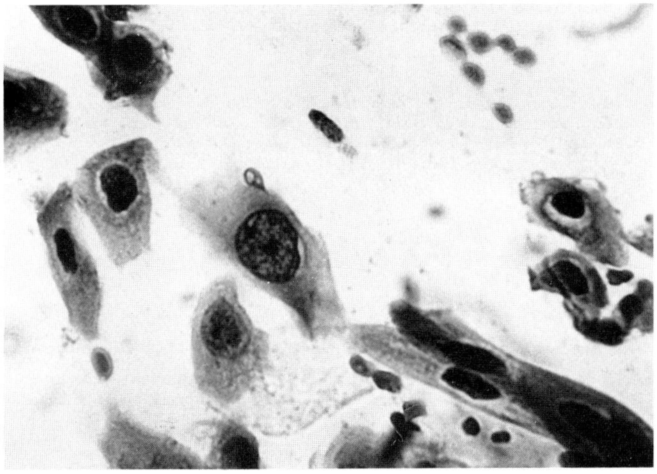

B

Fig. 3-7. Malignant cells from surface of squamous carcinoma. **A,** Group of malignant cells (M), and two mature squamous cells (S). For size comparison, note polymorphonuclear leukocytes (P). **B,** High-power view of malignant cells. Note altered nuclear-cytoplasmic ratio, pleomorphism, enlarged nuclei, irregular nuclear membrane, and hyperchromatism.

Table 3-3. REPORT OF SMEAR

Positive	Criteria for malignant cellular change are observed.
Negative	No malignant cells are observed in the specimen. These cells may appear atypical but do not demonstrate malignant criteria. In the event of continued clinical suspicion or persistence of a lesion, a negative report should not be taken as conclusive. This is particularly true in hyperkeratotic lesions.[8–11]
Suspicious or inconclusive	Cells seen that do not fulfill the malignant criteria adequately to allow a positive report, yet reveal enough deviation from normal to indicate follow-up studies should be performed.
Inadequate	Either cellular morphology is not preserved adequately for interpretation, or the presented material is too scanty to be a representative specimen.

BIOPSY

No tumor should be treated without confirmation of the diagnosis by histologic examination (Figs. 3-8 and 3-9). For intraoral malignancies, there is no good evidence from human studies that a properly performed biopsy will encourage the spread of tumor locally or by lymphatic or blood vessels. However, studies in animals have shown this to be a possibility.[12] The biopsy specimen should be adequate and be obtained from a representative portion of the tumor so that the pathologist can examine the tissue appropriately.

It doesn't matter whether the biopsy procedure is carried out by a dentist or a physician, provided he or she is well qualified in recognizing the potentialities of the lesion and is capable of obtaining an appropriate and adequate specimen. In general, the most satisfactory biopsy of an intraoral lesion is the incisional biopsy (removal of a small portion). However, incisional biopsy of a small lesion may distort its appearance and consistency, rendering proper evaluation of its extent almost impossible. If cancer is suspected in a very small lesion whose gross appearance would be altered by the biopsy, it is of utmost importance that the clinician who will apply the definitive treatment should see the lesion before the biopsy specimen is taken in order to judge the extent of resection or irradiation to be instituted.

Although biopsies of intraoral lesions ordinarily present no difficult technical problems, tumors in such areas as the base of the tongue, the pyriform fossa, and the nasopharynx may be difficult to obtain and may escape detection even by an experienced examiner. For tumors in these sites, it is frequently necessary to examine the patient and perform the

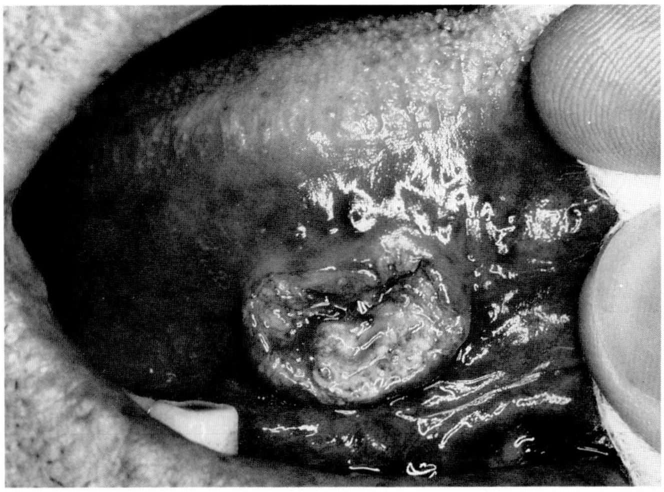

A

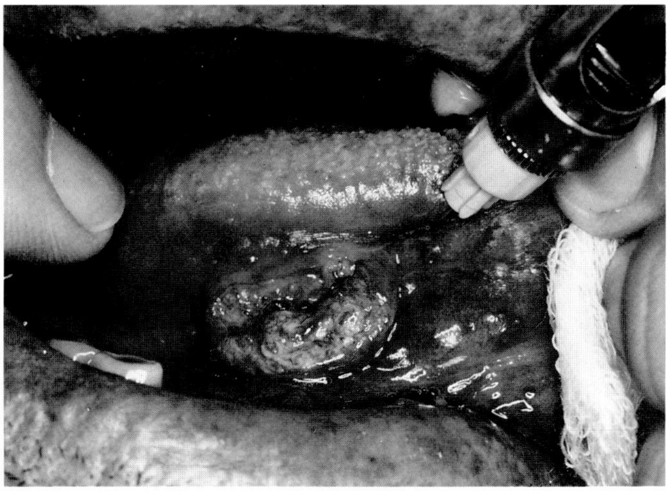

B

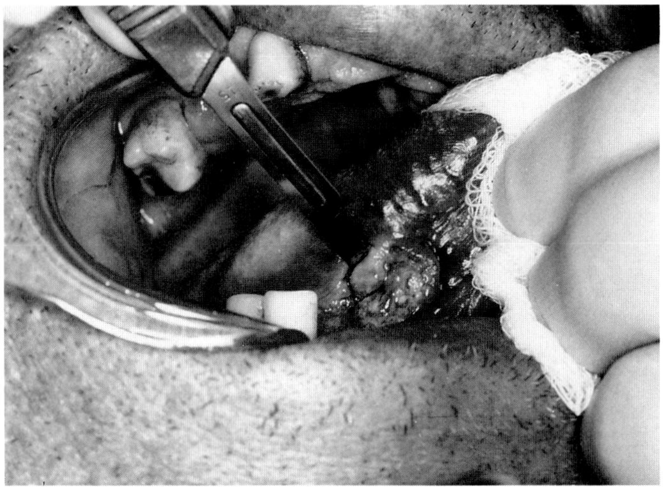

C

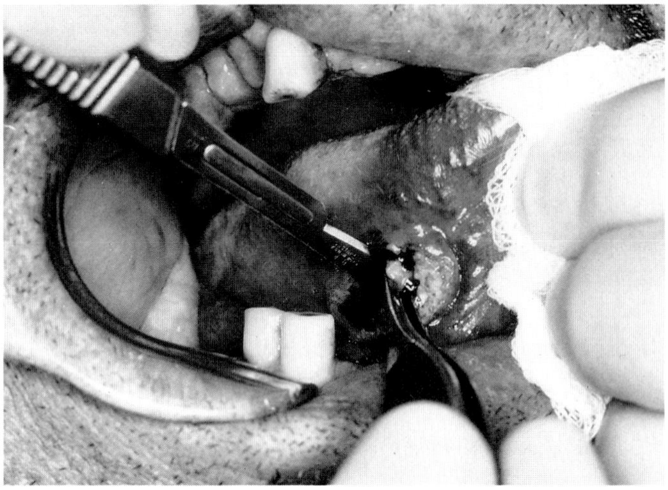

D

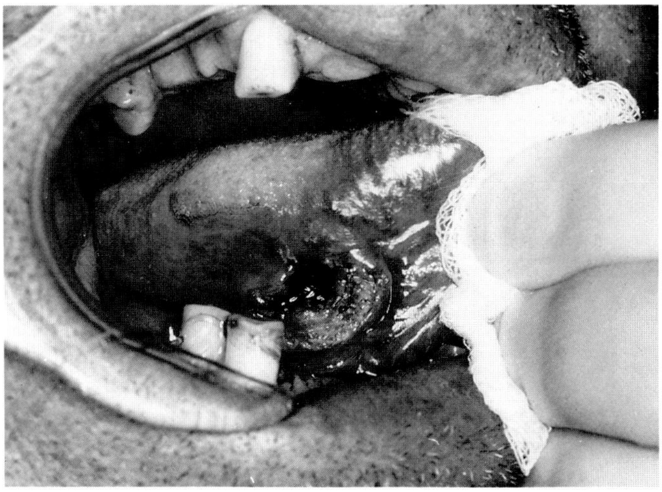

E

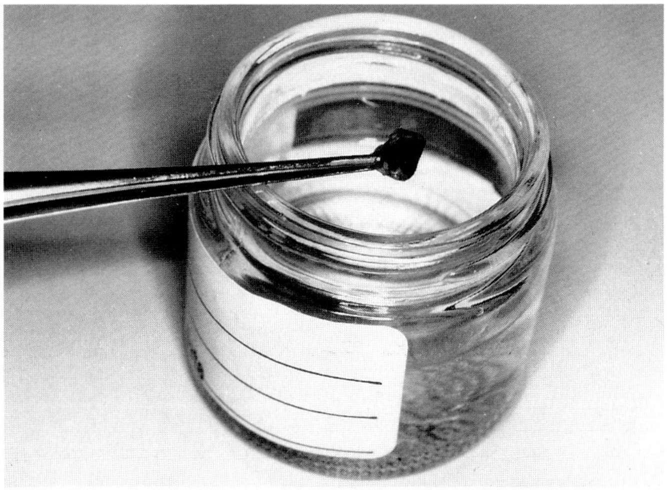

F

Fig. 3-8. Incisional biopsy technique. **A,** Squamous carcinoma of right tongue. **B,** Local anesthetic is infiltrated away and deep from the tumor so that tumor is not violated by needle. **C,** Incision is made with scalpel. **D,** Specimen is removed by gently grasping the forceps and excising the base. **E,** Excision site minutes after biopsy, showing hemostasis by use of pressure alone. **F,** Specimen is placed in 10% normal buffered formalin for histologic processing.

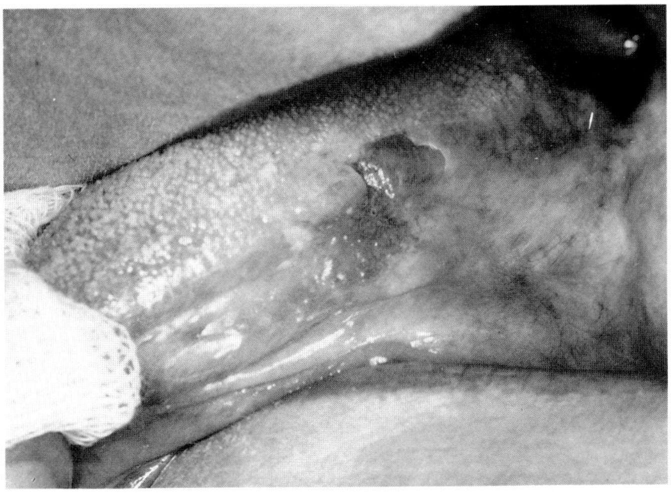

A

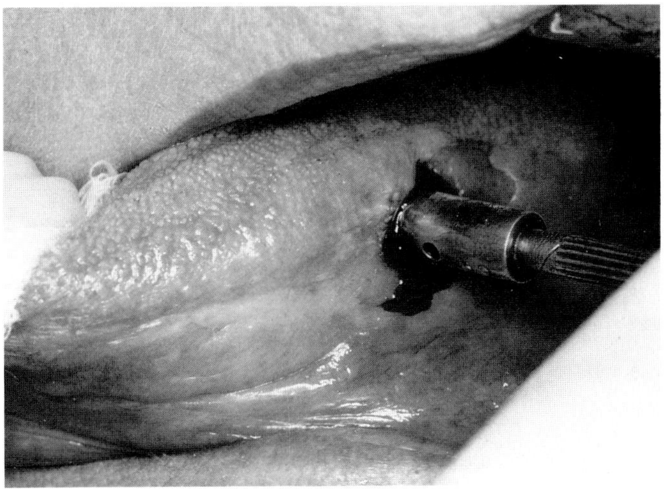

B

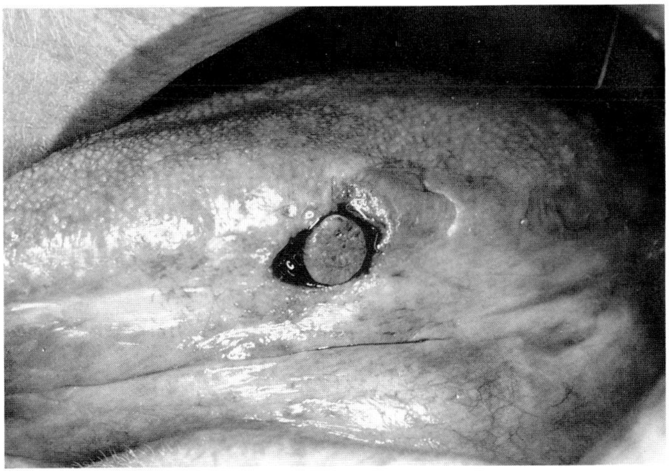

C

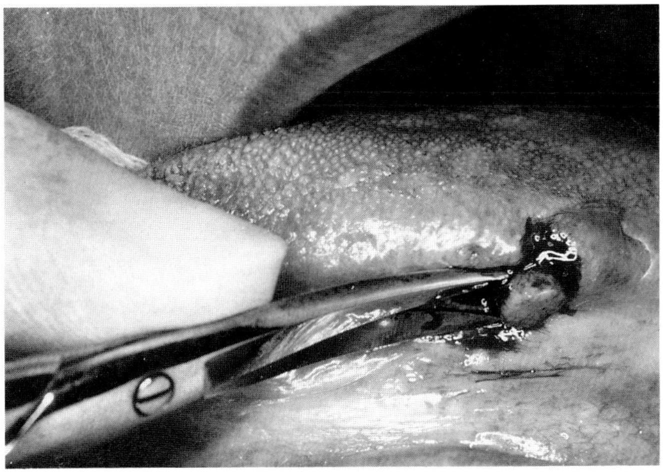

D

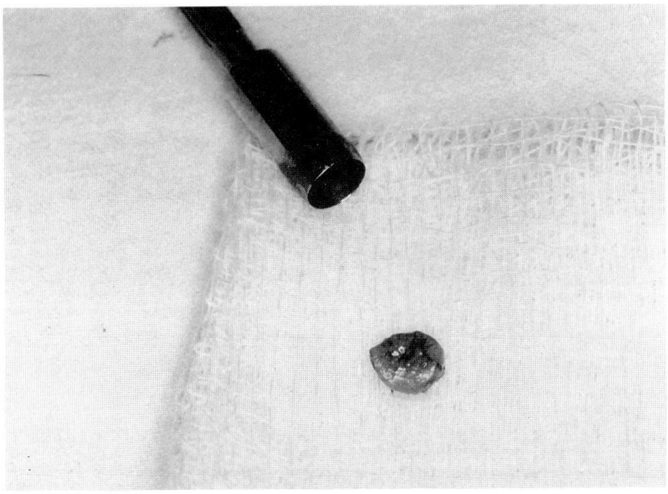

E

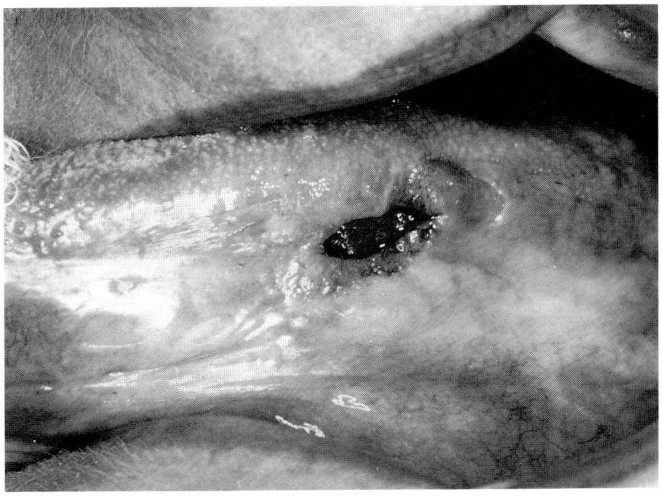

F

Fig. 3-9. Punch biopsy technique. **A,** Asymptomatic erythematous lesion on left lateral tongue, thought to be due to denture irritation. **B,** After administration of local anesthesia, the 5-mm punch biopsy instrument is inserted to obtain margins. **C,** Note clean margins obtained by twisting an incision of the punch instrument to a depth of about 2-3 mm. **D,** Without the specimen being touched by forceps, the base is excised with scissors. **E,** Biopsy specimen, unharmed by any instrument trauma. **F,** Incision site minutes after biopsy, where bleeding has been controlled by gauze packs. In most instances suturing is unnecessary.

biopsy with the patient under general anesthesia. Even if the cervical lymph nodes are palpable and suspected of being involved in metastatic carcinoma, the biopsy specimen should always be obtained from the primary lesion.

Lymph node biopsy is carried out only when the primary lesion cannot be identified or in diseases such as lymphoma and carcinoma of the thyroid. In such instances the entire lymph node should be excised (excisional biopsy) if at all feasible. Incisional biopsy of a suspicious lymph node should be avoided to prevent contamination of the biopsy site by tumor cells. Such a spillage of cells might worsen the prognosis in patients who otherwise might be curable.

In patients with cervical lymphadenopathy in whom a primary tumor cannot be identified, the location in the neck of the enlarged lymph node is of considerable help in identifying the site of origin of the metastasis (Fig. 3-10). However, it must be remembered that tumors can metastasize to almost any node (see Chapter 4).

Fine Needle Biopsy

The fine needle aspiration biopsy is a highly acceptable and accurate techique for differentiating benign from malignant lesions involving lymph nodes.[13-15] Use of this minimally invasive technique accelerates diagnosis and treatment as well as improves overall management. This technique also has greatly aided the evaluation of salivary gland lesions (see Chapter 9). Thus, it is a safe, quick, and reliable procedure that can immediately differentiate inflammatory, reactive, cystic, and neoplastic processes.

Unlike the incisional biopsy, fine needle biopsy is indicated in lymph nodes and salivary glands because it does not tend to spread tumor or disrupt the field for ideal surgical dissection.

The armamentarium includes a 22-gauge needle and a special holder for a 10- or 20-ml syringe to get optimal suction. Anesthesia is usually not required, and specimens are prepared by cytologic technique (Fig. 3-11).

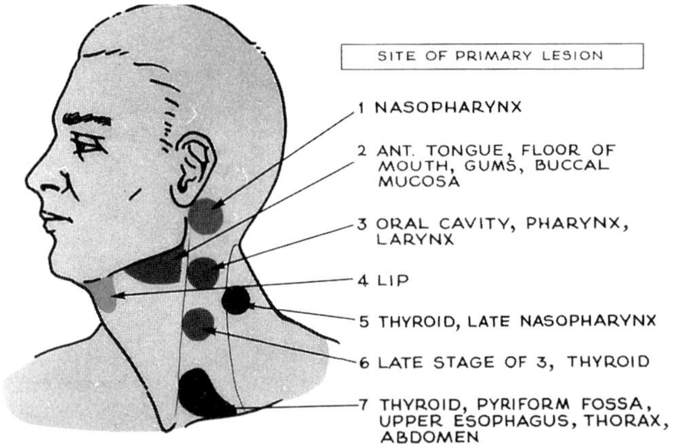

Fig. 3-10. Likely sites of lymph node metastases.

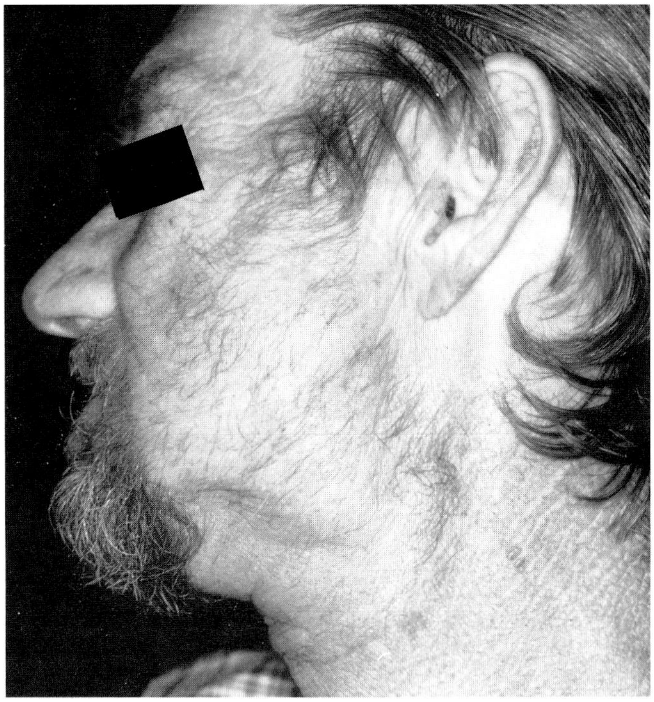

A

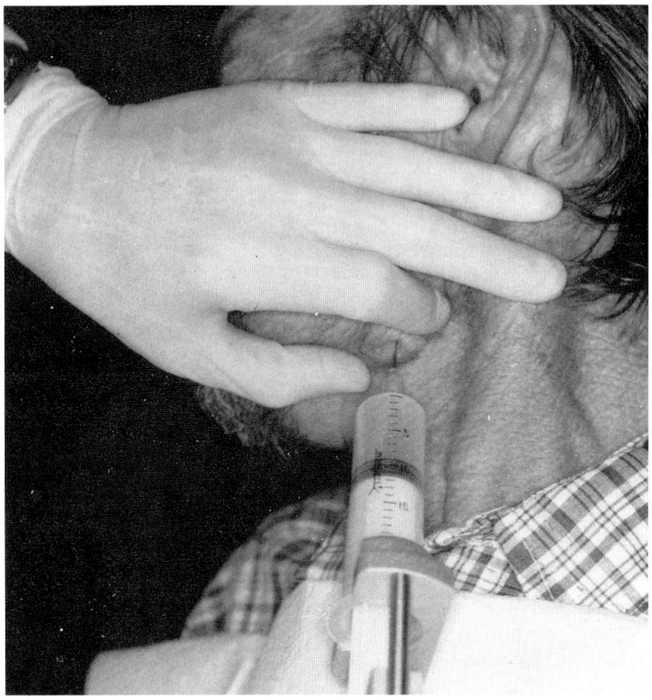

B

Fig. 3-11. Fine needle biopsy of a suspected malignancy of either salivary gland or lymph node origin. **A,** Slow growing, mildly painful submandibular lump. **B,** Fine needle (22 g) aspiration biopsy.

TOLUIDINE BLUE

Because epithelial dysplasia and early squamous cell carcinoma vary considerably in appearance and often resemble certain benign lesions, clinical identification is difficult and biopsy is frequently delayed by atempts at empirical remedies. Vital staining with toluidine blue has been shown to aid early recognition and accelerate biopsy, diagnosis and treatment.[16–20] Toluidine blue is a metachromatic dye of the thiazine group that has been effectively used as a nuclear stain because of its binding with DNA.

In the University of California, San Francisco, Oral Medicine Clinic, the reliability of this vital staining technique was tested in 132 consecutive patients suspected of having malignant or precancerous oral lesions, by comparing clinical toluidine blue dye uptake with results of a simultaneous biopsy (Figs. 3-12 and 3-13)[21] The histopathologic diagnosis confirmed 57 squamous carcinomas, 42 epithelial dysplasias, and 33 benign mucosal changes (Table 3-4). Overall accuracy of the toluidine blue uptake was 91%.

The accuracy of the toluidine blue technique supports its clinical use to further confirm clinical impressions regarding tissues at risk for malignancy as well as to assist the clinician to choose biopsy sites and surgical margins. Clinicians should, however, be aware that false positive reactions can result from dye retention by filiform papillae and ulcerations (Fig. 3-14). The mechanism for this reaction is unknown, but it might be related to a high rate of protein synthesis and/or binding by sulfated mucopolysaccharides. Since toluidine blue is regarded as a nuclear stain, selective dye uptake by

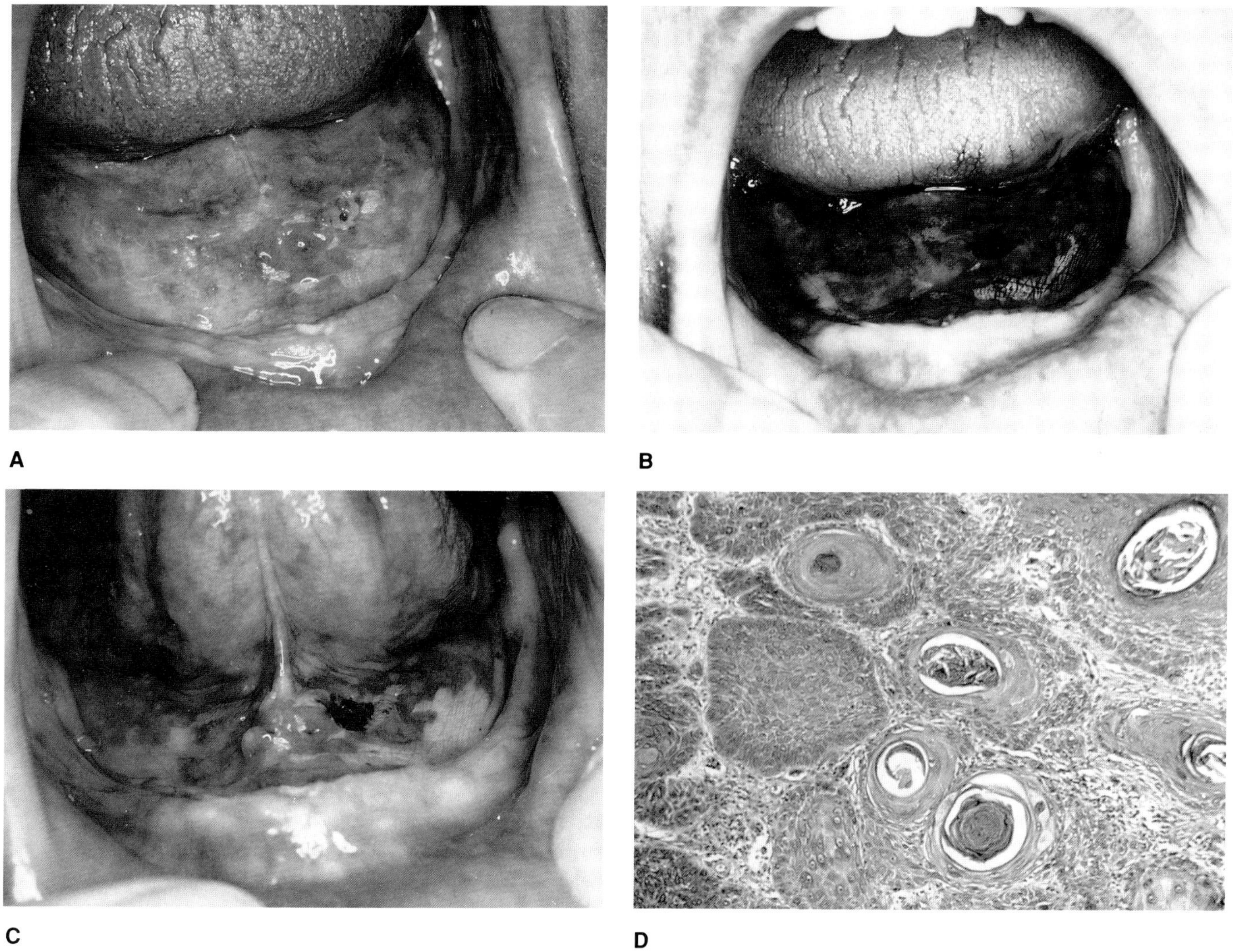

Fig. 3-12. Toluidine blue staining technique to identify dysplastic or malignant tissue. **A,** Small squamous carcinoma in left floor of mouth, thought to be an aphthous or a traumatic ulcer. **B,** Dye is applied to floor of mouth. **C,** After decoloration with 1% acetic acid, dye is retained in malignant site but not in leukoplakic areas. **D,** The biopsy confirmed squamous carcinoma.

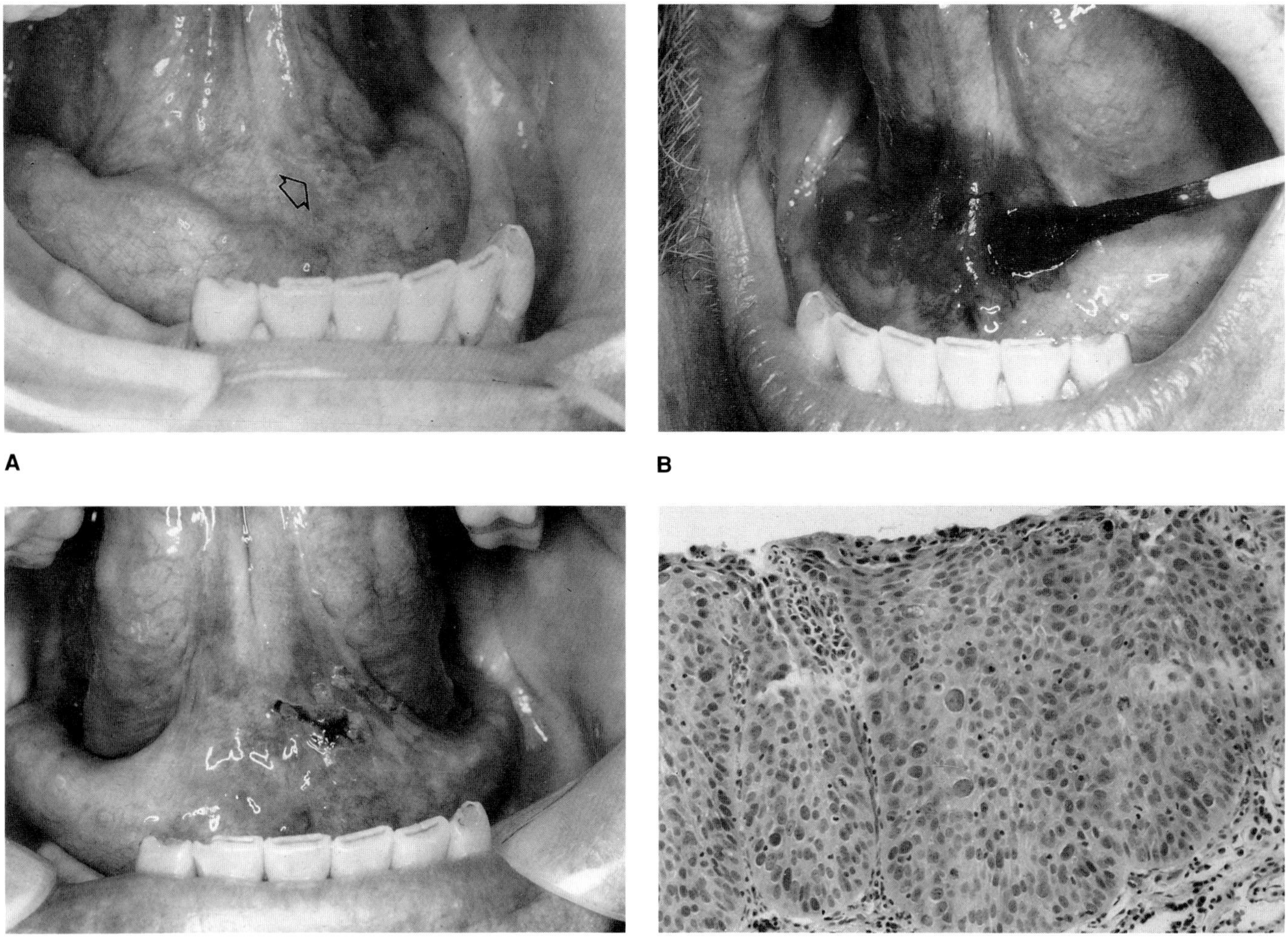

A B C D

Fig. 3-13. Intraepithelial carcinoma in a 43-year-old man who had had an "irritation" of the mouth floor for several months. **A,** Note the mild keratotic change that was soft to palpation and nonulcerated (arrow). **B,** Application of 1% aqueous toluidine blue dye. **C,** Note the residual area of tissue affinity for the dye after decoloration with 1% acetic acid. **D,** A biopsy from the dye-positive area revealed intraepithelial carcinoma (carcinoma in situ).

Table 3-4. COMPARISON OF TOLUIDINE BLUE UPTAKE WITH MICROSCOPIC DIAGNOSIS IN 132 CONSECUTIVE CASES*†

Microscopic Diagnosis	Toluidine Blue		
	No. Lesions	Uptake	Error
Benign	33 (25%)	10 (30%)	30% false positive
Dysplasia	42 (32%)	42 (100%)	none
Carcinoma	57 (43%)	55 (96%)	4% false negative

*Data from Silverman, Migliorati, and Barbosa, 1983.[21]

†Overall error: 12/132 = 9%.

dysplastic and malignant cells, which contain quantitatively more nucleic acids than normal tissue, is plausible. However, the most probable explanation of binding in vivo by precancerous and cancerous tissue is the immediate binding by sulfated mucopolysaccharides, which are found in higher quantities in tissues that are actively growing, such as tumors and tissues that are healing.[22,23]

It can be concluded that toluidine blue staining is a useful adjunct to careful examination, clinical judgment, and biopsy.

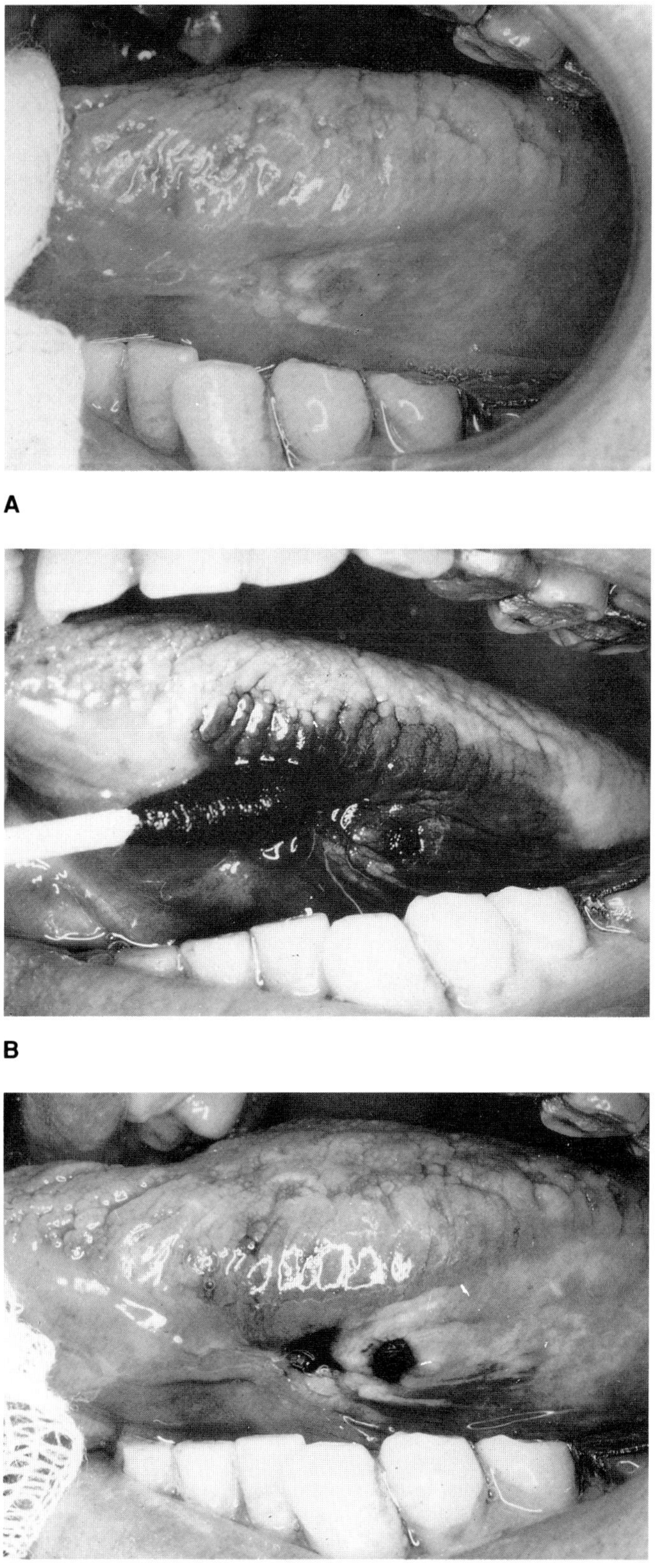

Fig. 3-14. False-positive result in toluidine blue staining. **A,** Suspicious ulcerated, keratotic lesion of left lateral tongue. **B,** Dye is applied. **C,** After decoloration, ulcer retains dye. Ulcer was actually a benign traumatic lesion; false-positive result was due to uptake of dye by fibrinous exudate in area of ulceration.

MONOCLONAL ANTIBODIES

No matter what diagnostic technique is utilized, the possibility of a false negative response exists. The development of monoclonal antibodies that have high sensitivity and specificity for epithelial dysplastic and malignant cells would enhance accuracy of diagnosis in some cases where the usual or typical cellular characteristics of precancer or cancer are not apparent. This technique could be applied to cytology as well as biopsy specimens.[24] Such antibodies could also possibly minimize errors regarding "tumor free" margins of surgical resections, thus reducing a potential source for recurrence. In addition, assuming the specificity of an antibody for cellular tumor antigen, binding of cytotoxic chemotherapeutic agents for tumor-killing and normal cell-sparing would be logical and possible sequelae for improving cancer control.

IMAGING THE ORAL CAVITY

Neoplasms of the oral cavity and oropharynx are usually discovered by clinical examination and confirmed by fine needle or surgical biopsy. Imaging studies are then employed to map the extent of tissue or bone invasion, detect the presence of non-palpable cervical adenopathy, and exclude carotid artery adherence by tumor. The two cross sectional techniques presently available are computed tomography (CT) and magnetic resonance imaging (MR). Both have limitations as well as advantages which make them complementary rather than competitive studies.

The soft-tissue contrast resolution of CT is relatively poor. This makes the distinction between tumor and normal muscle difficult (Fig. 3-15A). CT also requires the administration of intravenous contrast material to differentiate vessels from lymph nodes which increases the risk of an allergic reaction (Fig. 3-15B). CT is also frequently degraded by dental appliance artifacts.[25] The advantages of CT include its rapid acquisition (2-3 seconds per section), patient tolerance, relatively low cost ($400-600 per examination), and superior osseous detail compared with MR.

On the other hand, MR has several advantages over CT and has evolved into a reliable alternative for imaging head and neck anatomy and pathology.[26-29] The superior soft-tissue resolution of MR allows high contrast definition between neoplasms and adjacent muscle (Fig. 3-15D). In addition, MR can be obtained in multiple orthogonal planes (sagittal, axial, coronal, and oblique) planes, which is often helpful in assessing tumor volumes during and after therapy (Fig 3-16). Patent vessels have absent signal, or "signal void," within their lumen which easily distinguishes them from surrounding soft tissue structures. This feature obviates the requirement for intravascular contrast administration (Fig. 3-17).

However, MR is not without its drawbacks. Since all of the images within a given MR sequence are obtained simultaneously and not sequentially, patient movement during MR acquisition is less well tolerated than with CT. At present, MR studies are expensive ($800-1100 per study) and access is limited in many communities. In addition, while the soft-tissue contrast is superb with MR, fine-bone detail is inferior to that obtained with CT.

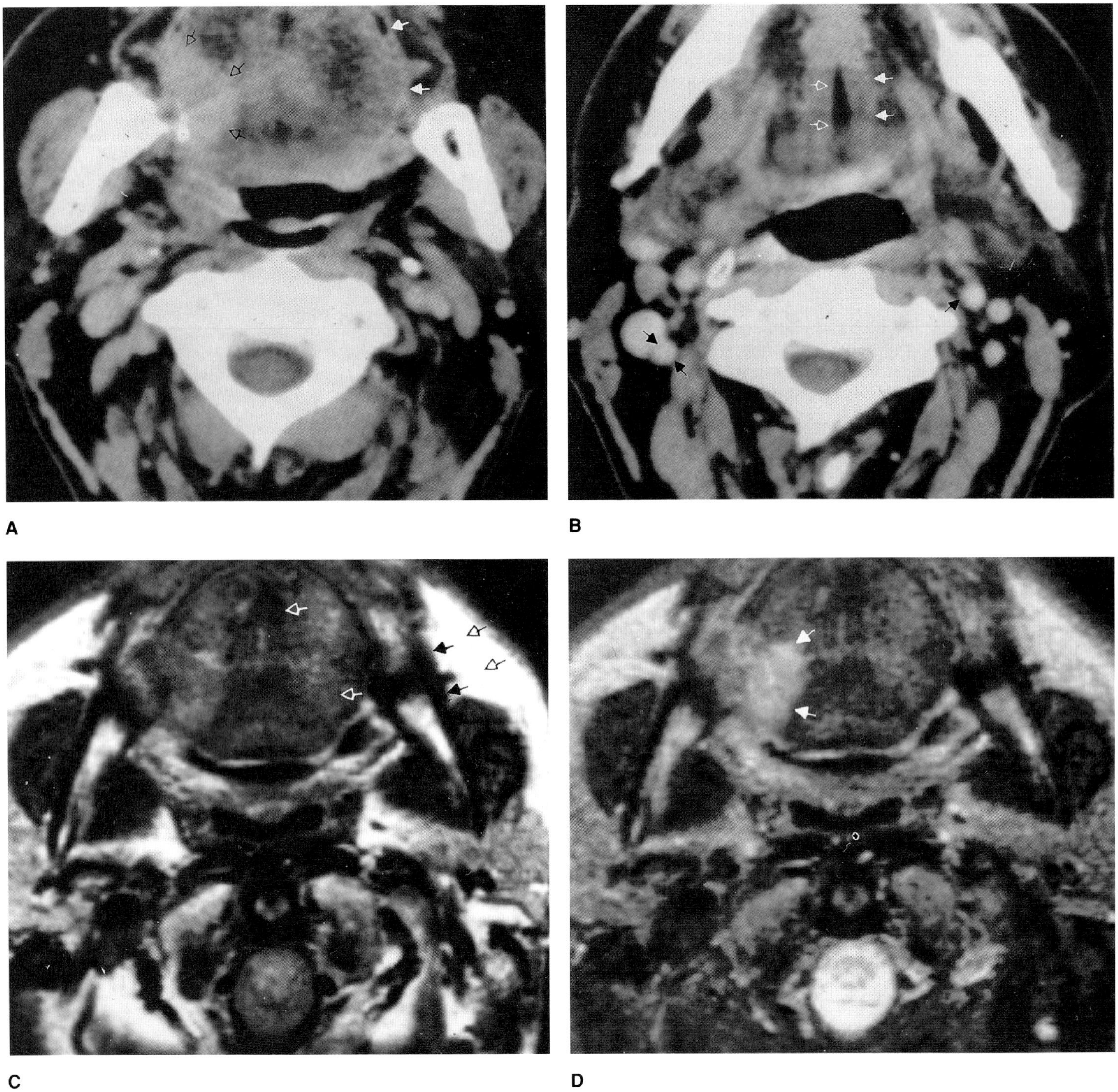

Fig. 3-15. Squamous cell carcinoma of the oral tongue. **A,** Axial CT section through the tongue and oropharynx. Note that the cortical bone of the mandible and vertebral body is of high density. The soft tissue of the tongue and surrounding muscles is of intermediate density, and the density of fat is low. The tongue has a mixed density consisting of peripheral higher density muscle (closed arrows) intermixed with low density fat. A right 2 cm lateral squamous carcinoma of the tongue is of similar density to surrounding muscle (open arrows). **B,** Axial CT section through the floor of the mouth. The mandible is seen lateral to the floor of the mouth musculature. A midline fatty septum (open arrows) separates the two paramedian genioglossus muscles (closed arrows). Intravenous contrast has been administered and enhances the normal carotid arteries and jugular veins (black arrows). This enhancement aids in separating reactive or metastatic nodes from vessels. **C,** Axial MR (T1-weighted) through the oral tongue. Note that the signal intensity of fat is high (open black arrows), muscle is low to intermediate (open white arrows), and cortical bone is very low (black arrows). The tumor is not well differentiated from muscle on the T1-weighted sequence. **D,** Axial T2-weighted sequence through the oral tongue (same patient as A through C). On this sequence, the carcinoma increases in signal intensity (arrows), providing good contrast between it and surrounding normal tongue. Note that the tumor stops short of the midline but extends posteriorly to involve part of the soft palate. While the tumor appears to abut the cortex of the right mandible, the marrow signal appears normal.

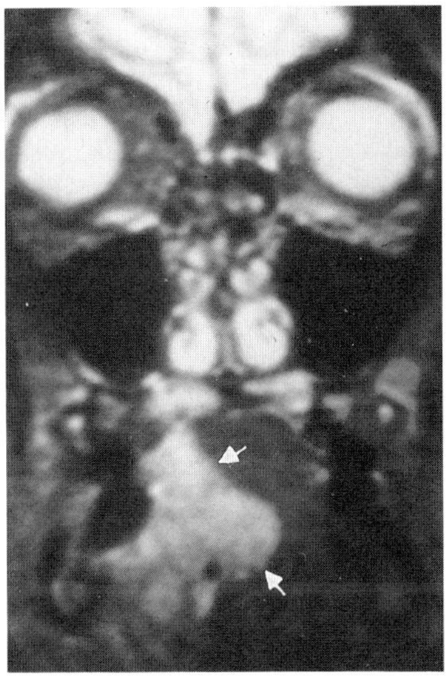

A

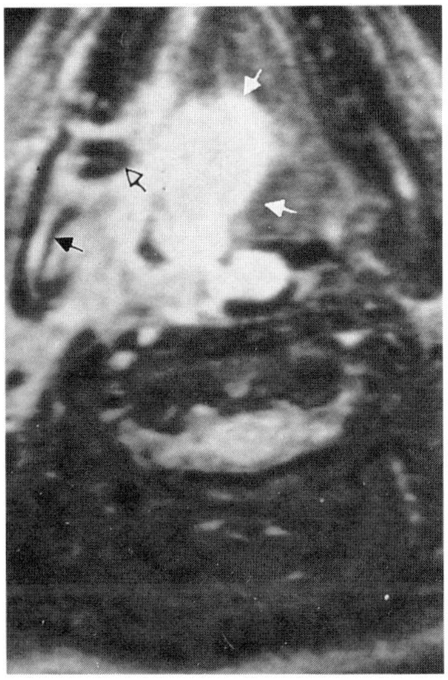

B

Fig. 3-16. Squamous cell carcinoma of the tongue (Stage 4), **A,** Coronal and **B,** Axial T2-weighted images. The tumor (white arrows) has high signal intensity and extends beneath the mucosa of the tongue, across midline, enveloping the right lingual artery. In addition, the tumor erodes the inner cortex of the mandible which is detected as a discontinuous dark cortical line (closed black arrow). The third molar "floats" within the tumor (open black arrow). Tumor extension can be seen to the soft palate and near the base of the tongue.

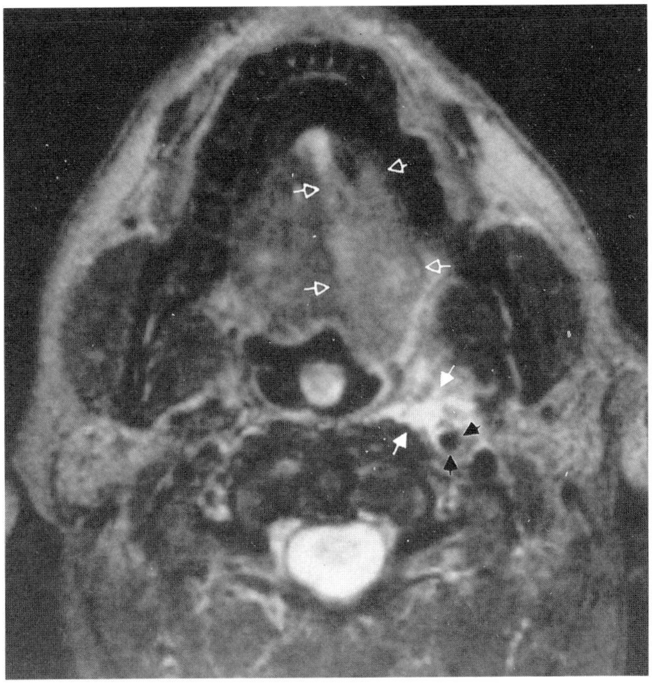

Fig. 3-17. Squamous carcinoma of the left base of the tongue with 12th nerve atrophy. Axial T2-weighted image demonstrates slight hyperintensity of the left half of the tongue due to denervation atrophy (open white arrows). The tumor is recognized by its high signal intensity near the tongue base (closed white arrows). Note that the carotid artery (black arrrows) is easily distinguished from surrounding tumor without the use of intravenous contrast.

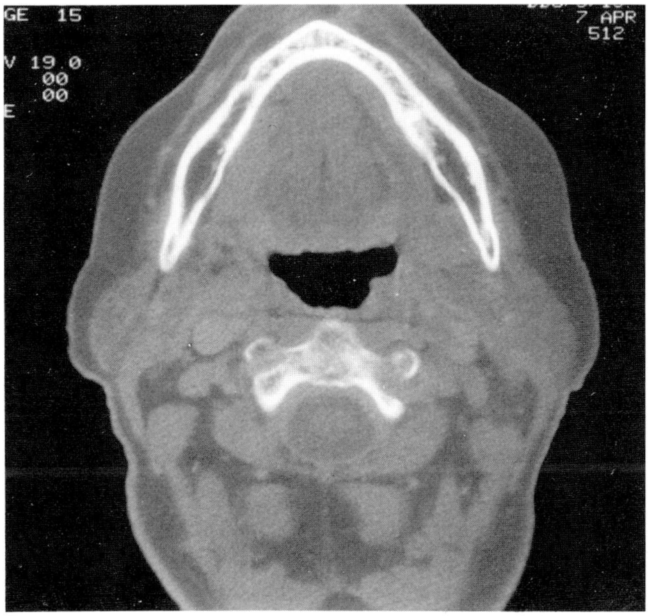

A

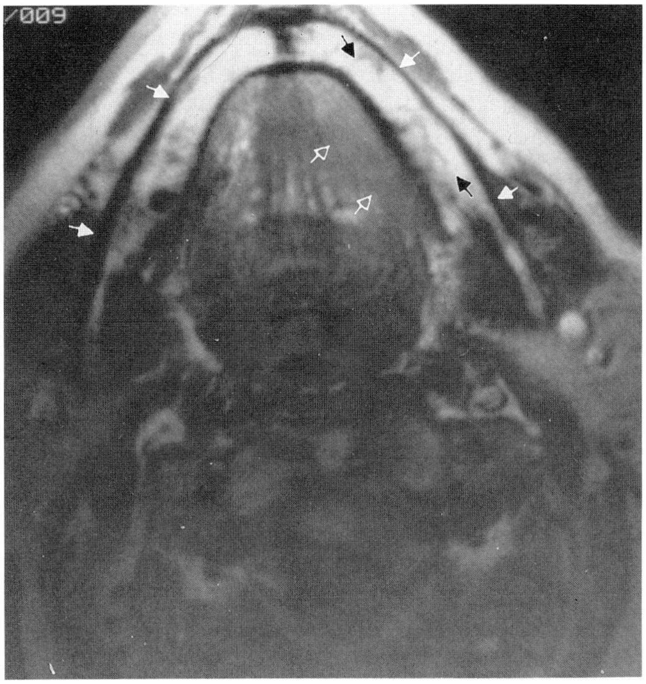

B

Fig. 3-18. Squamous carcinoma of the anterior floor of the mouth. **A,** CT scan with bone windows through the mandible. Excellent osseous detail is demonstrated on this high resolution CT scan of both the cortical and medullary portions of the mandible. No erosion is detected from the left anterior floor of mouth carcinoma. **B,** T1-weighted MR scan of floor of mouth. The mandible is demonstrated on this surface coil T1-weighted study as an area of bright signal intensity representing fat within the medullary cavity (black arrows) surrounded by low signal intensity cortical bone (closed white arrows). The anterior left floor of mouth carcinoma obliterates the fat near the genioglossus muscle (open white arrows). The intensity of the tumor is similar to muscle on this T1-weighted image.

TECHNICAL FEATURES OF MR AND CT

Both CT and MR are digital display techniques which depict anatomic sections as an array of pixel (*pic*ture *el*ements) signals or intensities. The signal generated with each pixel is dependent on both the physical parameters of tissue and the method of acquisition employed. With CT, the density of the pixel represents the relative x-ray attenuation by the structures within the pixel. The greater the attenuation of x-ray, the fewer number of x-rays traverse the tissue to interact with the detectors surrounding the patient. The attenuation of x-ray is directly related to the density of a given object or tissue.

Bone, which strongly attenuates x-rays, has the greatest density on the CT study. Soft tissue, such as muscle, attenuates x-ray less than bone and is accorded a lower density. Fat and air have the lowest attenuation coefficients and have the lowest density on CT scans (Fig. 3-15).

Similar to CT, the MR image is also composed of a matrix of pixel intensities. However, the intensity of each pixel depends on multiple tissue characteristics including the hydrogen or "proton" density, the T1 and T2 relaxation times of the tissue, and blood flow within the tissue. MR is actually a map of hydrogen protons over a given area. In order to return an MR signal, a tissue must have hydrogen protons which can be stimulated by the applied radiofrequency pulse. Some tissues have more available water for this interaction than others. For example, cortical bone contains few mobile water protons and has a low MR signal compared to other tissues (Figs. 3-15C, 3-15D, and 3-18). The most important factor influencing the MR signal is the inherent response of the hydrogen protons within a given tissue to the applied radiofrequency pulse. The response is characterized by the "T1" and "T2" relaxation rate of the tissue. These two phenomena describe the evolution of the MR signal within a given tissue. The images that result can be obtained so that soft tissue contrast depends primarily on the T1 or T2 relaxation rate of the tissues. These are referred to as T1 or T2 "weighted" sequences. They are obtained by varying the repetition rate (TR) of the applied radio-frequency (RF) pulse and the time (TE) at which the signal or echo is sampled after the RF pulse. At least two sets of images at the identical anatomic level are usually obtained, each demonstrating anatomic structures with different signals based on the intrinsic T1 and T2 relaxation times of that tissue (Fig. 3-15C and 3-15D). The shorter the T1 relaxation time, the brighter the signal on T1-weighted images. On T2-weighted images, the longer the T2 relaxation time, the brighter the signal intensity of the tissue. Water has a long T1 and T2 relaxation time and therefore will appear low in signal on T1-weighted images and bright on T2-weighted images. Certain tissues have similar relaxation values and appear similar in signal intensity. Other tissues differ markedly in their proton density, T1 and T2 relaxation times, and appear quite different on MR.

MR and CT Anatomy of the Oral Cavity and Oropharynx

Three major types of soft tissue are present in the oral cavity and oropharynx: muscle, lymphoid tissue, and fat. They exhibit different MR and CT signals, depending upon the intrinsic properties mentioned above the MR parameters selected. In general, fat has a short T1 relaxation time and has high signal intensity on T1-weighted images (Fig. 3-15C). Most soft tissue structures, such as the muscle of the tongue, have an intermediate signal intensity on both T1- and T2-weighted images. Tumors generate increased amounts of water protons which prolong relaxation times and result in higher signal T2-weighted images (Fig. 3-15D).

Lymphoid tissue, present in the palatine and lingual tonsils, as well as on the interior surface of the soft palate, has a signal intensity similar to that of muscle and most tumors on T1-weighted images (Fig. 3-19). Lymphoid tissue has a relatively long T2 relaxation time and therefore increases in signal intensity relative to muscle on T2-weighted images (Fig. 3-20). T1-weighted sequences (TR = 600 msec, TE = 20 msec) afford the best contrast between fat and muscle while T2-weighted sequences (TR = 2000 msec, TE = 80 msec) demonstrate the best contrast between muscle and lymphoid tissue.

The oral portion of the upper aerodigestive tract is divided into two major components: the oral cavity and oropharynx. The oral cavity contains the anterior two-thirds of the tongue, the buccal mucosa, the floor of the mouth, and the supporting mandible and maxillary bones. The oropharynx is that region posterior to the circumvallate papilla of the tongue and includes the posterior one-third of the tongue (tongue base), the palatine tonsils, the soft palate, and the

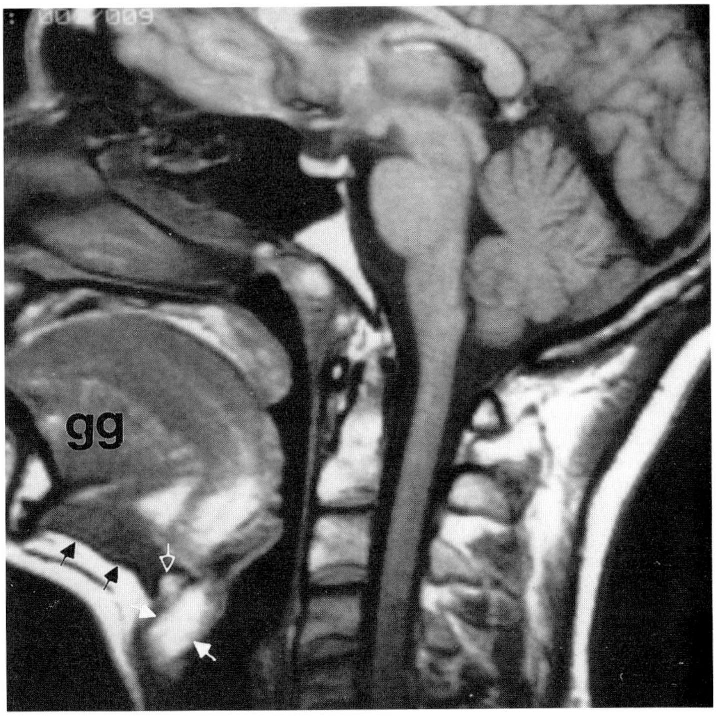

Fig. 3-19. Sagittal T1-weighted image of the normal tongue. The genioglossus muscle (GG) emanates from the genu of the mandible to insert in the intrinsic tongue muscles. The fat-filled preepiglottic space (closed arrows) is located just beneath the hyoid bone (open white arrows). The muscle connecting the genu of the mandible to the hyoid bone is the geniohyoid muscle (black arrows). Obliteration of the normal fat planes can be used as a marker of infiltrated tumor.

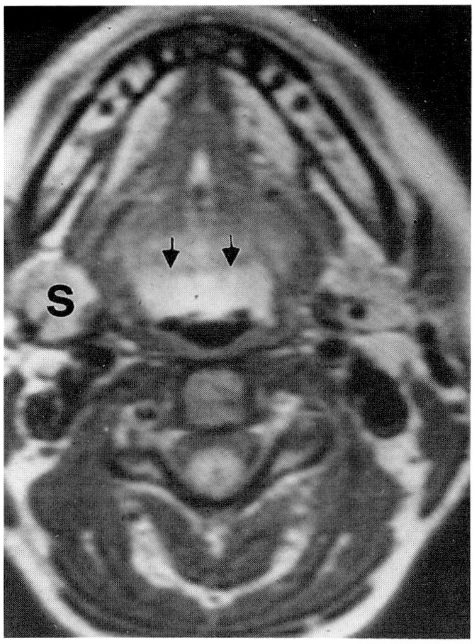

A

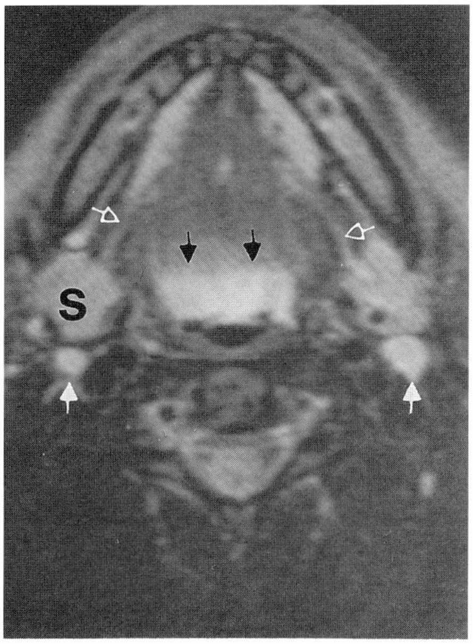

B

Fig. 3-20. Normal axial MR through the floor of the mouth. **A,** T1-weighted image. **B,** T2-weighted image. The midline septum is shown as a high signal intensity structure separating the genioglossus muscles. Of note at the posterior tongue base, lymphoid tissue increases in signal intensity on the T2-weighted image (black arrows). The signal intensity of this tissue is quite similar to that of neoplastic tissue. On either side of the floor of the mouth, submandibular glands are noted (S). The ducts of the submandibular glands (open arrows) can be seen emanating from the deep portion of the submandibular gland. It courses between the mylohyoid muscle and the hyoglossus muscle. Note the reactive submandibular adenopathy (closed white arrows) posterior to the submandibular glands.

oropharyngeal mucosa and constrictor muscles from the level of the soft palate to the top of the epiglottis.

The extrinsic muscles in the floor of the mouth are separated by normal fat planes. T1-weighted axial and coronal images demonstrate this anatomy most clearly (Fig. 3-20). The most prominent landmark in the floor of the mouth is the midline fat-filled lingual septum separating the paramedian genioglossus muscles. Deviation or obliteration of this septum is abnormal. The submandibular gland, located inferior to the mylohyoid muscle and beneath the mandible, has an intermediate signal intensity between muscle and fat on T2-weighted images (Fig. 3-20). The proximal 3-4 mm of the submandibular duct may normally be seen on T2-weighted images as a high signal intensity structure leaving the deep portion of the gland, just medial to the mylohyoid muscle. The sublingual gland occupies the anterior one-third of the lateral floor of the mouth, in a position medial to the mylohyoid muscle. It has a signal intensity which is similar to lymphoid tissue and can be difficult to separate from tumor. The lingual vessels, branches of the external carotid arteries, supply each half of the tongue and floor of mouth. They course within the fat plane between genioglossus muscles and hypoglossus muscles, sending perforating branches to the tongue.

The oral tongue is supported by the floor of the mouth. This large muscle is formed by three intrinsic muscles which interdigitate on either side of the midline. The tongue contains both muscle and fat which can be visualized on both CT and T1-weighted MR scans (Figs. 3-15A and 3-15C). On T2-weighted images, the tongue decreases in signal intensity in a homogeneous fashion (Fig.3-15D).

The oropharynx consists of the pharyngeal constrictor muscles surrounding the airway, the palatine and lymphoid tissue at the base of tongue, and the oral surface of the soft palate. The dominant fat plane deep to the airway, the parapharyngeal space, is best defined on T1-weighted sequences. Displacement of the parapharyngeal space often indicates deep-tissue invasion of neoplasm (Fig. 3-21A). Tumor which abuts lymphoid tissue in the palatine and lingual base cannot be differentiated on the basis of signal intensity.

Neoplasms

The most common tumors involving the oral cavity and oropharynx are squamous cell carcinomas and mixed cell tumors of minor salivary gland origin. These tumors have T1 relaxation times similar to those of lymphoid tissue and muscle and, therefore, may be difficult to differentiate from these structures on T1-weighted images (Figs 3-18B and 3-21A). However, displacement of fat planes by these infiltrating neoplasms facilitates a diagnosis on CT or T1-weighted MR studies. On T2-weighted sequences, the signal intensity of neoplastic tissue increases due to increased water (edema) production which accompanies these lesions. This affords good contrast between the tumor and the muscle it infiltrates (Figs. 3-15D, 3-16, and 3-17).

The intrinsic musculature of the oral cavity and oropharynx offers little resistance to the spread of carcinoma. Therefore, both measurement of surface extension and palpation of induration often underestimates the pathologic extent of squamous cell carcinoma. Improved radiologic delineation

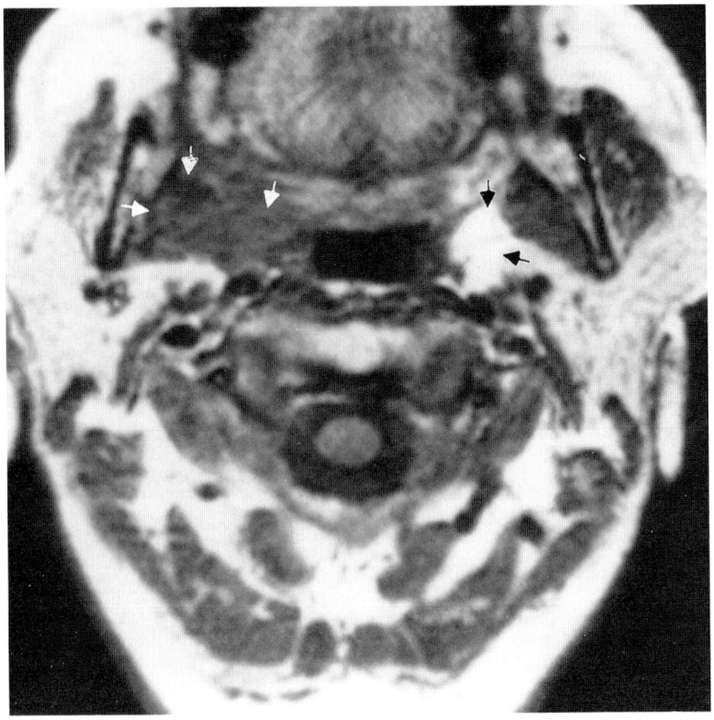

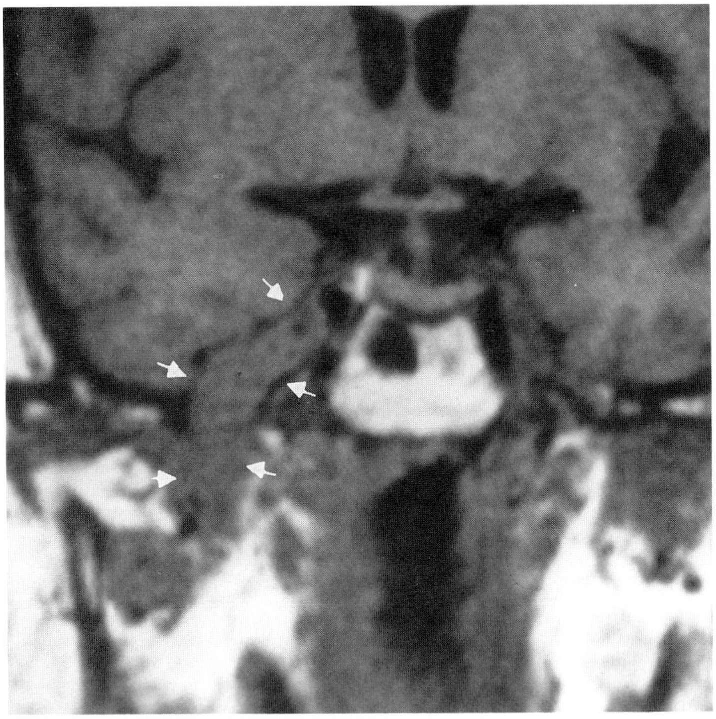

Fig. 3-21. Squamous carcinoma of the right tonsil. **A,** Axial T1-weighted image through the tonsil and oral tongue. The normal left parapharyngeal space is a high signal intensity fat-filled structure (black arrows). On the right, a carcinoma of the tonsil has invaded the parapharyngeal space and infiltrated the right pterygoid musculature (white arrows). **B,** Coronal T1-weighted view of the skull base and cavernous sinuses. The carcinoma has extended along a branch of the third division of the trigeminal nerve, infiltrating this structure and causing an enlargement of the foramen ovale and invasion of the cavernous sinus (arrows). Perineural tumor extension is common among squamous carcinomas of the head and neck.

of tumor extent and nodal involvement prior to surgery offers some key advantages in planning therapeutic possibilities and tailoring the margins of surgical and radiation therapy treatment.

CT has served as the staging modality of choice in evaluating tumors of the oral cavity and oropharynx. With the advent of high resolution MR, the optimal imaging modality is now in question. MR offers several advantages over CT in assessing tumors of the oropharynx and oral cavity. First, MR provides superior contrast between soft tissue normal anatomy and pathology without the need for intravenous contrast agents. This allows accurate detection of tumor extent across the midline of the tongue and into the tongue base, floor of mouth, and deep fascial spaces. The delineation of vascular structures without intravenous contrast agents permits easy differentiation of vessels from surrounding tumor and cervical adenopathy (Figs. 3-17 and 3-22). This is particularly helpful for assessing carotid artery invasion by tumor, a finding which, in most instances, prohibits routine radical neck surgery. In the tongue, the anatomic proximity of tumor to the contralateral lingual artery is particularly important in planning surgical or radiation therapy. Multiplanar MR imaging improved the estimation of tumor volume with sagittal and coronal images (Figs. 3-16 and 3-19). Finally dental artifacts produced by CT scans through the oral cavity are greatly diminished by MR in most instances, as dental amalgam is generally not ferromagnetic.[25]

A drawback of MR and CT imaging in the upper aerodigestive tract is the lack of contrast between tumor and lymphoid tissue. This is particularly true in and around the soft palate, base of the tongue, and the palatine tonsils where the signal intensity is similar to most malignant tumors on both T1- and T2-weighted images (Fig. 3-20). Close examination may demonstrate subtle intensity differences. However, morphologic changes such as asymmetric enlargement of the soft palate or tonsil or deep infiltration of the surrounding deep fat planes is probably the most useful way to detect a lesion adjacent to lymphoid tissue. In our experience, neither CT nor MR is accurate in detecting the interface of tumors with lymphoid tissue.

Both T1- and T2-weighted images are necessary in the evaluation of all lesions of the oral cavity and oropharynx. Axial and sagittal MR planes are the most useful in delineating oropharyngeal pathology. Axial images define the posterior and lateral extent of pathology, while sagittal images are helpful in defining invasion of the tongue base, preepiglottic space, and the posterior pharyngeal wall (Fig. 3-19).

The role of MR and CT in tumor diagnosis is limited. Most of these lesions are discovered by the patient or clinician and are frequently biopsied by the time a radiologist sees the patient for imaging studies. Unfortunately, the depth or extent of a lesion cannot always be predicted on the basis of clinical examination. MR and CT are, therefore, required to make this assessment. If a biopsy is performed prior to

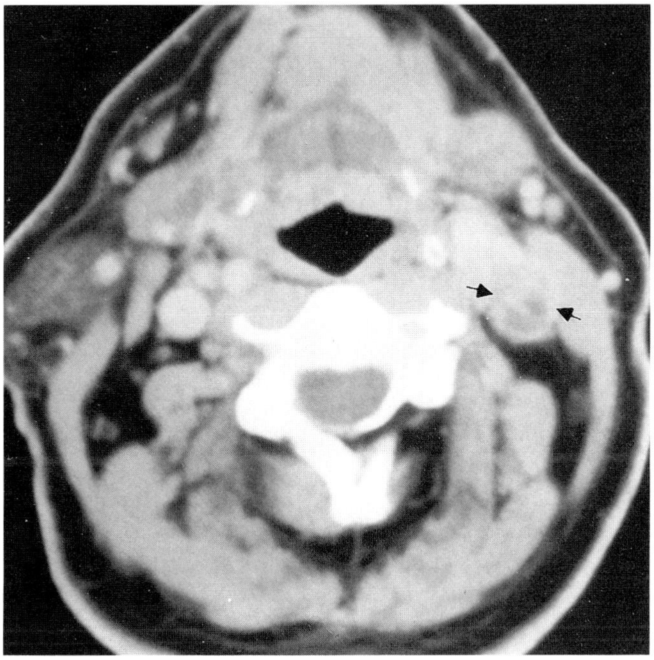

A

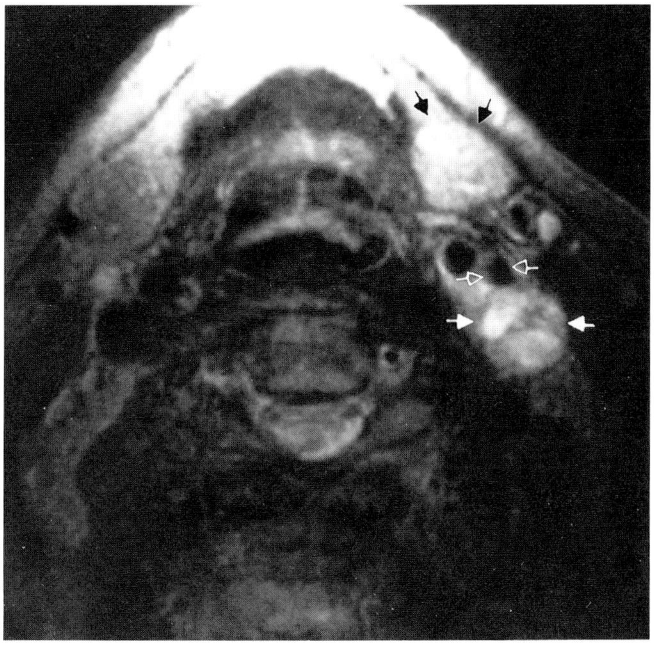

B

Fig. 3-22. Squamous carcinoma metastatic to cervical nodes. **A,** Axial CT section through the base of tongue and neck. A metastatic node is noted in the left posterior cervical region (arrows). Note its inhomogeneous central area. This is typical of metastatic nodes on CT. **B,** T2-weighted image of the same patient. The metastatic node is also inhomogeneous in this T2-weighted image which demonstrates with focal areas of bright and low-signal intensity (closed white arrows). It can be easily differentiated from the low-signal intensity lumen of the carotid artery bifurcation (open white arrows). The submandibular gland is located anterior to the carotid artery (black arrows).

imaging, the edema generated by the biopsy may simulate tumor infiltration on the imaging study. Therefore, if the patient is to have an imaging study, particularly in search of an unknown primary lesion, it is most important that it be performed prior to biopsy.

The pathways of extension of a neoplasm usually are predictable. A careful search for subtle tumor extension along regional nerves, muscles, and into regional nodes is necessary in order to derive the most information from the MR or CT study. Skull-base erosion or infiltration of the CNS may secondarily occur if perineural tumor reaches the sphenoid bone (Fig. 3-21B). Adenoidcystic carcinoma is notorious for extending along the regional nerves which are a distance away from the primary lesion. However, all soft-tissue tumors have this potential and a detailed search for this pathway of spread is necessary in every case. In the oral cavity, mandibular involvement by tumor will drastically alter the patient's management or surgical procedure. Both MR and CT have advantages over plain film assessment of the mandible. While MR is more sensitive to tumor extension into the medullary cavity, CT probably offers greater sensitivity to cortical bone erosion than any other modality and should be utilized when doubt exists regarding the integrity of the mandible adjacent to a neoplasm.

The detection of metastatic adenopathy is most important in the treatment of patients with oral cavity tumors. The presence of metastatic adenopathy from an oral tongue carcinoma decreases the 5-year survival rate by 50%.[29] Metastasis involves draining nodes in an orderly fashion, infiltrating the more proximal regional nodes prior to the more distal nodes in the chain. Therefore, a careful search can be directed at nodes in a specific region. Up to 30% of metastatic nodes are nonpalpable at the time of diagnosis due to their position beneath the sternocleidomastoid muscle or adjacent to the submandibular glands. These nodes can be evaluated easily by CT or MR. On CT, metastatic nodes are generally greater than 15 mm in diameter or have a low-density center surrounded by an enhancing rim (Fig. 3-22A). On MR, metastatic nodes often (but do not always) have an inhomogeneous signal intensity on both T2- and T1-weighted images (Fig. 3-22B). However, small reactive and metastatic nodes may appear similar in their MR signal. The introduction of a new contrast agent for MR, gadolinium DTPA, may increase the specificity of MR in the detection of these small metastatic nodes by providing the same appearance as on CT. Initial work with this does not indicate any improvement over unenhanced MR in the assessment of primary neoplasms.

Finally, the role of MR and CT in the setting of the unknown primary tumor is still undecided. Only one study to date has examined the sensitivity of CT in this setting.[30] The authors of this study concluded that CT was useful in locating the tumor or directing a biopsy in 30% of the 15 patients studied. A similar study of MR has not been published. However, the potential for even greater detection rates exists. For this reason, at the University of California, San Francisco, high resolution MR is utilized prior to biopsy in the patient with the unknown primary tumor. This does not retard the diagnostic or therapeutic work-up and has greater potential to direct biopsies during subsequent panendoscopy.

REFERENCES

1. Cole WH: Opening address: Spontaneous regression of cancer and the importance of finding its cause. *Natl Cancer Inst Monograph* 44:5, 1976.
2. Silverman S Jr, Bilimoria KF, Bhargava K et al: Cytologic, histologic and clinical correlations of precancerous and cancerous oral lesions in 57,518 industrial workers of Gujarat, India. *Acta Cytol* 21:196, 1977.
3. Sandler HC: Reliability of oral exfoliative cytology for detection of oral cancer. *J Am Dent Assoc* 68:489, 1964.
4. Hayes RL, Berg GW, Ross WL: Oral cytology: Its value and its limitations. *J Am Dent Assoc*79:649, 1969.
5. Folsom TC, White CP, Bromer L et al: Oral exfoliative cytology. Review of the literature and report of a three-year study. *Oral Surg Oral Med Oral Pathol* 33:61, 1972.
6. Allegra SR, Broderick PA, Corvese N: Oral cytology. Seven-year oral cytology screening program in the state of Rhode Island. Analysis of 6,448 cases. *Acta Cytol* 17:42, 1973.
7. Silverman S Jr: The cytology of benign oral lesions. *Acta Cytol* 9:287, 1965.
8. Sandler HC: Errors of oral cytodiagnosis: Report of follow-up of 1,801 patients. *J Am Dent Assoc* 72:851, 1966.
9. Stahl SS, Koss LG, Brown RC Jr et al: Oral cytologic screening in a large metropolitan area. *J Am Dent Assoc* 75:1385, 1967.
10. Shklar G, Cataldo E, Meyer I: Reliability of cytologic smear in the diagnosis of oral cancer. A controlled study. *Arch Otolaryngol* 91:158, 1970.
11. Rovin S: An assessment of the negative oral cytologic diagnosis. *J Am Dent Assoc* 74:759, 1967.
12. Safour IM, Wood NK, Tsiklakis K et al: Incisional biopsy and seeding in hamster cheek pouch carcinoma. *J Dent Res* 63:1116, 1984.
13. Frable WJ, Frable MAS: Thin-needle aspiration biopsy. The diagnosis of head and neck tumors revisited. *Cancer* 43:1541, 1979.
14. Kline TS, Kannan V, Kline IK: Lymphadenopathy and aspiration biopsy cytology. Review of 376 superficial nodes. *Cancer* 54:1076, 1984.
15. Scher RL, Oostingh PE, Levine PA et al: Role of fine needle aspiration biopsy in the diagnosis of lesions of the oral cavity, oropharynx, and nasopharynx. *Cancer* 62:2602, 1988
16. Niebel HH, Chamet B: In vivo staining test for delineation of oral intraepithelial neoplastic change: Preliminary report. *J Am Dent Assoc* 68:801, 1964.
17. Strong MS, Vaughn CW, Incze JS: Toluidine blue in the management of carcinoma of the oral cavity. *Arch Otolaryngol* 87:527, 1968.
18. Mashberg A: Reevaluation of toluidine blue application as a diagnostic adjunct in the detection of asymptomatic oral squamous carcinoma: A continuing prospective study of oral cancer III. *Cancer* 46:758, 1980.
19. Mashberg A: Tolonium (toluidine blue) rinse—a screening method for recognition of squamous carcinoma. Continuing study of oral cancer IV. *JAMA* 245:2408, 1981.
20. Rosenberg D, Cretin S: Use of meta-analysis to evaluate tolonium chloride in oral cancer screening. *Oral Surg Oral Med Oral Pathol* 67:621, 1989.
21. Silverman S Jr, Migliorati C, Barbosa J: Toluidine blue staining in the detection of oral precancerous and malignant lesions. *Oral Surg Oral Med Oral Pathol* 57:379, 1983.
22. Nader HB, Dietrich CP: Determination of sulfate after chromatography and toluidine blue complex formation. *Anal Biochem* 78:112, 1977.
23. Dietrich CP, Sampaio LO, DeOrca HM, et al: Role of sulfated mucopolysaccharides in cell recognition and neoplastic transformation. *An Acad Bras Cienc* 52:179, 1980.
24. Ranken R, Kaplan MJ, Silverman S Jr et al: A monoclonal antibody to squamous cell carcinoma. *Laryngoscope* 97:657, 1987.
25. Hinshaw DB, Holshouser BA, Engstrom HI, et al: Dental material artifacts on MR images. *Radiology* 166:777, 1988.
26. Mancuso AA, Hanafee WN: *Computer Tomography and Magnetic Resonance Imaging of the Head and Neck* (2nd ed). Baltimore, Williams & Wilkins, 1985.
27. Unger JM: The oral cavity and tongue: Magnetic resonance imaging. *Radiology* 155:151, 1985.
28. Schaefer SD, Maravilla KR, Suss RA, et al: Magnetic resonance imaging vs computed tomography: Comparison in imaging the oral cavity and pharyngeal carcinomas. *Arch Otolaryngol* 111:730, 1985.
29. Batsakis JG (ed): *Tumors of the head and neck: Clinical and pathological considerations* (2nd ed). Baltimore, Williams & Wilkins, 1979.
30. Muraki AS, Mancuso AA, Harnsberger HR: Metastatic cervical adenopathy from tumors of unknown origin: The role of CT. *Radiology* 152:749, 1984.

4

Spread of Tumor

KAREN FU
SOL SILVERMAN, JR.

Squamous cell carcinoma of the oral cavity spreads primarily by local extension and by lymphatic permeation. Hematogenous spread (by blood vessels) occurs rarely with oral malignancies, but is important in the development of distant metastases.

LOCAL EXTENSION

Local direct extension into surrounding tissue depends a great deal upon the anatomic location of the tumor. Muscle is easily invaded. The periosteum offers a good barrier, but eventually it is destroyed and the tumor may proceed into the osseous tissue (Fig. 4-1). Obviously, the unknown biologic characteristics that determine tumor aggressiveness (i.e., the differentiation, mitotic index, and biochemical properties of the neoplastic cells, as well as the efficacy of the host immune response) are major determinants.

LYMPHATIC SPREAD

Lymphatic spread is the most important as well as the most frequent pathway for spread of tumor (Fig. 4-2). The tumor usually involves the lymphatic channels by embolization. The lymph node gradually becomes replaced by tumor tissue and may attain a considerable size before tumor breaks through the capsule and ulcerates into the surrounding tissue (Fig. 4-3). The involved lymph nodes are freely movable at first, but as the tumor breaks through the capsule, the nodes become fixed to vital structures such as the carotid artery. The degree of lymph-node involvement has been categorized in a staging system which, in turn, is related to survival. (See Chapter 7.) Infection in the primary lesion may also give rise to an enlargement of the lymph nodes (lymphadenopathy) which become palpable even though they do not contain even microscopic deposits of cancer.

The usual pattern of findings from palpation of enlarged lymph nodes is described in Table 4-1, however the clinician must realize that various combinations may exist. These findings are helpful in patient management, but they are not diagnostic. Sometimes it is extremely difficult to distinguish an infected enlarged submaxillary salivary gland secondary to obstruction of the Wharton's duct from a metastatically involved submaxillary lymph node by palpation only. Ultrasonography, computed tomography (CT), magnetic resonance imaging (MRI), and fine needle aspiration may help to establish the diagnosis. (See Chapter 3.)

The frequency of metastatic involvement of lymph nodes is correlated with the size and depth of invasion, the site of origin, and the degree of differentiation of the tumor. In general, the frequency of lymph-node metastasis increases with the size and depth of penetration of the lesion.[1] This, however, does not preclude the occasional involvement of lymph nodes from a very small primary tumor. The risk for lymphatic spread appears greater the more posterior the location of the primary lesion in the oral cavity and pharynx (Table 4-2). This may be attributable to delay in diagnosis as well as to richer lymphatic drainage. More poorly differentiated tumors also have greater risk.

Lymphatic spread of intraoral carcinoma usually occurs in an orderly manner, involving first the uppermost, then the middle, and finally the lower cervical nodes. A study of 2,044 patients with head and neck carcinoma treated at the M.D. Anderson Hospital in Houston indicated that more than 50% had clinical evidence of metastatic cervical nodes upon admission.[2] The most commonly involved node is the subdigastric node (Table 4-2).

When lymph nodes are only microscopically involved by metastatic carcinoma, they may not be detectable clinically. The risk of subclinical disease in the lymph nodes in a patient with no clinical evidence of lymphadenopathy may be determined by studying the number of patients with necks that are initially negative, then become positive when the neck is not treated. Risk may also be evaluated by examining the incidence of positive nodes found in elective neck dissection specimens. The incidence of subsequent lymphadenopathy in patients with untreated necks that were initially negative is in the range of 20% to 35% for carcinoma of the floor of the mouth, 38% to 52% for the oral tongue, 17% for the gingiva, 22% for the hard palate, and 16% for the buccal mucosa. The incidence of positive nodes in elective neck dissection is in the range of 40% to 50% for carcinoma of the floor of the

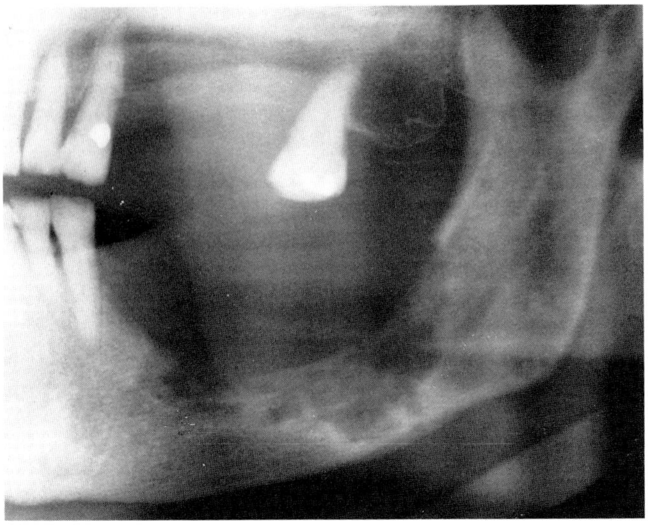

A

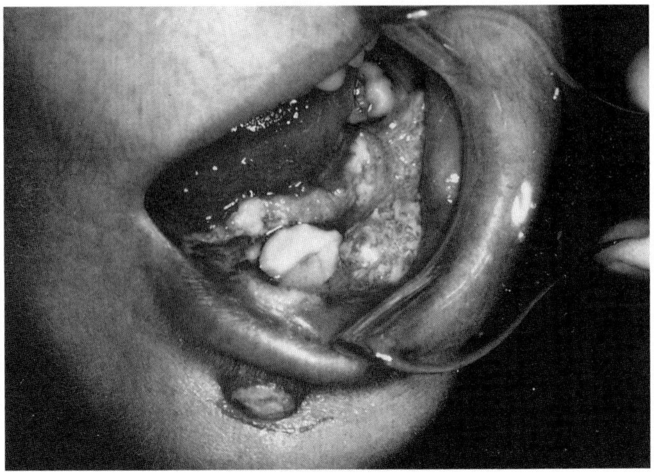

B

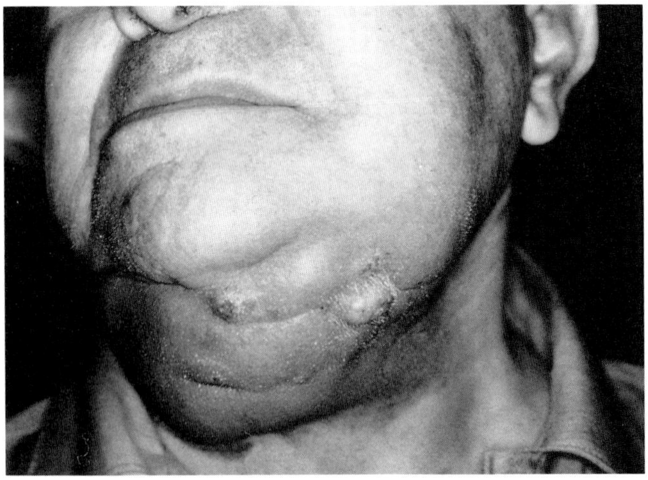

C

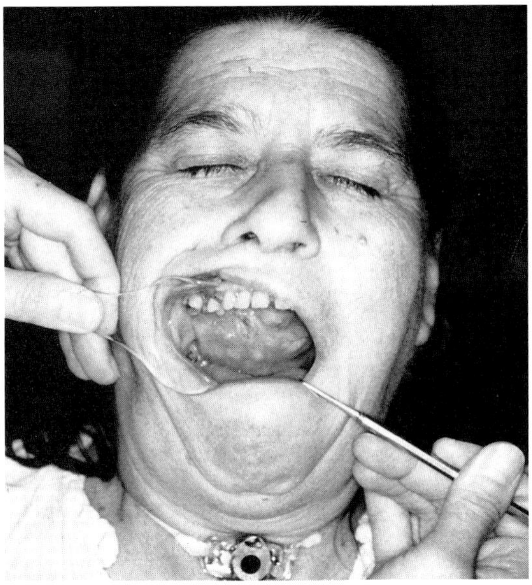

D

Fig. 4-1. Local extension. **A,** Mandibular alevolar bone is being destroyed by extensive carcinoma of the mouth floor, extending into gingiva and violating the periosteal barrier. **B,** Floor of mouth squamous carcinoma, present for 8 months, extending to tongue, gingiva, lip, and skin of chin. **C,** Local extension of squamous carcinoma into submental area and neck. The tumor was not responsive to radiation therapy. **D,** Local extension of an adenocarcinoma of the palate obstructing the oropharynx and requiring a tracheotomy to maintain the patient's airway.

mouth, 25% to 54% for the oral tongue, and 19% for the gingiva.[3] Since the incidence of occult lymph node metastases increases with the size of the primary lesion, elective irradiation of the neck may be indicated in patients presenting with advanced disease but without clinically palpable lymphadenopathy.

Occasionally a positive node in the neck for which a primary site cannot be found is diagnosed. Most lymph-node metastases from an unknown primary node occur in the neck.[4] The primary tumor will eventually be found in about one third of the cases, and in about 60% of these the location will be in the head and neck area (nasopharynx, thyroid, tonsil, base of the tongue, or hypopharynx).

HEMATOGENOUS SPREAD

Manipulation of a malignant tumor, for example during palpation and biopsy, often causes hematologic dissemination of tumor cells.[5] However, studies to evaluate the relationship between prognosis and the appearance of tumor cells in venous blood after manipulation have been equivocal.

In a Stanford University study of distant metastasis in head and neck cancer, 14% of 217 patients with oral carcinoma were found to have distant metastases clinically or at autopsy.[6] Most of these patients had advanced tumors. Lungs, bone, and liver were the most common metastatic sites. Data

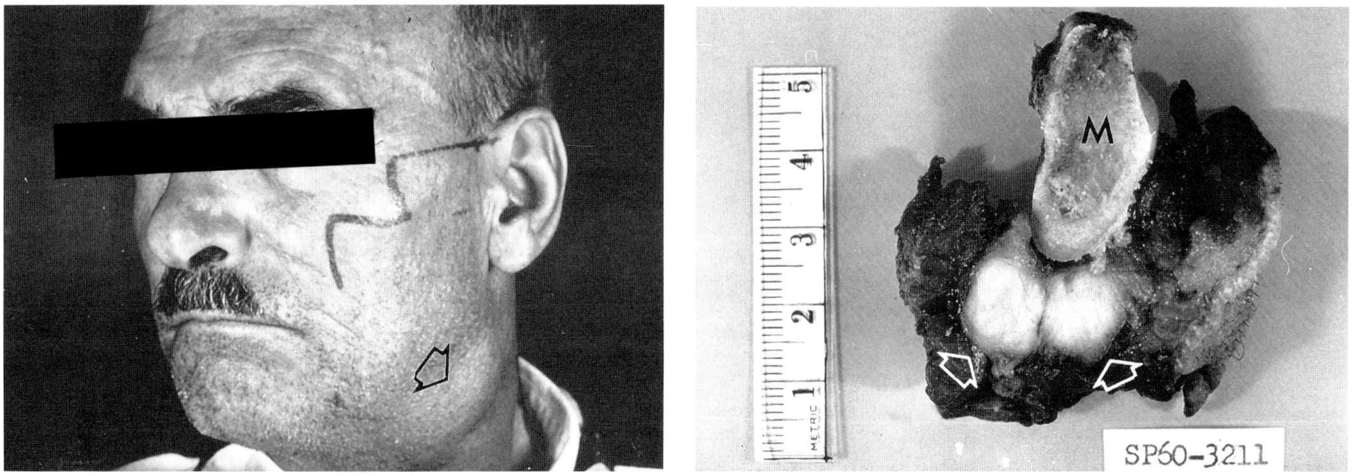

A B

Fig. 4-2. Lymphatic spread. **A,** Note large left cervical subdigastric node (arrow). **B,** Surgical specimen from this lesion shows still-encapsulated tumor-filled nodes (arrows). Various adjacent connective tissues are seen in cross-section through mandible (M).

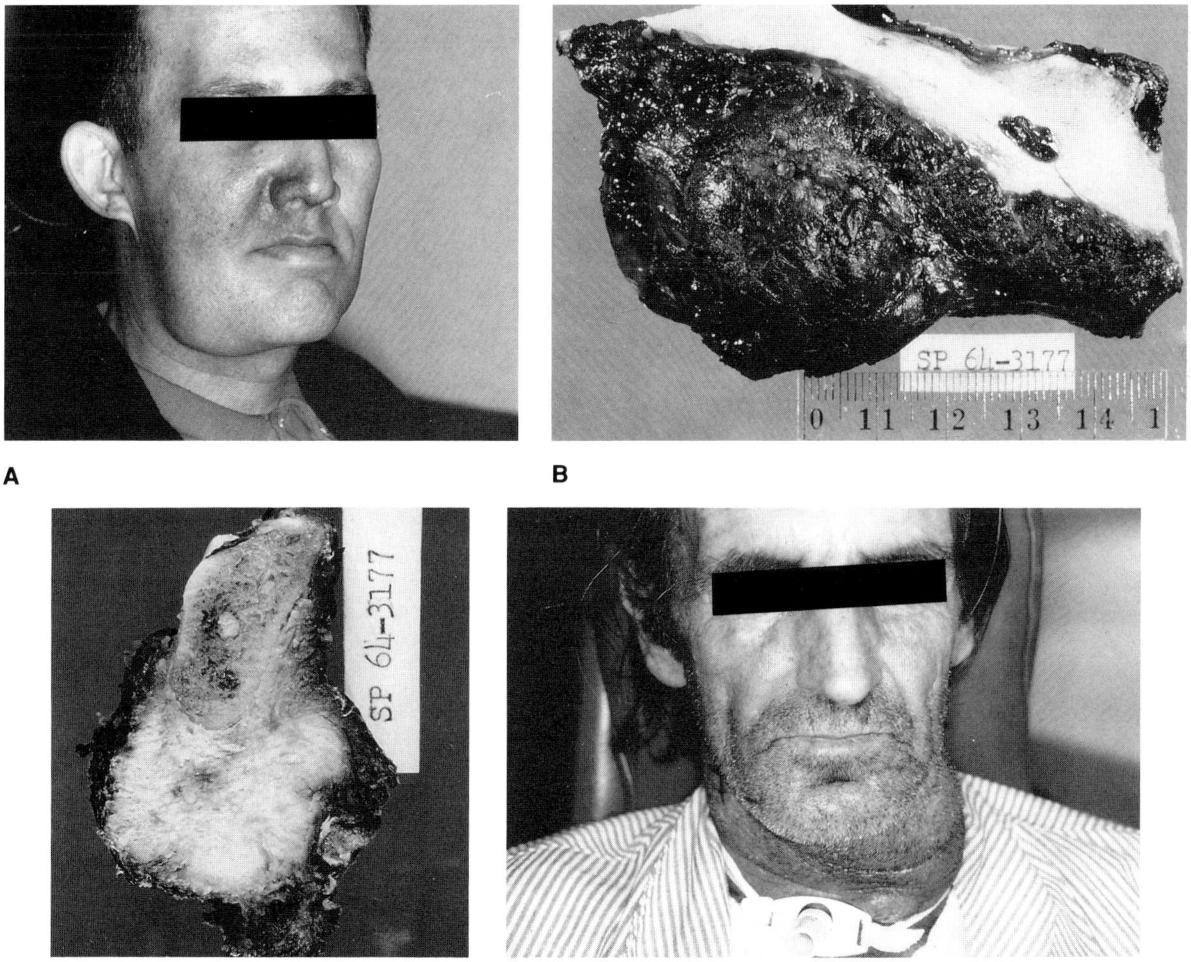

A B C D

Fig. 4-3. Capsular erosion of lymph nodes. Capsular erosion may be due to rapid growth of tumor or to delay in treatment. **A,** Uncontrolled node; tumor has broken through capsule and involved mandible. **B,** Surgical specimen, showing lymph node attached to mandible. **C,** Cross-section of same specimen, showing extension of tumor (white tissue) breaking the capsule and involving the mandible. **D,** This patient ignored the lump in his neck. By the time diagnosis was established, malignant cells had invaded vital structures in the neck and the mass was not resectable. A tracheotomy had to be performed. Radiation was ineffective in controlling tumor.

Table 4-1. LYMPH NODE PALPATION FINDINGS

Cause of Lymphadenopathy	Texture	Sensitivity	Mobility
Acute infection or malignancy	soft	tender	movable
Malignancy	firm	nontender	movable or fixed

Table 4-2. DISTRIBUTION OF CERVICAL LYMPH NODE METASTASES IN 1,155 PATIENTS WITH OROPHARYNGEAL SQUAMOUS CARCINOMAS*

Site of Primary Tumor	Regional Lymph Nodes Involved (%)	Nodal Regions Most Commonly Involved	
		First	Second
Nasopharynx	87	Subdigastric	Postcervical
Base of tongue	78	Subdigastric	Midjugular
Tonsillar fossa	76	Subdigastric	Midjugular
Oropharynx	59	Subdigastric	Midjugular
Retromolar pillar	45	Subdigastric	Submaxillary
Soft palate	44	Subdigastric	Midjugular
Oral tongue	35	Subdigastric	Submaxillary
Floor of mouth	31	Submaxillary	Subdigastric

*Data from Lindberg, 1972.[2]

from the M.D. Anderson Hospital (1948–1973) revealed that 11% of 5,019 patients with squamous carcinomas of the upper respiratory and digestive tracts developed distant metastases.[7] In a Connecticut study of 169 patients with advanced head and neck cancer who were observed from 1968 to 1982, the overall frequency of metastasis was 25%.[8] It was relatively low for the floor of the mouth (12%), tongue (14%), and oropharynx (19%), but more common in tonsillar fossa (26%), hypopharynx (30%), and larynx (59%). For carcinoma of the nasopharynx, the incidence of distant metastasis is relatively high, especially in patients with lymphoepitheliomas. The overall incidence of distant metastasis has been reported in the range of 18 to 34%,[9–12] 50% in patients with N2 and N3 disease,[1] and 80% in a small autopsy series.[13] The most common metastatic sites were lung and bone. The median time for occurrence was 7 months.

The risk for distant metastasis increases significantly with advanced lesions. Since it appears that the disease remains localized above the clavicles for a period of time and thus remains accessible to the surgeon or radiotherapist, the institution of early treatment is of utmost importance.

METASTASIS TO THE MOUTH

The oral cavity is infrequently the site of spread from other primary foci. When this occurs, it is chiefly from breast cancers, and the mandible is the most common metastatic site.[14] Oral signs and symptoms from a metastatic lesion may precede recognition of a distant primary site. Both white and black women who have had cancer of the cervix have been observed to have an increased rate of developing a subsequent cancer of the oropharynx during the first five years after their treatment. (See Chapter 9.)[15]

REFERENCES

1. Moore C, Flynn MB, Greenberg RA: Evaluation of size in prognosis of oral cancer. *Cancer* 58:158, 1986.
2. Lindberg R: Distribution of cervical lymph node metastases from squamous cell carcinoma of the upper respiratory and digestive tracts. *Cancer* 29:1446, 1972.
3. de Braud F, Heilbrun LK, Ahmed K et al: Metastatic squamous cell carcinoma of an unknown primary localized to the neck: Advantages of an aggressive treatment. *Cancer* 64:510, 1989.
4. Krementz ET, Cerise EJ, Ciaravella JM Jr et al: Metastases of undetermined source. *CA* 27:289, 1977.
5. Roger V, Brennhoud I, Hoeg K: Tumor cells in blood. The prognostic significance of tumor cells in blood during palpation and biopsy. *Acta Cytol* 16:557, 1972.
6. Probert JC, Thompson RW, Bagshaw MA: Patterns of spread of distant metastases in head and neck cancer. *Cancer* 33:127, 1974.
7. Merino OR, Lindberg RD, Fletcher GH: An analysis of distant metastases from squamous cell carcinoma of the upper respiratory and digestive tracts. *Cancer* 40:145, 1977.
8. Papac RJ: Distant metastases from head and neck cancer. *Cancer* 53:342, 1984.
9. Bedwinek JM, Perez CA, Keys DJ: Analysis of failures after definitive irradiation for epidermoid carcinoma of the nasopharynx. *Cancer* 45:2725, 1980.
10. Hoppe RT, Goffinet DR, Bagshaw MA: Carcinoma of the nasopharynx: Eighteen years' experience with megavoltage radiation therapy. *Cancer* 37:2605, 1976.
11. McNeese MD, Fletcher GH: Retreatment of recurrent nasopharyngeal carcinoma. *Radiology* 138:191, 1981.
12. Moench HC, Phillips TL: Carcinoma of the nasopharynx: Review of 146 patients with emphasis on radiation dose and time factors. *Am J Surg* 124:515, 1972.
13. Lynn TC, Huang SC, Tu SM: Treatment of nasopharyngeal carcinoma. *Excerpta Med Int Congr Ser* 571:408, 1982.
14. Meyer I, Shklar G: Malignant tumors metastatic to mouth and jaws. *Oral Surg Oral Med Oral Pathol* 20:350, 1965.
15. Newall GR, Krementz ET, Roberts JD: Excess occurrence of cancer of the oral cavity, lung and bladder following cancer of the cervix. *Cancer* 36:2155, 1975.

5

Treatment

MAURICE GALANTE • Surgery
THEODORE L. PHILLIPS • Radiation Therapy
IVAN J. SILVERBERG and KAREN FU • Chemotherapy

The appropriate and adequate treatment of intraoral malignancies is a complicated procedure that requires the cooperation of experienced and fully qualified specialists from several disciplines: surgeons, radiation oncologists, medical oncologists (chemotherapy), dentists, and paramedical/paradental professionals (social workers, nurses, hygienists). Often this cooperation is initiated by pretreatment conferences (tumor boards), which are routinely held at treatment centers in order to formulate the best possible treatment plan for individual patients and their specific tumors. Even at this stage, rehabilitation is an important consideration in the attempt to minimize morbidity and mortality. Since cancer ordinarily does not progress with the fulminating rapidity of some infections, there is always time for proper consultation and planning.

Several factors contribute to the poor overall results and unsatisfactory survival rates associated with oral cancer. These are malnutrition, alcoholism, tobacco, infection, and most important, the fact that lesions are usually seen in an advanced stage.

It is important that an enriched diet is maintained throughout the pretreatment, treatment, and posttreatment phases. Inordinate weight loss complicates recovery because patients become less active, owing to weakness, and less resistant to intercurrent infections. Since alcoholism and smoking are common in patients with intraoral malignancies, the elimination of these factors, though difficult, contributes significantly to a successful outcome.

Infection frequently accompanies large, ulcerated lesions of the oral cavity. It may at times be so severe as to mask the real extent of a lesion by increasing the area of induration and reaction. Often it is impossible to assess the size and spread of a lesion adequately without first clearing the inflammatory and infectious processes. Conversely, sometimes subtle dysplastic or malignant epithelial transformations are mistaken for benign inflammatory or infectious changes. Also, cervical lymph nodes may be enlarged as a result of inflammation rather than involvement with cancer. Therefore, the proper use of antibiotics is sometimes indicated before definitive treatment is instituted.

Definitive treatment, whether surgical or radiotherapeutic, should not begin before a histologic diagnosis of malignancy is unequivocally established by biopsy. (See Chapter 3.) There are very few exceptions to this rule.

Three forms of treatment are used today in the management of intraoral malignancies: surgery, radiation therapy, and chemotherapy. Surgery and radiation therapy are the only modalities employed, alone or in combination, in the curative treatment of intraoral malignancies. They can also be used, under proper indications, for palliative purposes. Chemotherapy is used primarily in the palliative management of intraoral malignancies, but it is occasionally used as an adjunct to radiation therapy of advanced tumors.

SURGERY

The surgical management of intraoral lesions entails the treatment of two entities: the primary lesion and the cervical lymph nodes. It is difficult to classify lesions as to whether primary surgery or radiation therapy is indicated. This decision most frequently depends upon the stage and site of the malignancy. When surgery is elected as the treatment of choice, it is used for permanent control ("cure") of the disease. Surgery is seldom used for palliative purposes alone. Two principal considerations are the possibility of obtaining adequate tumor-free margins and enabling a satisfactory postsurgical quality of life.

For many oral cancers, radiation and surgery achieve similar cure rates. In these instances, the selection of treatment modality is influenced by the patient's choice or by available facilities or specialists. Surgery is indicated under certain circumstances: (1) for tumors that are not radiosensitive, (2) for recurrences in already irradiated areas, (3) for situations in which the side effects of radiation are likely to be more severe than the surgical defects, and (4) for neoplasms involving bone, lymph nodes, and salivary glands.

Surgery has the advantage of affording an opportunity to examine all the significant margins and thus predict, to some degree, the eventual outcome. Once the lesion is removed with adequate margins, it is reasonable to assume that the

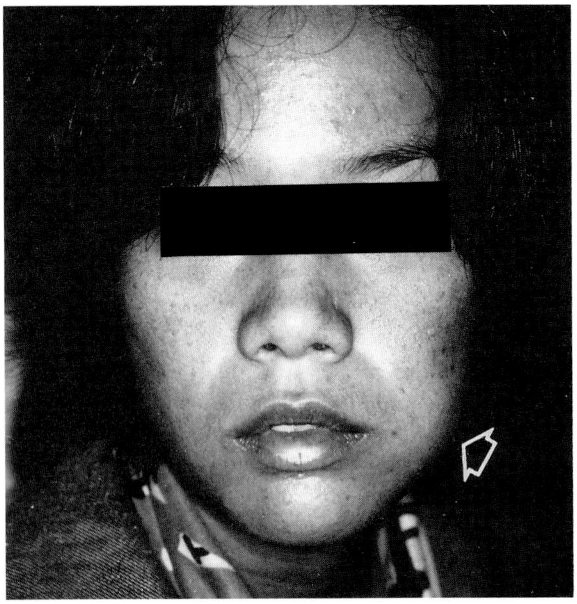

A

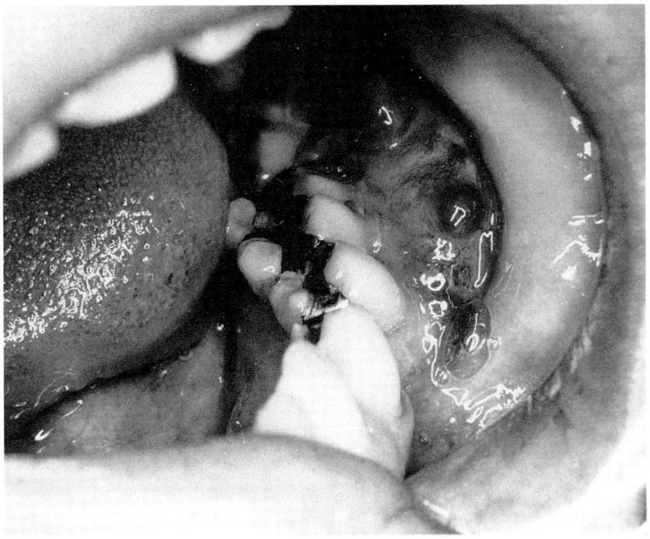

B

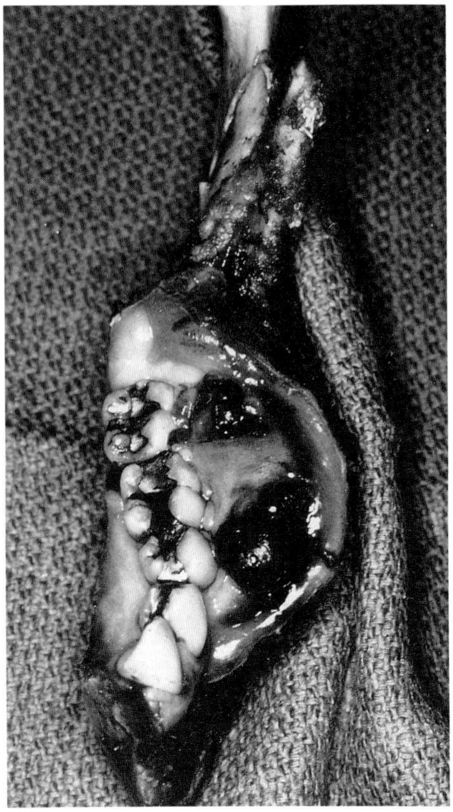

C

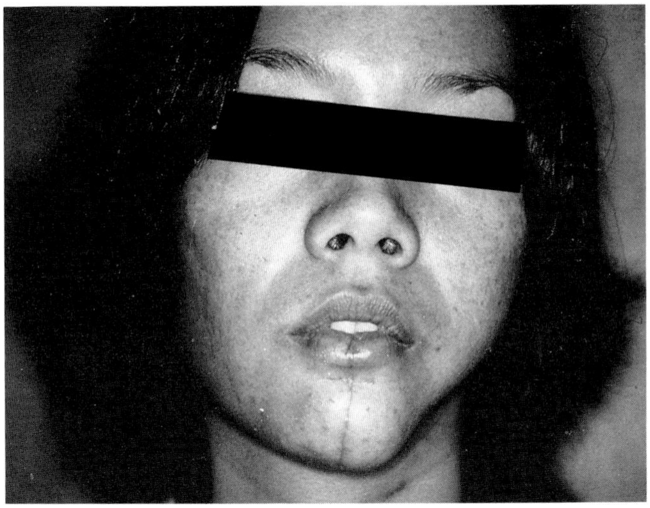

D

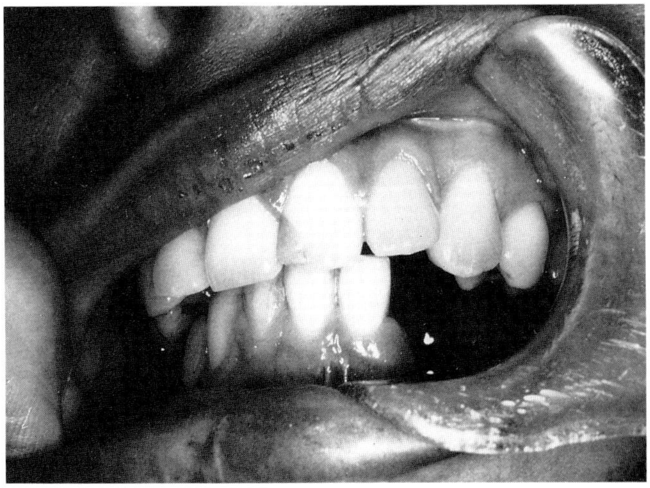

E

Fig. 5-1. Surgical resection of osteogenic sarcoma. Patient, 25 years old, had noticed asymptomatic lump in left mandible for 2 months. **A,** Patient at first examination. Note slight swelling of left face (arrow). **B,** Intraoral view of tumor which had expanded and eroded through mandibular cortical plate. **C,** Resection specimen. **D,** Patient 2 months after surgery. **E,** Good postsurgical occlusion of remaining mandible and intact maxilla.

patient is cured. However, multifocal cancer sites, as well as normal-appearing cells that have malignant potential, render assumptions that must be guarded. Careful and close follow-up is still mandatory.

Of necessity, surgery has the disadvantage of sacrificing cosmetically and functionally important structures such as the lip, tongue, mandible, and in some special cases, the eye. In addition, the intraoral location seldom permits a tumor to be removed with margins larger than 1 to 2 cm, whereas in other locations malignant tumors are excised with margins of normal tissue measuring at least several centimeters.

PRIMARY LESION

The extent of resection of a lesion depends entirely on its size and on the adjacent structures presumably involved. Thus the local resection of a segment of mandible might be sufficient to eradicate a lesion arising in the mandible (Fig. 5-1). Similarly, the local excision of a 1 cm lesion on the tip of the tongue might be sufficient to completely eradicate this type of carcinoma. Radical surgery is not always necessary (Fig. 5-2).

CERVICAL LYMPH NODES

Whereas the primary lesion ordinarily is best treated either by surgery or by radiation therapy, cervical nodes involved with squamous cell carcinoma almost always constitute a surgical problem. Although radiation therapy may permanently eradicate squamous cell carcinoma in an isolated lymph node, the dose of radiation needed for the entire neck would be prohibitive. Surgical removal of the involved nodes is a simpler method of dealing with this problem.

Neck Dissection

The lymph nodes in the area of primary drainage of the lesion are removed by means of a cervical lymphadenectomy (ordinarily known as a "neck dissection"). This is an operation whereby all the lymph nodes are removed from the level of the mandible superiorly to the clavicle inferiorly, and from the trapezius muscle posteriorly to the midline anteriorly, sacrificing the sternocleidomastoid muscle, the jugular vein, the omohyoid muscle, and the submaxillary gland.

When the lymph nodes are clinically palpable and presumed to be involved, the neck dissection is called "therapeutic." When the lymph nodes are not clinically palpable, regardless of whether they are or are not involved microscopically, the neck dissection, if done, is called "prophylactic." In some situations the neck dissection is limited to the upper neck (suprahyoid dissection).

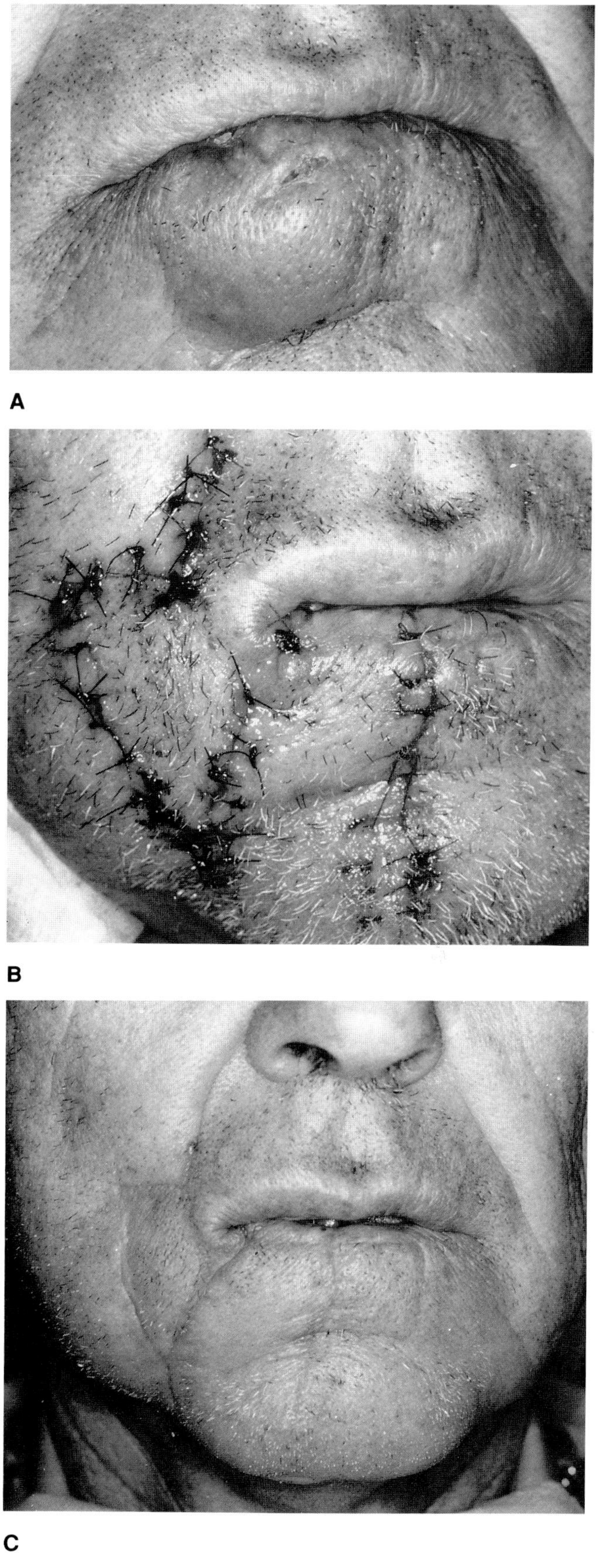

Fig. 5-2. Surgical management of carcinoma of lower lip. **A,** Patient gave 5-month history of firm and increasing, but not painful, swelling of lower lip. **B,** One week after excision and plastic revision. **C,** Three months after surgery, patient has slightly diminished oral opening but no loss of function.

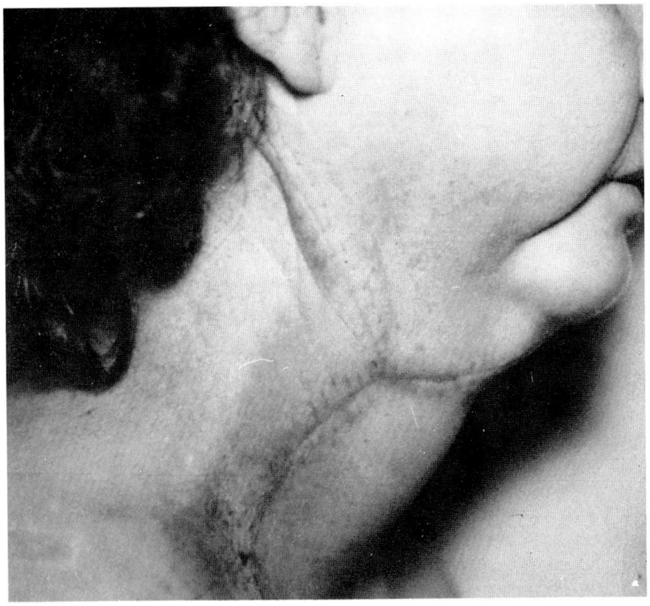

A

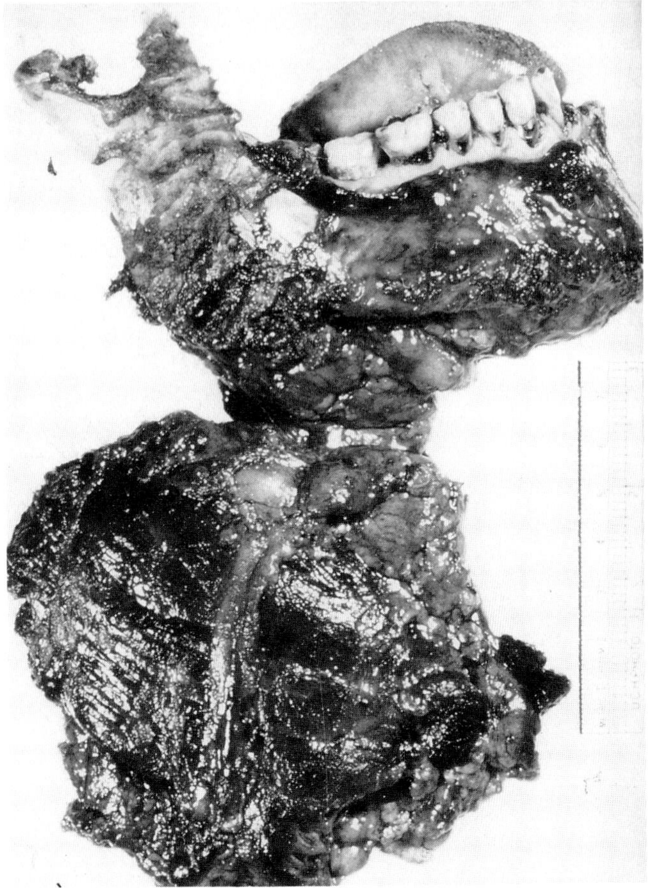

B

Fig. 5-3. Combined resection of carcinoma of right floor of mouth, involving tongue, mandible, and cervical lymph nodes. **A,** One month after surgery. Note lines of incision and closure. **B,** Surgical specimen, including tongue, right hemimandible, and contents of right neck.

COMBINED RESECTION

Large lesions that involve adjacent structures and are likely to have metastasized to the regional lymph nodes are best treated by an extensive type of resection whereby the primary tumor and adjacent tissues are removed in continuity with the contents of a neck dissection. Thus, a carcinoma of the floor of the mouth that extends medially to the tongue and laterally to the periosteum is best treated by a "combined resection" entailing a hemiglossectomy, removal of the floor of the mouth, a hemimandibulectomy, and a radical neck dissection in continuity (Fig. 5-3). This operation is ordinarily called a "Commando."

The functional and cosmetic results of such operations are usually satisfactory, especially if there is adequate preoperative preparation of the patient and expert postoperative rehabilitation. (See Chapter 10.) The extent of bone to be sacrificed depends on the likelihood or the extent of involvement of osseous tissue. Cancer can spread to the mandible from the primary tumor by direct extension or by metastasis, or from metastatically involved lymph nodes by direct extension.

LASER SURGERY

Laser surgery has been particularly useful for control of precancerous oral lesions (leukoplakia and erythroplasia) as well as localized cancerous lesions (Stage I and II).[1–5] The results have been impressive, owing to certain properties of the laser beam that minimize some of the difficulties usually encountered in surgical resections. (Figs. 5-4 and 5-5.)

For head and neck surgery, the carbon dioxide laser beam has been used. The laser emits visible monochromatic light waves (10.6 μm in length) which are strongly absorbed by the water in biologic tissue and can be used effectively for precision cutting or for limited destruction (evaporation) of tissue. The mechanism of action is that the absorbed energy causes the temperature of the tissue to rise, leading to vaporization of cells. The current and movement of the beam control the speed and depth of cutting or evaporation.

Laser energy seals lymphatic and small blood vessels, thus maintaining an almost bloodless surgical field with excellent visibility and preventing dissemination of dysplastic or malignant cells. The laser beam also sterilizes the field by its viricidal, bactericidal, and fungicidal properties.

The utility of the laser is further enhanced by its ease of operation, precise control, and lack of complications, allowing the patient a shorter hospital stay, immediate resumption of diet, and excellent healing with minimal functional liabilities.

Although the biologic explanations for these advantages are not completely clear, the properties that offer the laser advantages over the knife, electrocautery, or cryosurgery seem to be real and reproducible.

MOHS TECHNIQUE

Microscopically frozen-section-oriented histologic surgery (MOHS technique) has been successfully utilized in the resection of primary carcinomas in the head and neck.[6] The advantage is an increased possibility of removing all tumor cells and obtaining "clear" margins. Disadvantages include operating time and expense, as well as the possibility of missing very fine tumor extensions or separate adjacent tumor foci ("field cancerization").

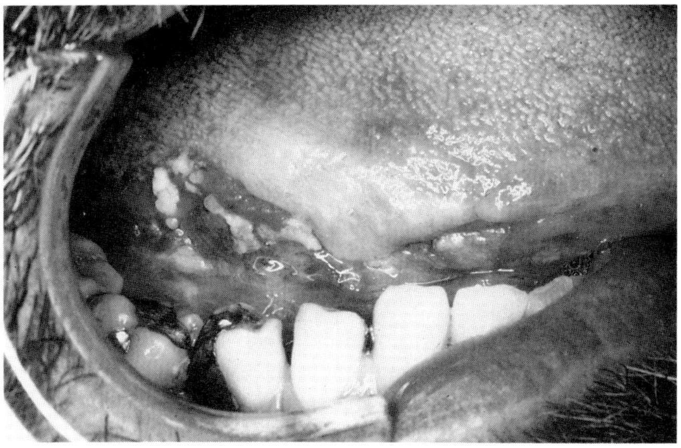

A

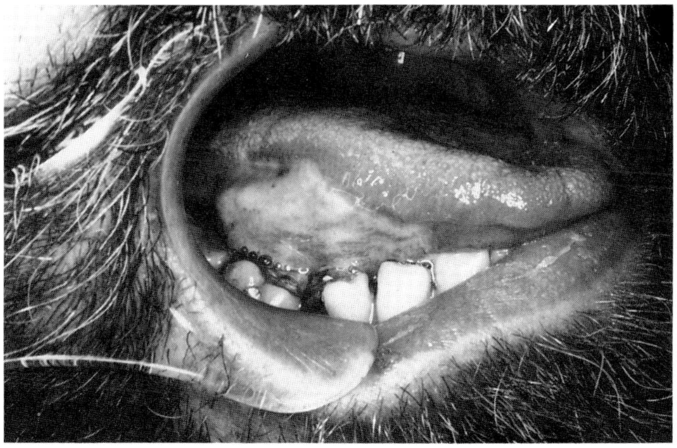

B

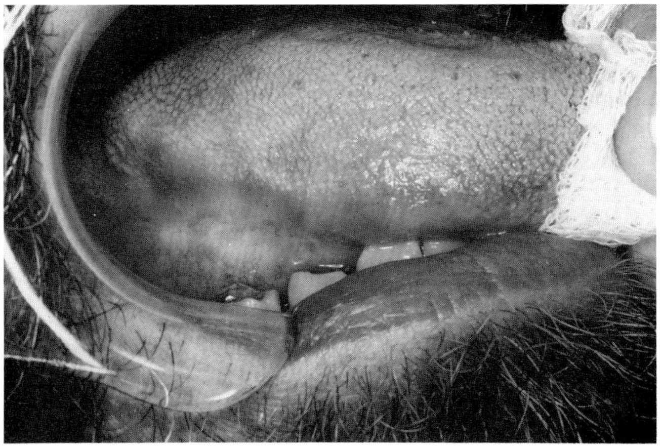

C

Fig. 5-4. Laser excision of carcinoma of the tongue. **A,** Painful, superficial squamous carcinoma, characterized by indurated, ulcerated erythroleukoplakic changes in a 45-year-old man. There was no clinically apparent lymph node involvement and no evident metastases. **B,** Three weeks after laser excision, the surgical defect is granulating and is covered by a yellowish pseudomembrane. The lesion was not closed by sutures and is approximately one-third healed. **C,** Six weeks after laser treatment the surgical defect is completely healed. The area is soft to palpation and there is no loss in speech or swallowing functions.

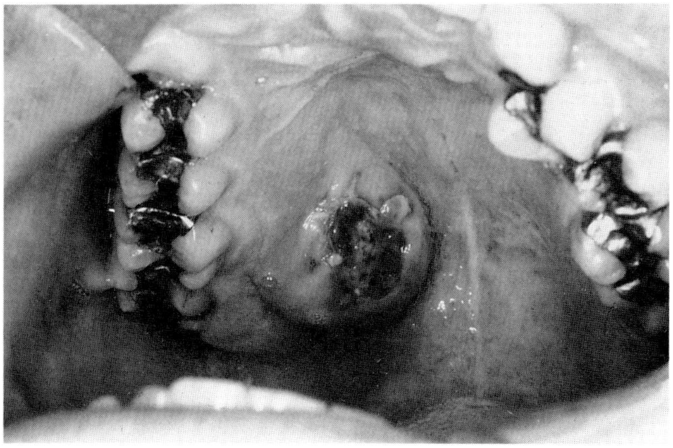

A

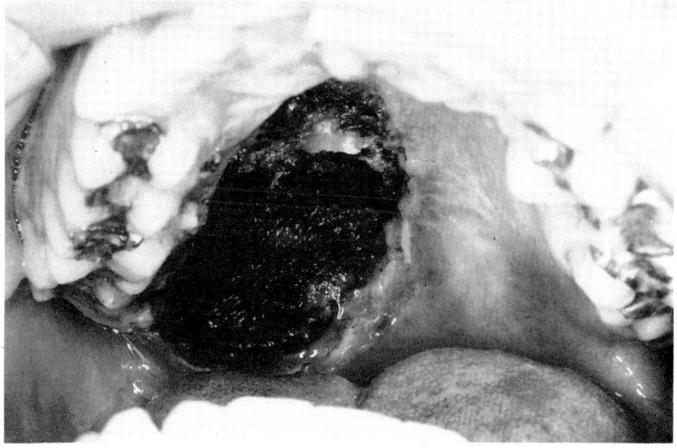

B

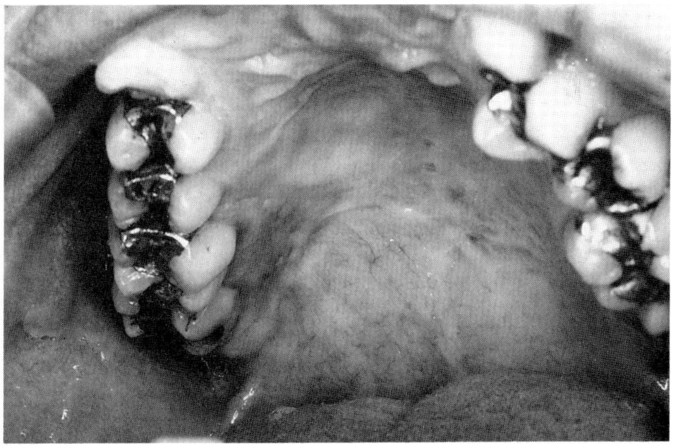

C

Fig. 5-5. Laser excision of malignant mixed tumor of minor salivary gland in the palate. **A,** Growth before surgery. **B,** Immediately after laser excision. Note excision site and laser charring of intact maxillary bone. **C,** Three months after surgery. Patient is asymptomatic and without evidence of tumor.

RADIATION THERAPY

CHOICE OF TREATMENT

In selecting between radiation therapy, surgery, or a combination of radiation with surgery for the treatment of oral cancer, it is necessary to understand the basic mechanisms by which radiation acts on tumor and normal tissues. If these basic mechanisms are clearly understood, a more rational choice of radiation in management of oral cancers can be made. As with any other cancer, the major factors influencing the choice of treatment are the following: (1) the relative cure that can be obtained with radiation as compared with surgery or another modality, (2) the relative morbidity associated with radiation treatment, and (3) the cosmetic and functional result of radiation versus surgery, or a combination of the two.

RADIOBIOLOGY

Basic Mechanisms

Ionizing radiation may be in the form of external beams of x-rays or gamma rays, external beams of electrons or heavy particles, or internally implanted sources of gamma rays. Radiation kills cells by primary and secondary interactions with the tissues. In general, the photons of x-rays or gamma rays dislodge electrons from the atoms of the tissue. These charged particles cause ionization along their tracks, which results in chemical changes in the water in the cell and in the critical macromolecules of the cell. The altered water atoms and molecules can also interact with the biologic macromolecules. It is now known that the major site of action of ionizing radiation on mammalian cells is in the nucleus where it causes breakage of chromosomes and disruptions in the DNA molecule.

Although many of the changes can be repaired, certain chromosomal and DNA breakages are not repaired normally and result in the inability of the cell to undergo more than a few subsequent divisions. In some types of cells, such as mature lymphocytes, radiation has a direct effect on the functioning of the nucleus and causes immediate cell death. In most cases the damage is to the DNA and chromosomes, and cell death results after several divisions. It should also be noted that cells themselves need not die to be mitotically dead; they may divide once or twice, but then remain as postmitotic giant cells that are no longer capable of causing tissue or tumor regeneration.

There is a constant relationship between the radiation dose and the fraction of cells that will survive this dose which can be expressed in the form of a survival curve. These curves are presented in terms of the logarithm of survival versus the dose and, in most instances, bend downward after a finite initial slope. In order to achieve complete tumor-cell sterilization, this exponential-type survival makes it necessary to use increasing doses of radiation as the number of cells in any given tumor increases. This usually requires the probability of less than one clonogenic cell surviving. Tumors vary in the percentage of cells that are clonogenic. Variation exists in the nature of the shape of the survival curve for various types of tumors and between tumor and normal tissue cells. Although these variations are relatively small after high doses of radiation, survival at a dose of 2 Gy (2000 cGy, 2000 rad), a common clinical dose, can vary from 20 to 80%, depending on tumor type. This may explain some of the differences in sensitivity of tumors to radiotherapy. The cellular repair and growth kinetic changes that take place during fractionated radiotherapy can become as important as the shape of the individual cell survival curve (as discussed below).

Differential Effects on Tumor and Normal Tissue

The events that cause cell death occur both in normal tissue and in tumor. The differential ability of ionizing radiation to sterilize a tumor without unacceptable damage to normal tissue is due to five major biological differences between tumor and normal tissue.

1. In general, the number of clonogenic cells present in the surrounding normal tissue is far greater than in the tumor. Thus, after complete sterilization of clonogenic cells in the tumor, there will be surviving surrounding epithelial cells and underlying vasculoconnective tissue cells which can repopulate the area formerly occupied by the tumor. In addition, normal cells may be recruited from areas outside the treatment volume. The fraction of cells surviving after irradiation is dependent on the dose: the higher the dose, the smaller the fraction surviving and, conversely, the larger the tumor, the greater the dose required to ensure sterilization of its cells.

2. Repair takes place in cells after radiation damage. This process is usually considered to be an intracellular repair of damage to the major nuclear components. Although this occurs in both tumor and normal tissue, it appears to be depressed in the portions of tumors that have poor vascularity and are hypoxic. In addition repair is depressed in certain tumor types, such as lymphoma. It may occur to a greater extent in slowly dividing normal tissues. Thus, when radiation is given in multiple doses, there can be more repair of damage in the normal tissue than in portions of the tumor.

3. Repopulation or proliferation of cells can occur after irradiation in both the tumor and normal tissue if viable clonogenic cells remain. Normal tissues seem able to respond to the radiation injury with more rapid cell proliferation. This homeostatic biologic mechanism does not appear to be available to tumors. In some cases, however, tumors may speed up their proliferation when they become smaller and better vascularized if all of their cells have not been killed.

4. Oxygenation plays an important role in radiation sensitivity; cells are three times more resistant when hypoxic. Although the centers of many tumors are hypoxic, making them more resistant to radiation, it is now known that some areas of tumors reoxygenate during treatment. This process can occur in a few hours to a few days. What otherwise would be resistant portions of tumors thus become more sensitive during a course of fractionated radiation therapy lasting over days or weeks. Reoxygenation seems to occur because of fluctuations in blood flow in tumor capillaries and due to tumor shrinkage.

5. Changes of cell position in the cell cycle can cause marked changes in cell and/or tumor radiosensitivity. Cell age or position in the cell cycle (resting, synthesis, mitosis)

can cause variations as great as a factor of three in cell sensitivity to radiation. If tumor cells are in a vulnerable position in their cycle while normal tissues are in a more resistant phase, a better differential between tumor and normal tissue damage may result. The use of halogenated pyrimidine sensitizers takes advantage of the fact that, for some tumors, more cells are in the S phase of their cycle than in some surrounding normal tissues (brain, soft tissue).

New Approaches

A number of experimental approaches are being employed to increase the tumor cell kill and decrease damage to normal tissue during radiotherapy. One approach is the use of neutrons or heavy charged particles that deposit their energy in dense patterns. These "high-LET" (linear energy transfer) radiations differ from conventional x-rays in that the damage they cause is less likely to be repaired and is less influenced by the concentration of oxygen. It is possible that these differences will yield greater tumor control for a given level of normal tissue damage in those cases where repair of tumor cells is unusually great or when hypoxia persists throughout treatment. Several trials have already shown that high LET treatment is more effective in salivary gland tumors.

A second approach to increasing the cell kill of hypoxic tumor cells is the use of radiosensitizers. Some of these chemicals have the ability to sensitize hypoxic cells to radiation much in the same way that oxygen does, but because they are inert and not metabolized by the tissue, they can reach the hypoxic centers of tumors. The best analog yet developed, etanidazole, is currently in active clinical trial using patients with head and neck cancer. Other radiosensitizers are analogs of thymidine (bromodeoxyuridine and iododeoxyuridine) which are incorporated into dividing cells, increasing their sensitivity.

A third method, which is just being introduced into the clinic, is the use of radioprotective compounds that selectively decrease the radiation injury to normal tissue. These compounds are particularly promising in head and neck tumors since they appear to be especially active in oral mucosa and in the salivary glands.

Hyperthermia, the induction of temperatures in the range of 42° to 45° C, is being applied to the treatment of oral cancer in conjunction with radiotherapy. Either external applicators using ultrasound or microwaves or interstitial needles heated by microwave antennas, local current fields, or ferromagnetic seeds can be used to induce elevated temperatures for 15 to 60 minutes. When this treatment is combined with radiation, the effect can be doubled or the necessary radiation dose reduced. Trials of this modality in curative therapy have just begun.

Cytotoxic chemotherapy is selectively used in combination with radiation. It can increase local tumor response and, in some instances, extend control rates in advanced squamous carcinoma.

Summary

Thus, we see that although radiation damages both tumor and normal tissue, a number of factors influence tumor response and that a fractionated, multiple-dose course of radiation therapy can effect complete sterilization of the tumor with adequate survival of normal tissue. Some basic principles are evident. The smaller the number of tumor cells present, the greater the probability of radiation sterilization and/or the lower the dose required for a given probability of sterilization. Certain tumor cell types, such as lymphomas, will have greater radiosensitivity and radiocurability. Large necrotic tumors with anoxic foci, particularly those deeply invading bone or muscle where reoxygenation may not occur, will be more resistant to radiation. Damage to normal tissue depends on dose as well, and the incidence of complications will increase with large tumors requiring higher doses.

SELECTION OF PATIENTS FOR RADIATION THERAPY

Based on the foregoing principles, the selection of patients for radiation therapy of cancer of the oral cavity can be approached rationally. Those lesions that are small (under 3 cm and superficial without necrotic areas) will be amenable to radiation sterilization (Fig. 5-6). The choice of radiation therapy versus surgery for such early, superficial lesions will depend on the functional and cosmetic results of the two modalities. If a regional excision can be accomplished without much morbidity, this would often be the treatment of choice since there would be no residual radiation injury. On the other hand, if the lesion involves large portions of the tongue, floor of mouth, or buccal mucosa and would result in morbidity if excised, then local irradiation would be the treatment of choice (Figs. 5-7 and 5-8).

With lesions that are large, deeply invasive, and particularly when bone is involved, radiation sterilization of the tumor is less likely without extensive normal tissue damage, therefore surgery, or a combination of irradiation and surgery, may be required (Fig. 5-9). When the histologic nature of the lesion is such that it is potentially extremely radiosensitive, as in various lymphomas, radiotherapy would be the treatment of choice.

If the location and clinical behavior of a lesion indicates significant lymphatic permeation, then radiotherapy is often advantageous, either alone or in combination with surgery, because a wider volume of the potentially involved lymphatic structures can be covered (Fig. 5-10). For example, in carcinomas of the tonsil or tongue, bilateral irradiation of the neck can prevent the development of lymph-node metastases in the neck that shows no clinical signs of involvement. In addition, prophylactic treatment of the lower neck when the upper neck is involved can prevent the involvement of lymph nodes in this region.

The availability of equipment and expertise is certainly a factor in treatment selection, and obviously surgery would be preferable if adequate radiotherapy equipment and personnel are not available.

The patient's medical condition probably has less influence on the selection of modality than is generally thought. A course of radiotherapy is debilitating, particularly so in the oral cavity region where mucositis and decreased taste and salivary function make it difficult to maintain weight and general condition. Thus, poor general condition is a contraindication for radiotherapy, although this modality may be selected for patients in whom extensive surgery and lengthy anesthesia are absolutely prohibited.

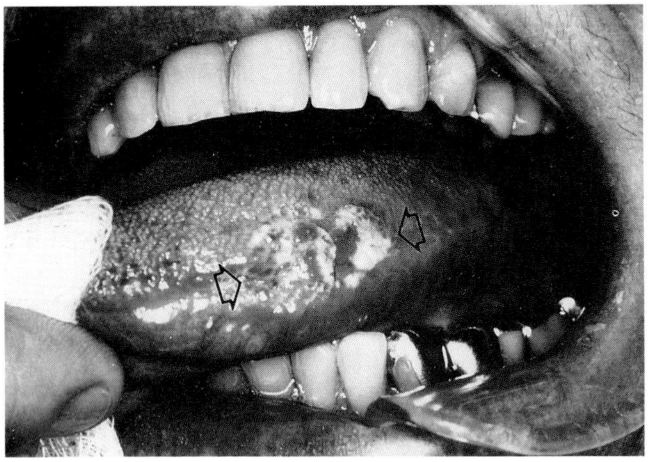

A

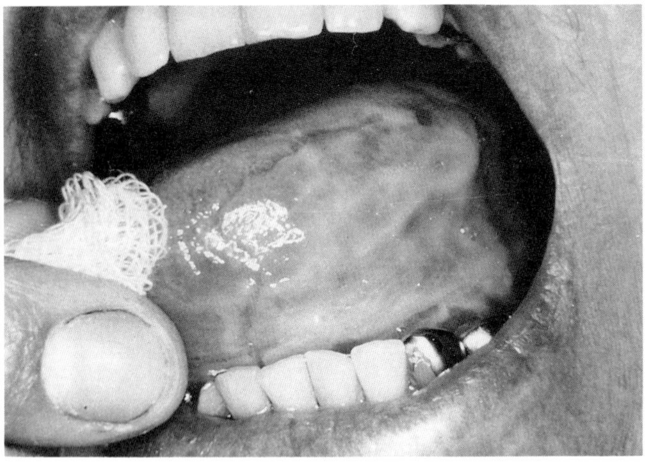

B

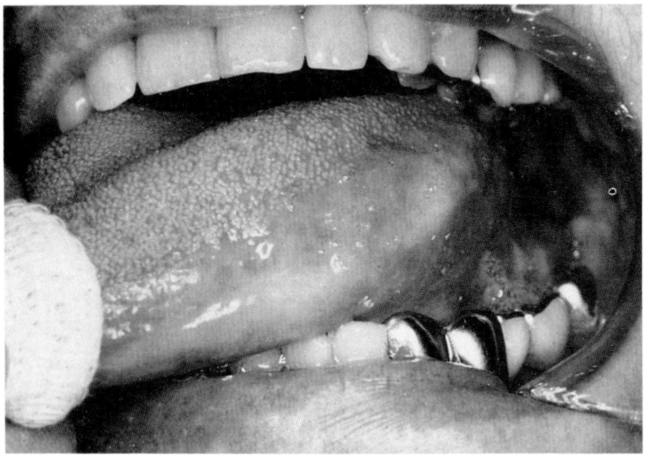

C

Fig. 5-6. Irradiation of carcinoma of the left tongue. **A,** Squamous cell carcinoma before treatment (arrows), mistaken for 4 months for a benign leukoplakia secondary to chronic irritation. **B,** Mucositis, appearing shortly after irradiation began and disappearing 1 month after it ended. **C,** One year after treatment, there is no evidence of tumor. Patient was asymptomatic and suffered no loss of function.

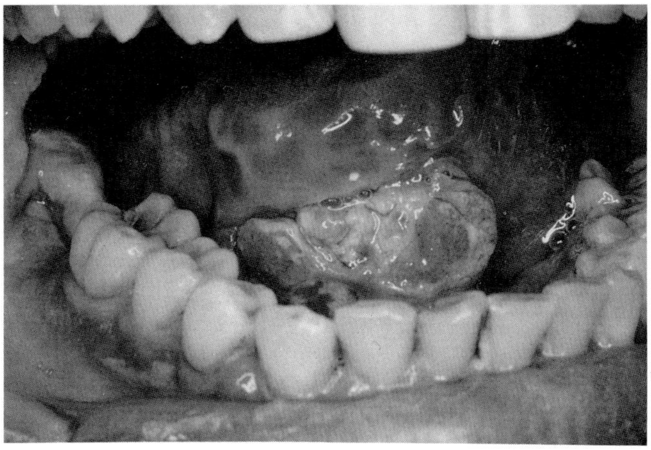

A

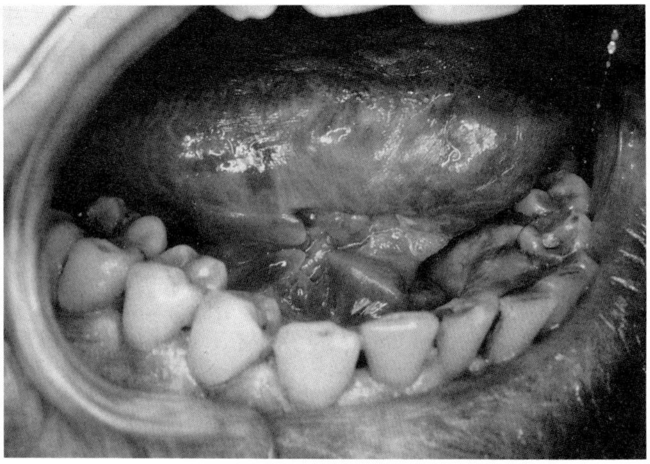

B

Fig. 5-7. Advanced (stage 3) squamous carcinoma of the tongue controlled by external radiation followed by an implant boost for a total of 7500 cGy. (**A,** before, and **B,** is after.)

Because of the wide number of variables indicated in the selection of treatment, it is necessary that a team approach be used in the management of oral lesions. The dentist, surgeon, radiation oncologist, and in some cases the medical oncologist should see and evaluate the patient jointly.

The decision on treatment will depend on all of the factors outlined above and will often be individualized for the exact histologic nature, extent, and depth of invasion of the lesion and the condition of the patient.

RADIATION TECHNIQUES

Radiation therapy for oral cancer is administered either by external beam or by interstitial sources. The low-energy external beam sources are referred to as orthovoltage (100 to 300 kilovolt [peak] (KVP) x-rays). These superficial x-rays are used for lip lesions or small to medium tumors in the oral cavity treated by means of an intraoral cone. Megavoltage

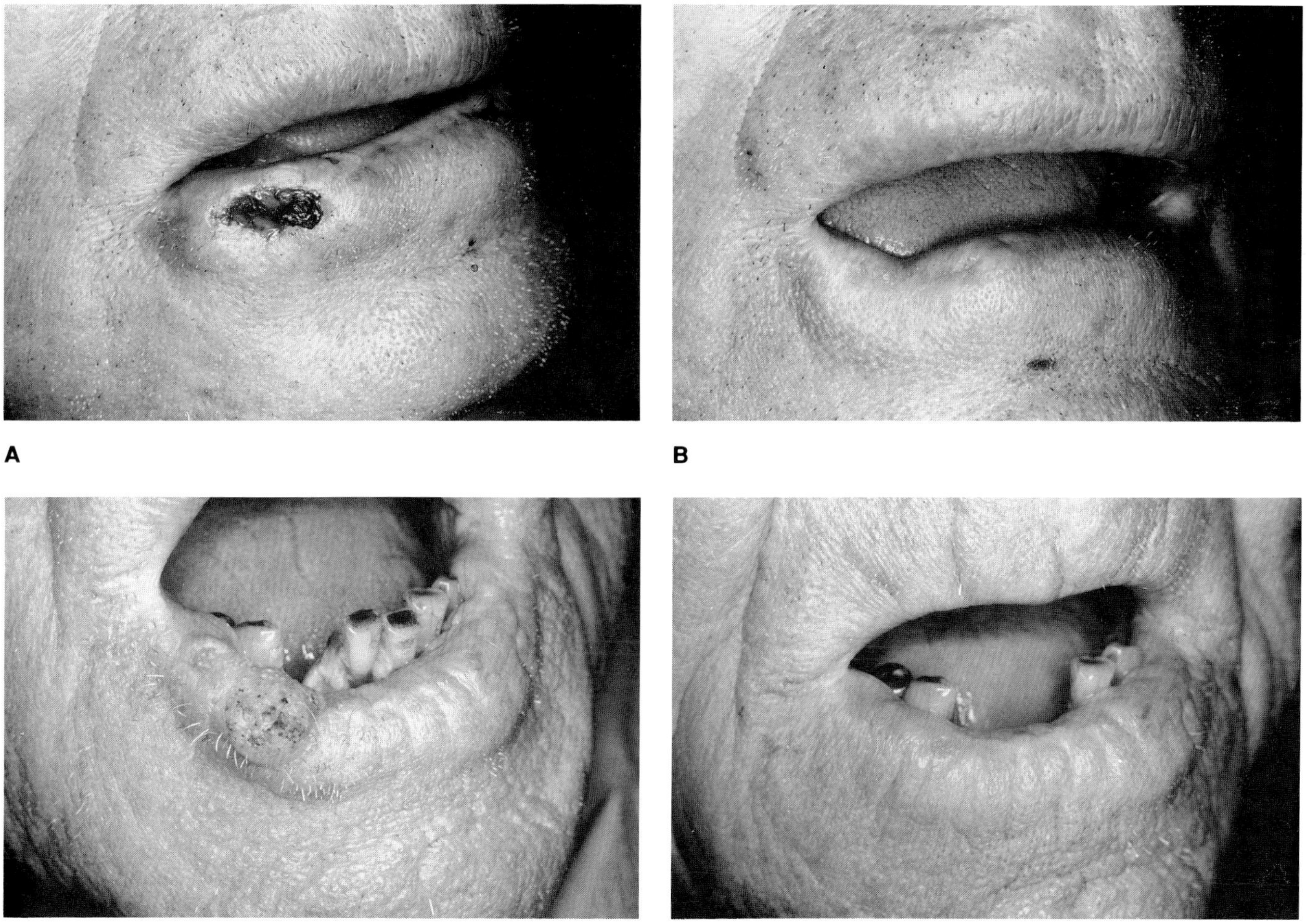

Fig. 5-8. Moderately large squamous carcinoma of lower lip, treated by irradiation. **A,** Tumor before treatment. Induration extended over 3 cm and appeared to infiltrate underlying muscle. **B,** Three months after irradiation, patient was asymptomatic, suffered no loss of function, and was not bothered by mild alteration in appearance. **C,** Superficial exophytic squamous carcinoma of the lower lip. **D,** The tumor disappeared after 6000 cGy without any cosmetic defect.

beams from cobalt-60 or linear accelerators of 4 million electron volts (meV) or higher are used for external beam treatment. These high-energy photons allow multiple beam treatment, often with wedges, shaping blocks, and compensating filters to protect uninvolved tissues. Complex treatment plans with these beams often allow delivery of a higher dose to the tumor volume than to the surrounding normal tissues.

Interstitial implant treatment is used commonly for delivery of a high dose to a limited volume (Fig. 5-11). Implants deliver the radiation in the immediate vicinity of the implanted isotope and also deliver it at a relatively low-dose rate which has certain biologic advantages in sparing the normal tissue. Interstitial sources can be placed directly or, preferably, afterloaded into tubes or needles. The sources most commonly used include ^{192}Ir, ^{137}Cs, ^{125}I, and ^{198}Au.

Electron beams may be used rather than x-ray or photon beams. They have the advantage of limited penetration in tissue so that a high dose may be given to superficial lesions with only minimal irradiation of underlying tissue. These beams are usually generated by linear accelerators of 12 meV or higher. Electrons are used in perioral cone treatment and in adding additional dose to cervical lymph nodes overlying the spinal cord.

COMBINATIONS OF SURGERY AND IRRADIATION

The extreme radiosensitivity of lymphomas makes combined treatment unnecessary. However, the need for doses exceeding normal tissue tolerance in larger squamous and adenocarcinomas of the oral cavity often necessitates a combination of radiation and surgery. Surgery is able to remove

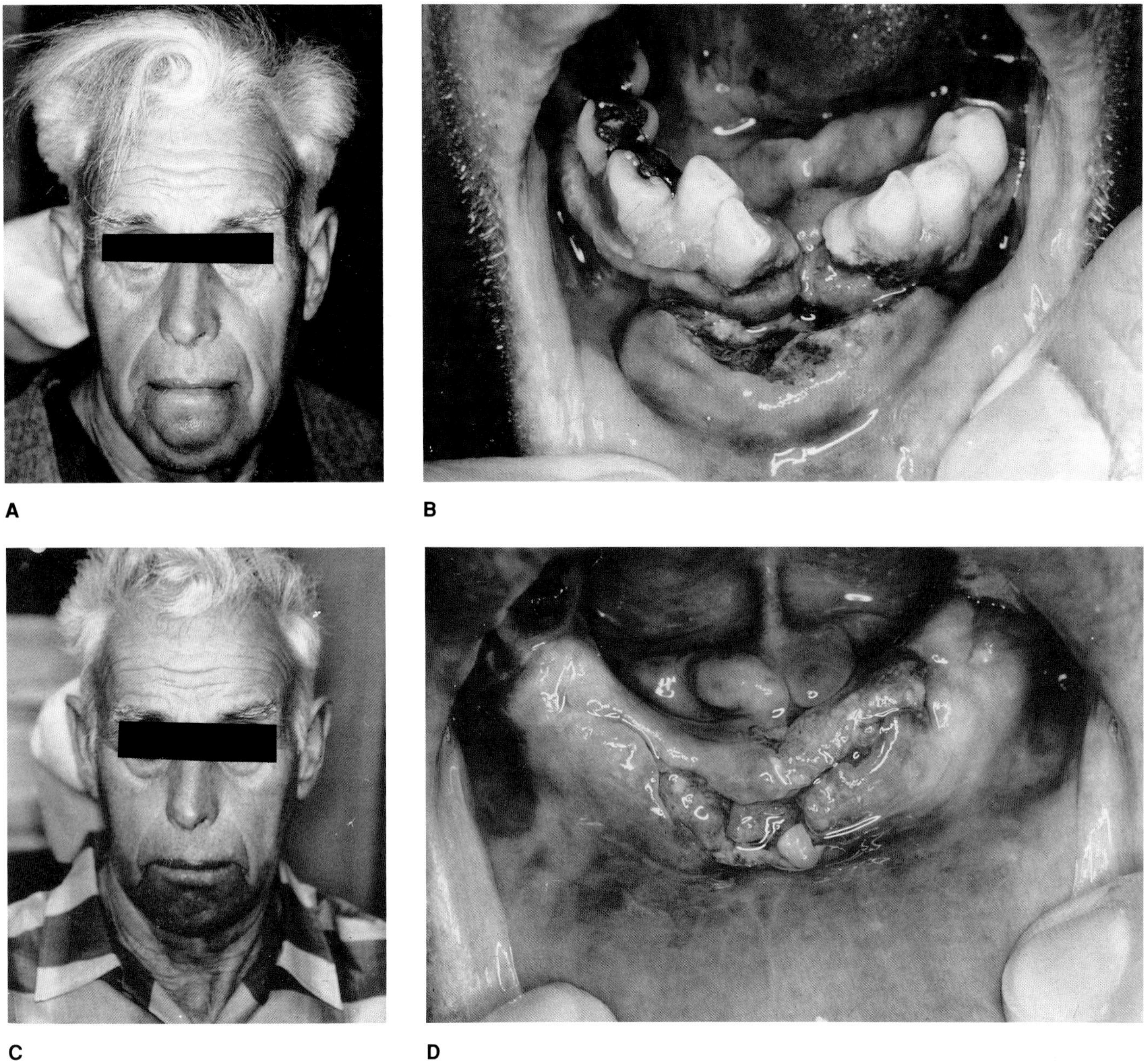

Fig. 5-9. Labiogingival carcinoma treated by preoperative irradiation and surgery. **A,** Patient before treatment. Note extraoral swelling. **B,** Intraoral view of lesion, which involves the labial mucosa, reflex, and gingiva. **C,** After radiation therapy, tumor has shrunk. Note skin pigmentation caused by radiation. **D,** Tumor shrinkage after radiation allowed better margins for later surgical resection. Teeth were extracted before irradiation.

the major bulk of the tumor and the resistant central portion. Radiation is then able to sterilize the microscopic routes of spread in the lymphatics and tissue planes not resected in the standard excisional procedures. Combinations of radiation and surgery are used in at least one third of all oral cancers.

Radiation can be administered preoperatively for squamous cell lesions to reduce the size of the tumor, sterilize the microscopic involvement of lymphatics and lymph nodes, and increase the margins of normal tissue resected. If the tissues are irradiated using proper fractionation and tissue compensation techniques, and if surgery is done by a well-trained head and neck surgeon, the rate of postoperative complications in patients undergoing preoperative irradiation is not much higher than that occurring in patients receiving surgery only.

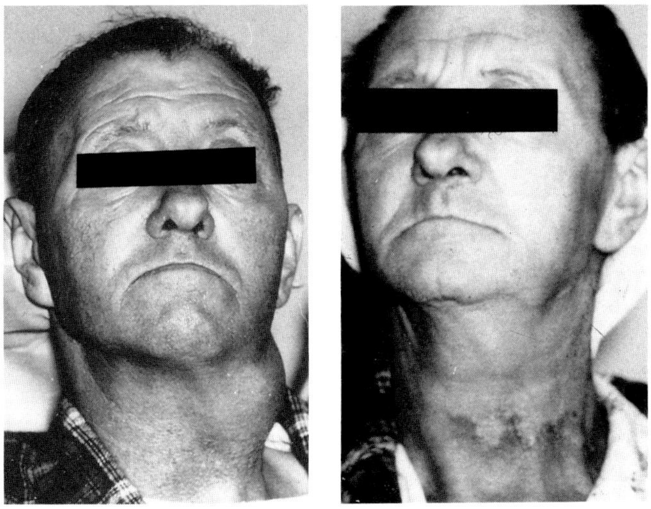

A **B**

Fig. 5-10. Radiation therapy for primary carcinoma and metastatically involved lymph nodes. **A,** Patient had primary carcinoma of left oropharynx. Lump in left neck brought him to clinician. **B,** After radiation therapy, tumor has resolved. Note skin changes (erythema and pigmentation) in irradiated field.

Postoperative irradiation is used extensively as well. Higher radiation doses can be given postoperatively and the surgeon can better judge margins. Postoperative irradiation can also sterilize the surgical field, residual disease, and those lymphatic draining regions not removed by surgery. The choice between preoperative and postoperative irradiation is complex and requires multidisciplinary coordination.

CHEMOTHERAPY

Both systemic and regional (perfusion, infusion) use of cytotoxic chemotherapeutic agents in head and neck cancer have been actively explored. Although chemotherapy by itself is not curative in head and neck cancer, it has been used for the palliation of patients with advanced or recurrent disease not amenable to surgery or radiotherapy. Chemotherapy has also been used as an adjuvant to surgery and radiotherapy in attempts to improve the local-regional control rate and survival. However, results of the majority of controlled clinical trials of combined modality treatment in head and neck cancer, thus far, have been negative.

Chemotherapeutic agents act by interfering with cell metabolism or replication. Toxicity is a prime problem, especially in tissue such as oral and gastrointestinal mucosa and bone marrow that grows rapidly. There may be severe toxic reactions—nausea, vomiting, oral and gastrointestinal ulcerations, bone marrow suppression, infections, bleeding, and even death. The generally debilitated state of head and neck cancer patients contributes substantially to the toxicity of chemotherapy, just as it contributes to problems with other therapeutic modalities.[7] These patients often have poor nutritional status because of swallowing defects caused by persistent local tumor, radiation-induced fibrosis, surgical defects, or orocutaneous fistulas. In addition, factors such as the high incidence of alcoholism in this patient population, the occurrence of distant metastases, and the general catabolic effects of a malignancy add to the debility. If at all possible, before chemotherapy is initiated nutritional status should be improved to lessen potential toxic reactions such as stomatitis. (A more detailed discussion of dental procedures and chemotherapy will be found in Chapter 8.)

CHEMOTHERAPEUTIC DRUGS

Four drugs dominate the literature on chemotherapeutic treatment of head and neck cancer: methotrexate, bleomycin, *cis*-platinum, and 5-fluorouracil. All four have been studied extensively as single agents or in combination with other drugs, and they have been given before or after radiotherapy, during radiotherapy, or following other treatment.

Methotrexate

Methotrexate, a folic acid antagonist or antimetabolite, is the most extensively studied drug in head and neck cancer (Figs. 5-12 and 5-13).[8,9] Although the data are extensive, there is controversy about how best to give this drug. Unresolved variables include the route of administration, the schedule of administration, the dosage, and the use of "rescue" with calcium leucovorin.

Methotrexate has been given extensively by intra-arterial (IA) and peroral (PO) routes. The rationale for intra-arterial infusion is that prolonged contact of the tumor cell population with the antimetabolite will result in sequential death of cells as the cells enter the vulnerable metabolic phase of cellular division. The arterial route can also be used to deliver a high concentration of drug to the tumor site.

This form of treatment has engendered much controversy. Data are difficult to compare because methods or techniques of treatment are not uniform, drug and dose schedules differ, and treatment durations vary. The IA route requires careful patient selection, expertise, and close follow-up. The cumulative response rate of about 50% is not markedly different from the cumulative response rates achieved with systemic methotrexate. It is not considered standard therapy.

Systemic methotrexate has been mainly given either in intermittent weekly or semiweekly IV injections of 40 to 60 mg/m^2 of body surface area, or in monthly courses. The data for the weekly or biweekly approach show that 50% of the patients achieve a greater than 50% reduction in tumor size, whereas 29% of those on a monthly course do so. This seems to indicate that weekly or semiweekly administration of methotrexate is superior.[10]

One approach that has been developed to increase the therapeutic index of methotrexate is "rescue" with leucovorin after administration of high doses of the drug.[11] The mechanism of action of methotrexate is the result of its tight binding to dihydrofolate reductase. This enzyme converts the biologically inactive dihydrofolate to tetrahydrofolate, the folate form needed to support nucleic acid synthesis. Without sufficient levels of intracellular tetrahydrofolate, cells are unable to synthesize DNA. Leucovorin (N^5N^{10}

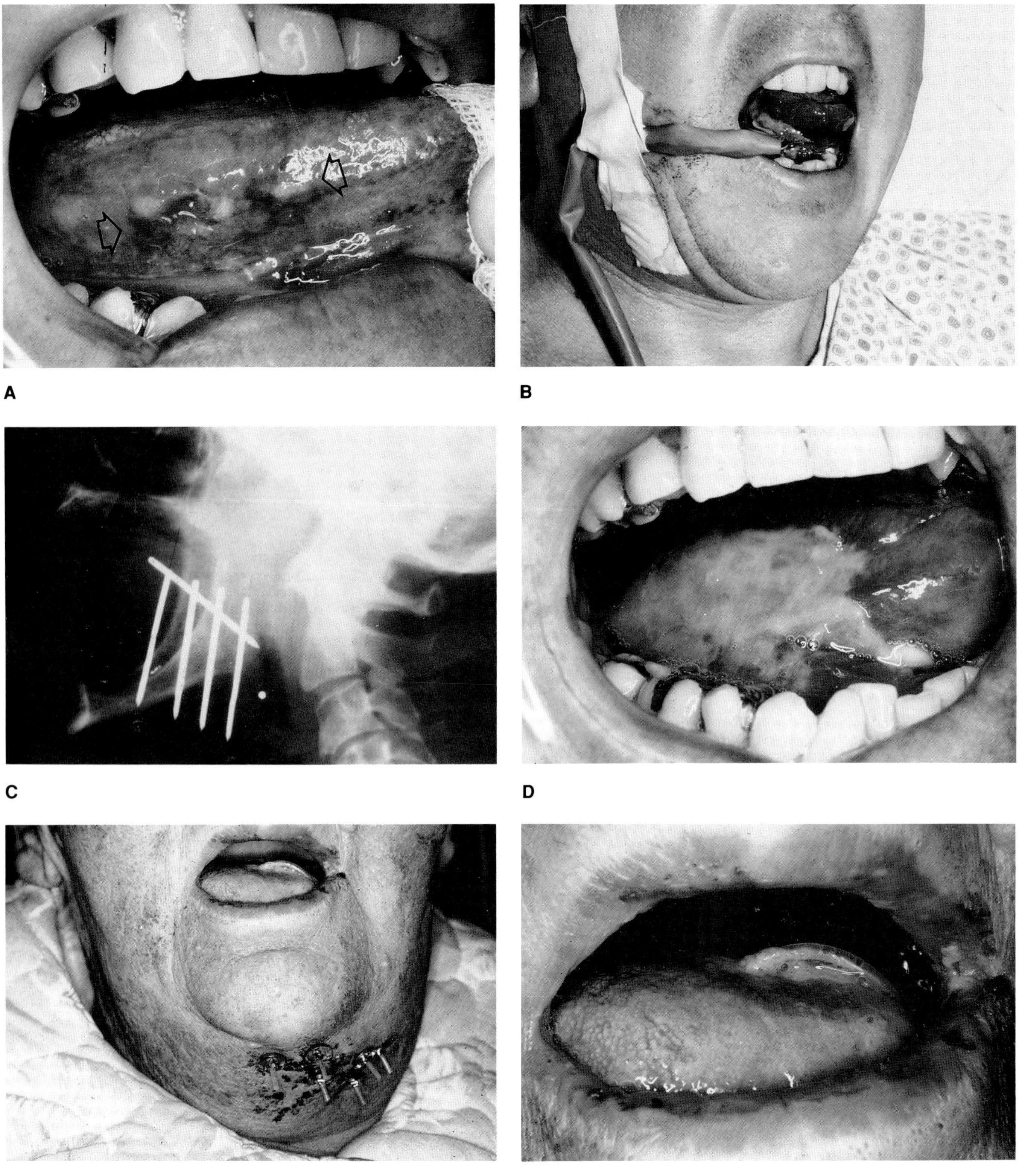

Fig. 5-11. Radiation therapy using interstitial implants. **A,** Superficial squamous cell carcinoma of the right tongue (arrows). **B,** Radium needles were implanted while patient was under general anesthesia. **C,** Radiograph showing needles in place (left in 6 days). **D,** Tongue 24 hours after needles were removed. Note mucositis caused by irradiation. Tumor has been completely controlled for 4 years. **E,** Patient with floor-of-mouth carcinoma had initial extraoral irradiation followed by iridium implant. Note polyvinyl tubes in place, seeded with radioactive seeds. **F,** Close-up view of plastic tube entering and leaving tongue.

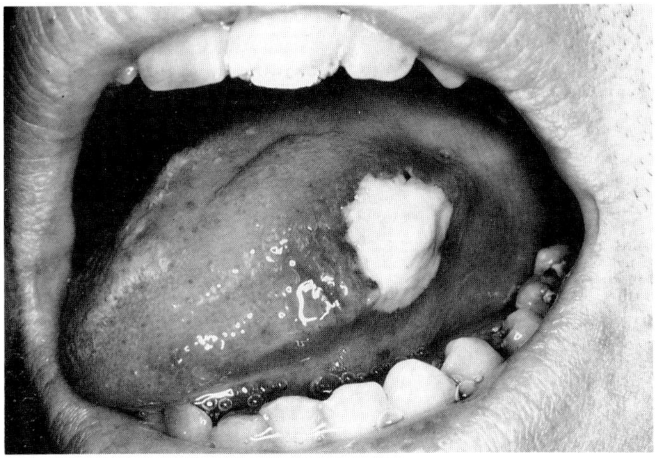

Fig. 5-12. Painful tongue ulcer after high-dose methotrexate therapy. Ulcers appeared during periods of transient neutropenia and disappeared after chemotherapeutic drugs were withdrawn.

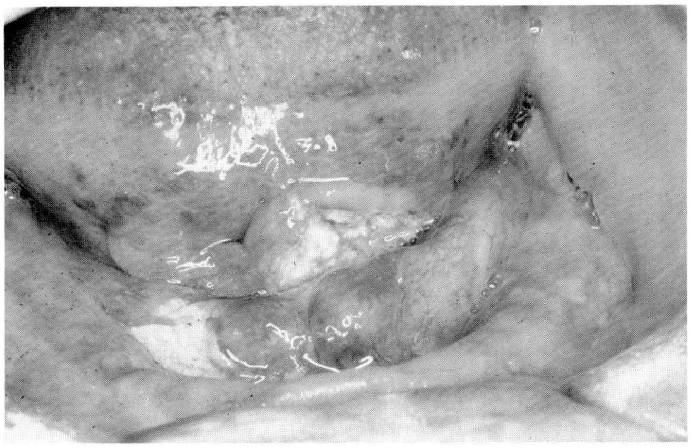

A

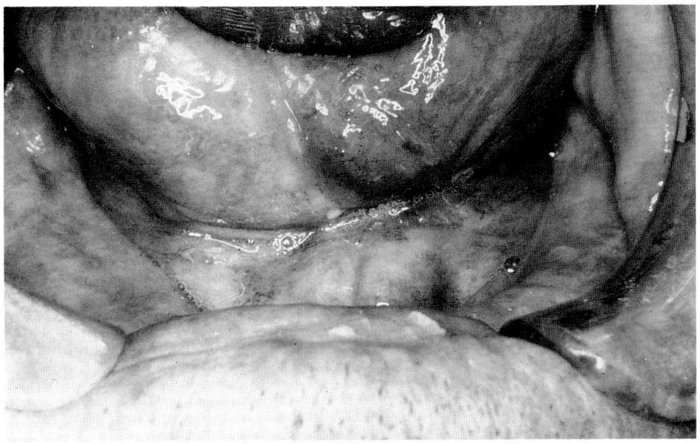

B

Fig. 5-13. Methotrexate therapy for tumor recurring after irradiation. Patient refused surgery. **A,** Indurated and ulcerated lesion on floor of mouth and ventral tongue. **B,** One month after weekly IV injections of 25 mg methotrexate, patient is asymptomatic and ulcer has healed. Patient continued on this regimen for 8 months without evidence of active tumor. After this period, tumor regrowth appeared and the patient subsequently died.

formyltetrahydrofolate) supplies the product of the reaction inhibited by methotrexate and thereby overcomes its major effects.

Normal cells possess a common carrier-mediated transport mechanism for folates and methotrexate, but some tumor cells may lack or have a less efficient transport mechanism. When the concentration of methotrexate exceeds 10^{-3} to 10^{-4} moles/liter, the drug will enter the tumor cells by diffusion. Leucovorin, however, can readily enter normal host cells since they contain the carrier transport mechanism, but it will not enter and "rescue" cancer cells because of the lack of transport sites.

Methotrexate combined with leucovorin has not produced reductions in tumor size that differ greatly from results of systemic methotrexate alone. However, toxicity may be less in patients given leucovorin in addition to methotrexate, thus making this treatment safer.

Studies[12–14] of the effect of high-dose methotrexate given with leucovorin rescue have yielded conflicting results with regard to response rate, but improved survival has not been demonstrated. One study using a dosage of 5000 mg/m^2 showed a significant drug-related death rate.[7] Thus, this form of treatment has not been shown to be superior to low-dose methotrexate and should not be considered standard therapy.

The site of tumor as a prognostic variable has been relatively neglected. When responses to methotrexate were examined as a function of tumor site, they were found to occur with highest frequency in lesions of the oral cavity and oropharynx, with intermediate frequency lesions of the larynx, and with lowest frequency in lesions of the nasopharynx and hypopharynx.[15] Response was of longest duration in alveolar ridge, posterior tongue, and laryngeal lesions, and of shortest duration in palatal, oropharyngeal, floor of mouth, and hypopharyngeal lesions.

Bleomycin

Bleomycin is the generic name for a group of antibiotics that was isolated in Japan from *Streptomyces verticillis*. This drug disrupts the cell by interfering with DNA function. In U.S. studies on file with the Bristol Pharmaceutical Company, 112 (38%) of 298 evaluable patients with squamous cell cancers of the head and neck region responded. Forty-eight showed tumor regression of 25% or more, 54 showed regression of 50% or more, and 10 had virtually complete regression.

The optimum dosage in the compiled data was 0.25 to 0.50 unit/kg, administered twice weekly or weekly. Responses were evenly divided between the IV and IM routes of administration. Total cumulative doses of bleomycin averaged 323 units for the 112 responders (range 105 to 845 units) and less for those patients who failed to respond. Pulmonary toxicity limited the total dose. Average response duration was 3.0 months; the longest lasted 11 months.

Presumably, the responding patients received an average total dose higher than that of the failures since their response encouraged continued therapy with bleomycin. Because of the risk of pulmonary toxicity, total doses exceeding 400 units are not recommended. If higher total doses are given, there is an increasing dose-related risk of pulmonary fibrosis and death.

Cis-platinum

Cis-platinum is the newest agent which has demonstrated activity in head and neck cancer. Structurally, it is an inorganic complex consisting of a central atom of platinum surrounded by chlorine and ammonia ions in the *cis* position in the horizontal plane. Although the mechanism of its antitumor action has not been fully elucidated, *cis*-platinum seems to act by altering DNA structure.

In early studies in which the drug was given by IV injections, toxicities included dose-related renal damage, myelosuppression, nausea and vomiting, and hearing loss. Although activity was observed in a range of solid tumors, renal toxicity, in particular, appeared to limit the drug's usefulness. However, it was later shown that in most patients, even high doses of *cis*-platinum are tolerated without significant renal impairment if care is taken to maintain adequate hydration before the drug is administered and if a vigorous osmotic diuresis with mannitol and half-normal saline is maintained during and after platinum administration.

An early review[16] found that the cumulative response rate for *cis*-platinum as a single agent was 28% in 83 cases. Since then, the therapeutic potential of this drug has been confirmed in several studies. A meeting abstract[17] reported a comparison of *cis*-platinum, given at 50 mg/m^2 on days 1 and 8 of every month, versus methotrexate, given at the conventional dosage of 40 to 60 mg/m^2/week. The response rates (28% versus 24%), duration of remission, and survival times were equivalent, but methotrexate was better tolerated. Other reports have shown *cis*-platinum to be slightly more active than methotrexate using different dose scheduling, but also still more toxic.[18] Very high doses of *cis*-platinum have not increased the number of responses.[19]

5-Fluorouracil

The anticancer drug 5-fluorouracil (5-FU) is specifically synthesized to interfere with cellular metabolism. Chemically, it is a thymine in which the 5-methyl group has been synthetically replaced by a fluoride atom. Biologically, it may work in two ways: either by being incorporated into RNA and interfering with its function, or by inhibiting synthesis of DNA.

Toxicity from 5-FU seems to be a function of how it is given. The main side effect of daily or weekly bolus injection is bone marrow suppression. Gastrointestinal tract symptoms, primarily stomatitis, are more often seen when the doses are increased. With continuous IV infusion, the degree of myelosuppression is much less than with a bolus injection of the same total dose of 5-FU. However, the gastrointestinal toxicity is greater with infusion therapy.

Given by conventional bolus injection in the past, 5-FU has been considered only minimally active in squamous cell head and neck cancers. Several studies have shown response rates of 10% and 20% with only a few months' duration of responses and no real impact on survival. It does have more utility in the much less common adenocarcinomatous lesions in the head and neck area such as salivary gland tumors.

Because of these unimpressive results, 5-FU is rarely used as a single agent. However, its effectiveness is dramatically increased when it is infused over several days, usually in combination with other drugs, especially *cis*-platinum. Toxicity in such combinations, even with very large doses of 5-FU (1000 mg/m^2/day), is in general quite manageable. With the combination of 5-FU infusion and *cis*-platinum, complete response rates of 30% to 50% in head and neck cancer have been reported.

MULTIDRUG COMBINATION THERAPY

Most of the possible two-, three-, and four-drug combinations of *cis*-platinum, methotrexate, bleomycin, and 5-FU have been or are now being studied. Much attention has been paid to the possibility that giving methotrexate one hour before 5-FU may augment the response. New biochemical studies, however, indicate that 24 hours would be an optimal interval between the administration of methotrexate and the subsequent administration of 5-FU.[20]

A bewildering collection of multidrug programs exists, involving the four most studied agents as well as less often used drugs. Each has certain advantages and disadvantages. A representative sampling appears in Table 5-1.[21–30] Many of these represent research still in progress. It is not yet clear how the response rates will translate into improved survival. At present, if response alone is considered, *cis*-platinum followed by a 5-day infusion of 5-FU seems to represent the best program, at least in terms of complete and overall response rates. This program has substantial toxicity, and because it requires hospitalization it is quite costly. The use of infusion pumps has allowed the administration of 5-FU in selected patients in an outpatient setting, reducing cost and morbidity.

ADJUNCTIVE CHEMOTHERAPY

Efforts have been made to use chemotherapy to potentiate the effects of radiation by treating patients with drugs during radiation therapy. The rationale for this is that chemotherapy may (1) control already disseminated tumor cells, (2) potentiate the killing effect of ionizing radiation, and (3) be more effective against the remaining tumor cell growth fraction once radiation has reduced tumor bulk.[31]

Various drugs and combinations of drugs have been given concurrently with radiation. Radiation given with concurrent *cis*-platinum as a single agent has been used with no clear impact on either response or survival.[32,33] Nonrandomized *cis*-platinum-based drug combinations together with radiotherapy have produced similar results.[34,35] Bleomycin at 5^U per week with concurrent full-course irradiation has produced a significant relapse-free survival, but as yet the data has not shown increased survival.[36] One study with close follow-up of patients has indicated that chemotherapy in some patients may obviate the need for surgery after irradiation.[37] That approach is being tested in a randomized trial by the Veterans' Administration Hospital cooperative group.[38] Response to chemotherapy has been shown to be predictive of subsequent responses to irradiation.[39]

Induction chemotherapy, the use of cytotoxic drugs as initial therapy prior to surgery or irradiation, is also receiving attention. The presumed advantages are that (1) drug deliv-

Table 5-1. RESPONSE RATES REPORTED IN MULTI-DRUG STUDIES IN HEAD AND NECK CANCER PATIENTS

Cis- Platinol	5-Fu	Methotrexate	Bleomycin	Velban	Vincristine	No. Treated	Complete Response (CR)	Partial Response (PR)	CR + PR	Investigators
	X	X				30	1 (3%)	4 (13%)	16%	Jacobs[21]
	X	X				35	4 (11%)	21 (60%)	71%	Pitman et al.[22]
	X	X				35	5 (14%)	20 (57%)	71%	Pitman et al.[23]
X	X					30	8 (27%)	13 (43%)	70%	Kish et al.[24]
X		X	X			86	14 (17%)	27 (32%)	49%	Vogl et al.[25]
X			X	X		191			24%	Williams et al.[26]
X			X		X	27			41%	Drelichman et al.[27]
		X	X		X	24	3 (12%)	5 (21%)	33%	Garusi et al.[28]
X		X	X		X	90	15 (16%)	30 (34%)	50%	Clavel et al.[29]
X	X	X	X			41	8 (20%)	13 (32%)	52%	Lester et al.[30]

ery to tumors whose vascularity is still intact will be improved, (2) patients whose general condition and nutritional status have not been weakened will be better able to tolerate intensive chemotherapy, (3) definitive local treatment will be more effective after cytoreduction of the primary tumor and nodal metastases, and (4) subclinical metastases will be eradicated.[31]

Methotrexate, *cis*-platinum, 5-FU, and bleomycin have been used, singly or in combination, for induction chemotherapy. The observed response rates are superior to rates in patients treated only by surgery and/or radiation, but randomized studies thus far have not shown a survival advantage for patients so treated.[31] Varying combinations of methotrexate, bleomycin, platinol, vincristine, and 5-FU are included here.[40–42] Three courses of infusion of *cis*-platinum followed by a five-day infusion of 5-FU, administered before definitive surgery and/or irradiation in 85 patients, gave 54% complete responses and 39% partial responses, for an overall response rate of 93%. An extension of this work with 164 patients showed that achieving a complete response with chemotherapy before definitive treatment resulted in a median survival of 24 months or more as compared with 13.5 months for partial responses. Long-term survival benefits from this program are not clear.

CANCER IMMUNOTHERAPY

Although immunologic intervention in cancer was conceived of nearly a century ago, it has only been scientifically evaluated during the past 20 years. While the immune system undoubtedly plays an important role in the development of cancer and its spread, the interrelationships are poorly understood. It is clear that the risk of developing cancer is much greater in immunosuppressed or immunodeficient individuals. For example, there is an increased evidence of oral malignancies in HIV-infected patients.

Cancer immunotherapy, in the broad sense, refers to attempts to control or prevent a cancerous process by stimulating the immune system. Either specific or nonspecific immunotherapy can be conferred by immunization which is either active (vaccine) or passive (immune serum and cells or their products), or by the use of general stimulants of the immune system such as interferon, BCG (Calmette-Guerin bacillus), or levamisole.

None of these modalities, whether experimental or clinical, has been effective to date in preventing or altering the course of head and neck cancer. Immunotherapy certainly is not standard clinical treatment at this time.

Summary

With all of the new drugs and delivery programs, there are certain points to observe. Subtle and poorly understood interactions may greatly change response rates for roughly similar drug combinations. Most chemotherapy programs assign patients according to stages but treat all advanced stages identically even though response rates vary as a function of the primary site. The site of recurrence or metastases will also influence outcome. In addition, prior treatment, which can influence outcome, often prevents adequate comparison of results. Lastly, response rates may reflect the experience of a patchwork of institutions whose patients may vary enormously in such characteristics as general medical health, exposure to alcohol, and compliance to follow-up.

In spite of these limitations, the general trend of results following the newer combined modality therapy in head and neck cancer has been increased response rates, more complete remissions, and longer disease-free survivals. As we learn more about the mechanism of drug action and the interaction of drugs with each other and with radiation therapy, clinical studies will be designed that should continue to improve the therapy for patients with these diseases.

REFERENCES

1. Strong MS, Vaughn CW, Healy GB et al: Transoral management of localized carcinoma of the oral cavity using the CO_2 laser. *Larygoscope* 89:897, 1979.
2. Rodenburg JLN, Panders AK, Vermey A et al: Treatment of superficial lesions of the oral mucosa with the carbon dioxide laser: A report of 58 cases, with 5 years follow-up. *J Exp Clin Cancer Res* 3:283, 1983.
3. Frame JW: Removal of oral soft-tissue pathology with the CO_2 laser. *J Oral Maxillofac Surg* 43:850, 1985.
4. Guerry TL, Silverman S, Dedo HH: Carbon dioxide laser resection of superficial oral carcinoma: Indications, technique, and results. *Ann Otol Rhinol Laryngol* 95:547, 1986.

5. Chu FWK, Silverman S, Dedo HH: CO_2 laser treatment of oral leukoplakia. *Laryngoscope* 98:125, 1988.
6. Davidson TM, Haghighi P, Astarita R et al: Microscopically oriented histologic surgery for head and neck mucosal cancer. *Cancer* 60:1856, 1987.
7. Amer MH, Al-Sarraf M, Vaitkevicius VK: Factors that affect response to chemotherapy and survival of patients with advanced head and neck cancer. *Cancer* 43:2202, 1979.
8. Goldsmith MA, Carter SK: The integration of chemotherapy into a combined modality approach to cancer therapy. V. Squamous cell cancer of the head and neck. *Cancer Treat Rev* 2:137, 1975.
9. Bleyer WA: The clinical pharmacology of methotrexate. New applications of an old drug. *Cancer* 41:36, 1978.
10. Carter SK: The chemotherapy of head and neck cancer. *Semin Oncol* 4:413, 1977.
11. Ambinder EP, Perloff M, Ohnuma T et al: High dose methotrexate followed by citrovorum factor reversal in patients with advanced cancer. *Cancer* 43:1177, 1979.
12. Woods RL, Fox RM, Tattersall MN: Methotrexate treatment of advanced head and neck cancers: A dose-response evaluation. *Cancer Treat Rep* 65 (Suppl 1):155, 1981.
13. Woods RL, Fox RM, Tattersall MH: Methotrexate treatment of squamous-cell head and neck cancers: Dose-response evaluation. *Br Med J* 282:600, 1981.
14. Kirkwood JM, Canellos GP, Ervin TJ et al: Increased therapeutic index using moderate dose methotrexate and leucovorin twice weekly vs. weekly high dose methotrexate-leucovorin in patients with advanced squamous carcinoma of the head and neck: A safe new effective regimen. *Cancer* 47:2414, 1981.
15. Bertino JR, Boston B, Capizzi RL: The role of chemotherapy in the management of cancer of the head and neck: A review. *Cancer* 36:752, 1975.
16. Prestayko AW, D'Aoust JC, Issell BF et al: Cisplatin (cisdiamminedichloroplatinum II). *Cancer Treat Rev* 6:17, 1979.
17. Hong WK, Schaefer S, Issell B et al: A prospective randomized trial of methotrexate versus cisplatin in the treatment of recurrent squamous cell carcinomas of the head and neck (Meeting abstract). *Proc Am Soc Clin Oncol* 1:202, 1982.
18. Campbell JB, Dorman EB, McCormick M et al: A randomized phase III trial of cisplatinum, methotrexate, cisplatinum + methotrexate and cisplatinum + 5-fluorouracil in end-stage head and neck cancer. *Acta Otolaryngol* (Stockholm) 103:519, 1987.
19. Veronesi A, Zagonal V, Tirelli U et al: High-dose versus low-dose cisplatin in advanced head and neck squamous carcinoma: a randomized study. *J Clin Oncol* 3:1105, 1985.
20. Browman GP, Archiblad SD, Young JE et al: Prospective randomized trial of one-hour sequential vs. simultaneous methotrexate plus 5-fluorouracil in advanced and recurrent squamous cell head and neck cancer. *J Clin Oncol* 1:787, 1983.
21. Jacobs C: Use of methotrexate and 5-FU for recurrent head and neck cancer. *Cancer Treat Rep* 66:1925, 1982.
22. Pitman SW, Kowal CD, Bertino JR: Methotrexate and 5-fluorouracil in sequence in squamous head and neck cancer. *Semin Oncol* 10:15, 1983.
23. Pitman S, Fischer D, Kowal C et al: Sequential methotrexate-5 fluorouracil (M-F) in squamous head and neck cancer: Prolonged survival in patients with recurrent disease (Meeting abstract). *Proc Am Soc Clin Oncol* 2:166, 1983.
24. Kish JA, Weaver A, Jacobs J et al: Cisplatin and 5-fluorouracil infusion in patients with recurrent and disseminated epidermoid cancer of the head and neck. *Cancer* 53:1819, 1984.
25. Vogl SE, Schoenfeld DA, Kaplan BH et al: A randomized prospective comparison of methotrexate with a combination of methotrexate, bleomycin, and cisplatin in head and neck cancer. *Cancer* 56:432, 1985.
26. Williams SD, Velez-Garcia E, Essessee I: Chemotherapy for head and neck cancer. Comparison of cisplatin + vinblasstine + bleomycin versus methotrexate. *Cancer* 57:18, 1986.
27. Drelichman A, Cummings G, Al-Sarraf M: A randomized trial of the combination of cis-platinum, oncovin and bleomycin (COB) versus methotrexate in patients with advanced squamous cell carcinoma of head and neck. *Cancer* 52:399, 1983.
28. Garusi GF, Jirillo A, Demicheli R et al: Combination chemotherapy (CT) with vincristine, bleomycin and methotrexate (VBM) in advanced squamous cell carcinoma of the head and neck (H and N) (Meeting abstract). UICC Conference on Clinical Oncology, Oct. 28–31, 1981. Lausanne, Switzerland: International Union Against Cancer, 1981.
29. Clavel M, Cognetti F, Dodion P et al: Combination chemotherapy with methotrexate, bleomycin, and vincristine with or without cisplatin in advanced squamous cell carcinoma of the head and neck. *Cancer* 60:1173, 1987.
30. Lester EP, Johnson CM, Lester JD et al: Head and neck advanced squamous carcinoma: Treatment with cis-platinum, bleomycin and sequential methotrexate/5-fluorouracil. *Proc Am Soc Clin Oncol* 3:182, 1984.
31. Hong WK, Bromer R: Chemotherapy in head and neck cancer. *N Engl J Med* 308:75, 1983.
32. Tobias JS, Smith BJ, Blackman G et al: Concurrent daily cisplatin and radiotherapy in locally advanced squamous carcinoma of the head-and-neck bronchus. *Radiother Oncol* 9:263, 1987.
33. McDonald S, Mills EE, Van der Merwe AM et al: Simultaneous radiation therapy and cisplatin chemotherapy in advanced cancer of the head and neck. A pilot study at Tygerberg Hospital, Parowvallei, South Africa. *Am J Clin Oncol* 10:410, 1987.
34. Shankar Giri PG, Taylor SA: Concurrent chemotherapy and radiation therapy in advanced head and neck cancer. *Am J Clin Oncol* 10:417, 1987.
35. Murthy AK, Taylor SG IV, Showel J et al: Treatment of advanced head and neck cancer with concomitant radiation and chemotherapy. *Int J Radiat Oncol Biol Phys* 13:1807, 1987.
36. Fu KK, Phillips TL, Silverberg IJ et al: Combined radiotherapy and chemotherapy with bleomycin and methotrexate for advanced inoperable head and neck cancer: Update of a Northern California Oncology Group randomized trial. *J Clin Oncol* 5:1410, 1987.
37. Jacobs C, Goffinet DR, Goffinet L et al: Chemotherapy as a substitute for surgery in the treatment of advanced resectable head and neck cancer. A report from the Northern California Oncology Group. *Cancer* 60:1178, 1987.
38. Hong WK, Wolf GT, Fischer S et al: A new strategy to preserve the larynx in the treatment of advanced laryngeal cancer: Preliminary report (Abstract). *Proc Am Soc Clin Oncol* 6:130, 1987.
39. Ensley JF, Jacobs JR, Weaver A et al: Correlation between response to cisplatin-combination chemotherapy and subsequent radiotherapy in previously untreated patients with advanced squamous cell cancers of the head and neck. *Cancer* 54:811, 1984.
40. Cognetti F, Pinnaro P, Carlini P et al: Neoadjuvant chemotherapy in previously untreated patients with advanced head and neck squamous cell cancer. *Cancer* 62:251, 1988.
41. Villar A, Pera J, Arellano A et al: Induction chemotherapy with cisplatin, bleomycin and methotrexate in advanced head and neck cancer—lack of therapeutic gain. *Radiother Oncol* 10:175, 1987.
42. Hansen HS, Rygaard J, Andersen AP et al: Bleomycin, methotrexate and vincristine before irradiation of stage III and IV laryngeal and pharyngeal squamous cell carcinoma. A study initiated by the Danish Society of Head and Neck Cancer. *Acta Oncol* 26:13, 1987.

6

Radiation Effects

SOL SILVERMAN, JR.

Ionizing radiation delivered in doses that will kill cancer cells induces unavoidable changes in the surrounding normal tissues, causing compromises in function and host defenses and severe complications (see Chapter 5). The degree of these changes is directly proportional to the volume of tissue irradiated and the total dose given, and is inversely proportional to the number of fractions and total time in which this dose is delivered. It is also related to the radiation energy, with radiation of less than one million electron volts causing greater damage to bone. These radiation changes are the direct result of the killing of normal tissue cells as expressed at the tissue level. The radiation damage to normal cells is the limiting factor in maximal treatment of many cancers.

The radiation changes associated with treatment of the oral cavity include acute skin reactions, or radiation dermatitis, and delayed skin and subcutaneous damage, including telangiectasis, fibrosis, and edema. Intraoral changes include acute mucositis (erythema, pseudomembrane-covered ulcerations, and hyperkeratosis) and delayed soft tissue necrosis. Damage to the bone can result in osteonecrosis and sequestration or progressive osteonecrosis. Radiation changes in the salivary glands result in abnormal saliva and secondarily increased caries and other dental defects. Radiation also directly damages the taste buds in the tongue and results in transient, or sometimes permanent, loss or alteration of taste.

It has been suggested, but not demonstrated statistically, that radiation effects on chromosomes (mutagenesis) may predispose cells to subsequent malignant behavior. A mechanism that could account for this could be the loss of salivary protection against carcinogens.[1] One study indicated that low-dose radiation is more likely to induce malignant changes than high-dose radiation.[2]

MUCOCUTANEOUS CHANGES

Unless intraoral or interstitial treatment is used, most patients will develop some erythema and moderate tanning of the skin in the treatment portal (Chapter 5, Fig. 5-9). Hair follicles are quite radiosensitive, therefore if hair is in the treatment beam it will cease to grow and will fall out. This is often transient.

The acute oral mucosal reaction (mucositis) is secondary to radiation-induced mitotic death of the basal cells in the oral mucosa. Because these cells require two weeks to mature, there is a delay of about this time between the onset of radiation therapy and the appearance of mucositis. If the radiation is delivered at a rate equivalent to the ability of the oral mucosa to regenerate, then only mild mucositis will be seen. When the weekly or daily dose is increased just slightly, destruction will outpace proliferation and a rather marked mucositis will develop (Fig. 6-1). This occurs at doses of between 180 and 220 cGy (1 cGy = 1 rad) per day, five days per week. Thus, patients receiving 170 cGy per day will rarely develop mucositis, and those receiving 220 cGy per day will always develop a rather marked confluent mucositis. The reason for a higher daily dose is the possibility of a greater killing effect on cancer cells. Acute mucositis is not related to late radiation-induced atrophy and telangiectasis of the mucosa (Fig. 6-2). However, this late change often increases the risk for pain and/or necrosis.

Management may sometimes require a one-week interruption of therapy. Topical anesthetics (viscous xylocaine) may be of some value, but the pain usually requires systemic analgetic drugs. Since infections may be associated, appropriate diagnoses and antimicrobial agents must be considered.

LOSS OF TASTE

Because of the irradiation of the taste buds, patients will develop a partial (hypogeusia) or complete (ageusia) loss of taste during treatment.[3] The alterations in taste for sweet, sour, bitter, and salt are variable and are caused by damage to the cells in the taste buds and/or their innervating nerve fibers.[4] These cells will regenerate within four months after treatment in most cases, although permanent impairment may result.

Dietary consultations regarding recipes with pleasing texture and perceptible and pleasing taste are essential to improve intake of food. Failure to eat is often associated with the loss of pleasure in eating and lack of imagination in food preparation. This is further complicated when surgery, often

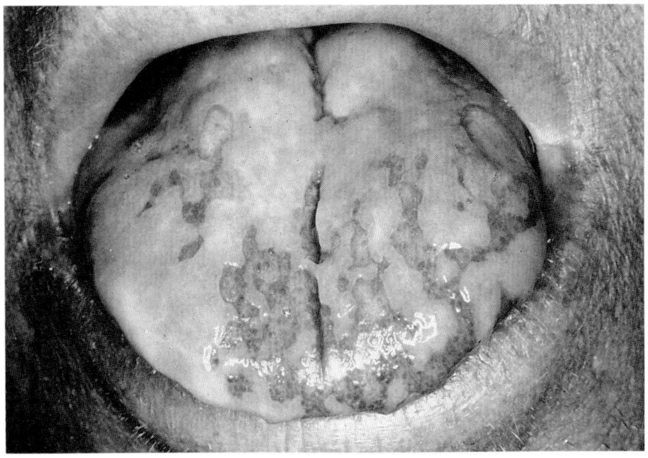

Fig. 6-1. Moderately severe mucositis 3 weeks after irradiation began. Yellowish-white pseudomembranes are covering areas of ulcerated mucosa.

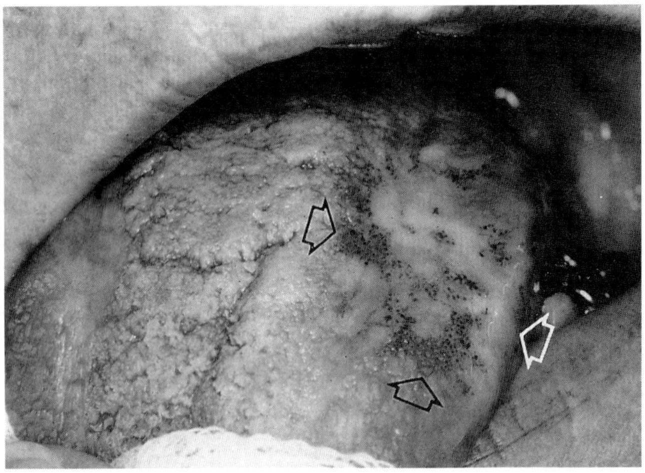

Fig. 6-2. Long-lasting radiation-induced changes in the tongue, including telangiectasia (black arrows), and fibrosis and atrophy (white arrow).

presenting problems in mastication and swallowing, has also been required as a part of treatment. Recent trials with zinc supplements far exceeding recommended daily doses appear to be promising (zinc sulfate capsules, 220 mg twice daily with meals; approximately 100 mg elemental zinc).[5,6] In addition to improving taste perception in some patients, zinc has occasionally improved saliva production.

SALIVARY FUNCTION

Exposure of the salivary glands to the field of ionizing radiation induces fibrosis, fatty degeneration, acinar atrophy, and cellular necrosis within glands. A critical dose level has not been identified.[7,8] The serous acini appear to be more sensitive than the mucinous. During irradiation, the glandular secretions are usually diminished, thick, sticky, and very bothersome to the patient. Some patients are unable to produce more than 1 ml of pooled saliva in 10 minutes. The duration of this depressed salivary function varies from patient to patient. In most patients, there is usually regeneration several months after treatment, and the undesirable signs and symptoms of xerostomia (discomfort, difficulty in speech and swallowing) are at least partially reversed. In some patients, recovery of adequate saliva for oral comfort and function may take from six to 12 months; in others the saliva remains inadequate indefinitely and is the source of major posttreatment complaints. When both of the parotid glands are exposed to the treatment beam, saliva diminution is most marked, and the prognosis for recovery is the worst.

Frequent sips of water and water rinses are essential for partial control of radiation-induced xerostomia. Sugarless chewing gum and tart candy may be helpful. In some patients, pilocarpine hydrochloride (solution or tablets) has been effective in stimulating saliva production.[9] Approximately 5 mg four times daily has been an optimal dosage for most patients. Side effects can include sweating and stomach discomfort, but this usually occurs only at higher dosages.

In a double-blind controlled study of 12 patients irradiated for head and neck cancer at the Oral Medicine Clinic, University of California, San Francisco, pilocarpine administration (15 to 30 mg daily) appeared to be beneficial.[10] All 12 patients had marked xerostomia which had failed to improve even though six months had elapsed since radiation treatment. After receiving pilocarpine, nine of 12 improved subjectively, nine of 12 had increased stimulated parotid flow rates, and six of 12 demonstrated improvement in whole saliva volume. While on placebo medication for three months, none of 12 showed objective or subjective benefit. Another salivary gland stimulant, bethanechol (Urecholine®), administered as tablets in divided doses varying from 25 to 200 mg daily, has been helpful in many xerostomic patients.

Synthetic saliva solutions and saliva substitute lubricants have been of limited help in the majority of patients with dry mouth,[11,12] although some favorable reports have been published.

NUTRITION

Because of the painful mucositis, loss of taste, and partial xerostomia, the lack of desire or frank inability to eat is a common and almost universal complaint in patients receiving external irradiation to the oral cavity. This is particularly the case when the field includes the oropharynx. These changes, in combination with difficulty in mastication and swallowing caused by the tumor and the treatment, will result in weight loss. A marked weight loss leads to weakness, inactivity, discouragement, further anorexia, and susceptibility to infection. Therefore, close attention is given to food intake and weight maintenance during treatment and follow-up. Dietary supplements, menu preparations, and encouragement to eat become important factors. Diets vary, depending upon patient attitude and effort, previous surgical intervention, saliva and taste status, food texture, and pain. There is usually very little change in the peripheral blood count before, during, or after head and neck treatment, either in response to poorer nutrition or to radiation.

DENTAL CARIES

Patients who have not shown any degree of caries activity for years may develop dental decay and varying degrees of disintegration after irradiation (Fig. 6-3). The cervical areas are most typically affected. This condition appears to be due to the lack of saliva as well as to changes in its chemical composition.[13–16] One result of radiation xerostomia is a pronounced shift toward a highly acidogenic, highly carinogenic oral microflora.[17–19] The protective influence of saliva has been demonstrated by the extensive dental destruction found in animals subjected to salivary gland ligation or removal and in patients with xerostomia caused by drugs (e.g., diuretics, antidepressants) or disease (e.g., Sjögren's syndrome).[20]

Radiation-induced dental effects depend upon salivary changes and occur when the glands are included in the field of treatment, not upon direct irradiation of the teeth themselves.[21] Whether direct irradiation of teeth alters the organic or inorganic components in some manner, making them more susceptible to decalcification, has not been shown clearly.[22,23] Remineralization of enamel by a salivary substitute has been reported.[24] There do not appear to be any clinical or histologic pulpal differences in noncarious human adult teeth, whether they have been in or out of the primary field of radiation. Studies in monkeys have also found no dental pulp damage.[25,26]

To prevent or at least minimize radiation caries, oral hygiene must be maximal, including intensive home care and frequent office visits for examination and prophylaxis.[27] Mouth rinsing is essential; hydrogen peroxide rinses (3% H_2O_2 and equal parts water) and/or antiseptic mouth rinses, if tolerated, are helpful in eliminating debris and controlling microbial flora. Daily topical fluoride applications, either as

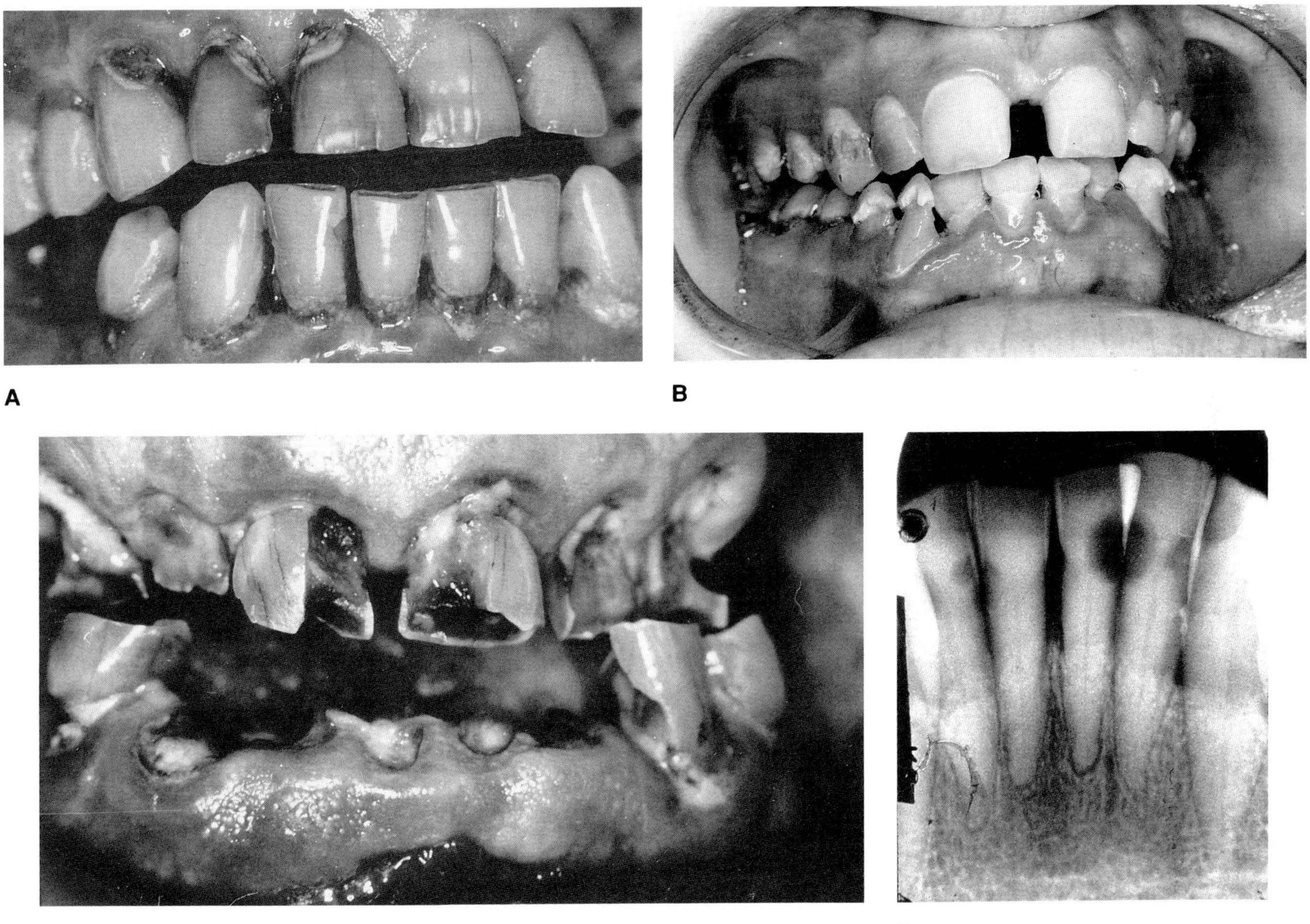

A B C D

Fig. 6-3. Rampant dental caries due to radiation-induced xerostomia. Irradiation of salivary glands eliminates protective effect of salivary lubrication and enzymes. **A,** Typical postradiation cervical caries. **B,** Flaking off of enamel (an infrequent consequence) predisposes teeth to widespread decalcification. **C,** Later stage of radiation caries when proper care is ignored. Teeth are disintegrating and fracturing off at cervical area. **D,** Characteristic radiographic appearance of radiation caries which is especially likely to attack the susceptible cervical areas.

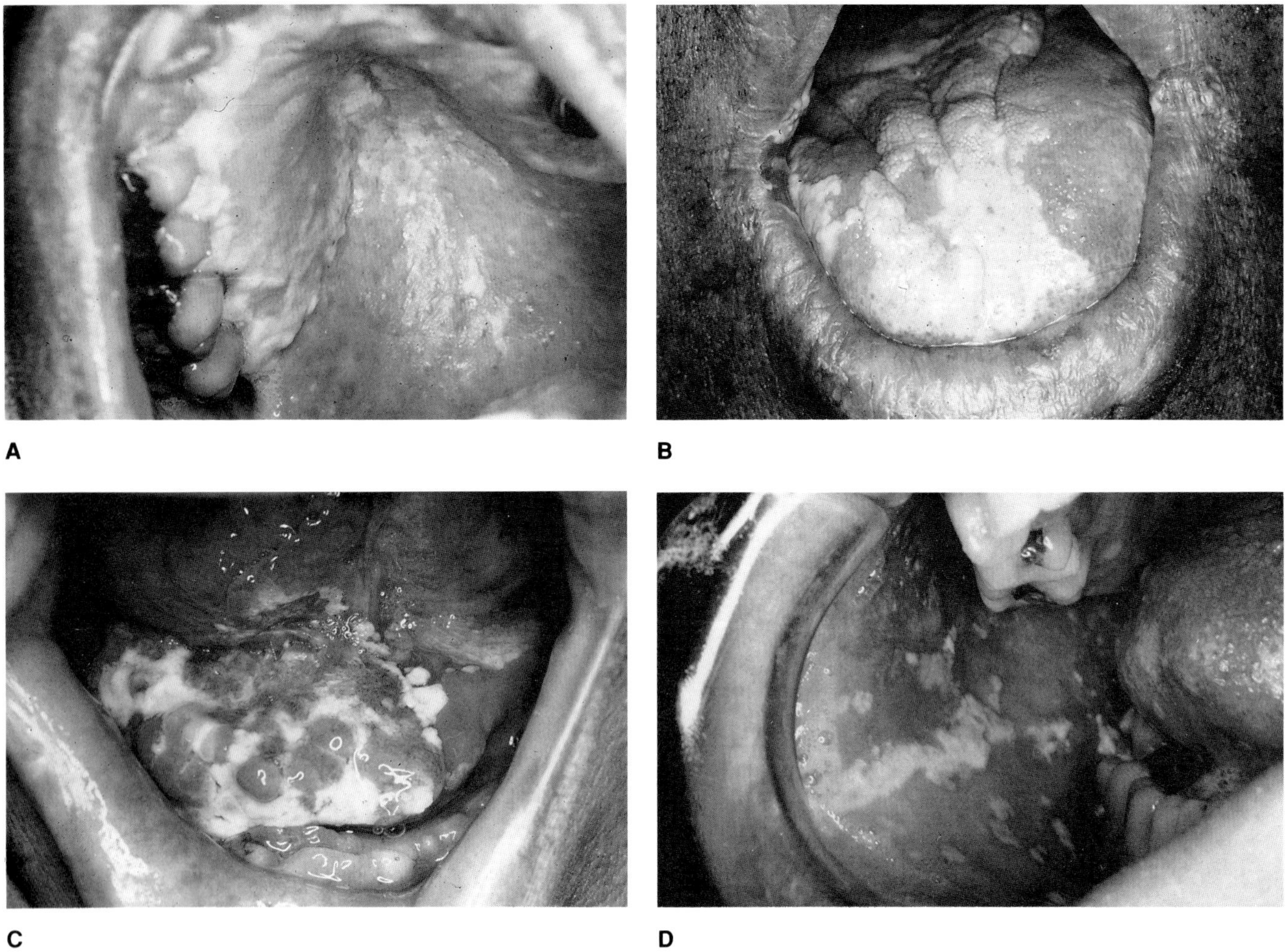

Fig. 6-4. Candidiasis following radiation-induced xerostomia. This infection can take many forms and is often confused with mucositis. **A,** Candidiasis of the palate after 4 weeks of irradiation. **B,** Lingual candidiasis at the end of radiation. Note angular cheilitis. **C,** Acutely painful candidiasis after 3 weeks of irradiation. **D,** Mucositis complicated by candidiasis at the end of the fourth week of radiation (approximately 3000 cGy). The patient also complained of dryness.

a solution for mouth rinsing or a gel delivered by means of a tray, are extremely effective.[28,29] Attempts should be made to increase salivary flow either by local or systemic means. Foods and beverages containing sucrose should be avoided as much as possible. If carious lesions develop, removal and restoration should take place immediately. Appropriate use of dental x-ray imaging is in order when indicated to monitor caries activity.[30]

CANDIDIASIS

Infections of the mouth by *Candida albicans* are commonly seen in irradiated patients (Fig. 6-4, Table 6-1), and are related to the alterations in saliva.[31,32] Clinically the signs may be confused with radiation mucositis or other sources of infection. Candidiasis is usually painful. Management is primarily with the use of antifungal drugs. Systemic administration (200 mg ketoconazole daily with food) is usually more effective for both response and compliance. Topical administration entails the use of nystatin or clotrimazole tablets dissolved orally. Because of pain from mucositis and dryness, patients may experience difficulty in dissolving tablets topically. Suspensions are another alternative form of treatment, but often this treatment is not as effective as the

Table 6-1. OCCURRENCE OF ORAL *CANDIDA* IN 109 IRRADIATED ORAL CANCER PATIENTS*

	Candida Culture		
Percent of Patients	**Before Therapy**	**End of Therapy**	**After Therapy†**
41	Negative	Negative	Negative
10	Negative	Negative	Positive
27	Negative	Positive	Positive
22	Positive	Positive	Positive

*Data from Silverman, Luangjarmekorn, Greenspan, 1984 (67 men, 42 women).[31]
†Mean time, 14 months.

tablets (possibly because of limited contact time between drug and fungus). These fungal-control approaches are often used in combination. Antiseptic mouth rinses similar to those used for caries control may be helpful if tolerated. In addition, topical (viscous xylocaine) or systemic analgetics may be required.

OSTEORADIONECROSIS

Osteonecrosis is one of the more serious complications of head and neck irradiation for cancer (Fig. 6-5). Bone cells and vascularity may be irreversibly injured (Fig. 6-6).[33,34] Fortunately, in many cases devitalized bone fragments will sequestrate and lesions will spontaneously heal. However, when radiation osteonecrosis is progressive, it can lead to intolerable pain or fracture and may necessitate jaw resection. The preventive and therapeutic use of antibiotics and hyperbaric oxygen can be effective, but reproducible beneficial results remain uncertain.[35–37]

The incidence of osteoradionecrosis varies depending upon the reporting institution, aggressiveness of radiotherapy, and follow-up time (Table 6-2).[38–42] The risk for developing a spontaneous osteoradionecrosis is somewhat unpredictable, but it is related to the dose of radiation delivered and bone volume. The risk is increased in dentulous patients, even more if teeth within the treatment field are removed after therapy. Spontaneous bone exposure usually occurs more than one year after radiation is completed.

Animal models to study the effects of ionizing radiation on jaw bones have demonstrated changes similar to those observed in human specimens: marrow avascularity and fatty degeneration; reduction of osteocytes, osteoblasts and osteoclasts; enlarged lacunae; and microfractures.

University of California Study

To assess the contributory factors in the development of osteoradionecrosis, the records of 100 patients irradiated for head and neck cancer at the University of California, San Francisco, between 1971 and 1977 were reviewed retrospectively.[38] The group comprised 60 men and 40 women whose average age was 65 years. At the time of diagnosis, 78 were dentulous and 22 were edentulous. All patients received megavoltage external beam radiotherapy and/or interstital radium or iridium implants. The maxilla and/or mandible were within the radiation fields. Special care was taken to calculate the bone dose as well as the tumor dose. The dose of external beam radiotherapy was in the range of 5000 to 7500 cGy, delivered at 180 cGy per fraction, five daily fractions per week. The total radiation dose included the dose from the external beam and from the interstital implant.

Osteoradionecrosis developed in 22 of these 100 patients. A higher percentage of dentulous patients developed osteonecrosis (24%, 19/78) than edentulous patients (14%, 3/22). All but one necrosis developed in the mandible. There was no correlation between tumor size and the incidence of osteonecrosis.

Thirty-nine of the 100 patients received a higher radiation dose to the bone than to the tumor. The incidence of osteonecrosis appears to be directly related to the radiation dose to the bone (Table 6-3). Osteonecrosis developed in 85% of the dentulous patients and 50% of the edentulous patients who received more than 7500 cGy to the bone. None of the patients who received less than 6500 cGy developed osteonecrosis.

All patients were observed for at least six months. The time at which osteoradionecrosis developed was variable. In 15 of the 22 cases it occurred more than one year after radiation treatment was completed. In the edentulous patients it appeared from one to 18 months (average ten months) after treatment; in the dentulous group it appeared from six to 72 months after treatment (mean 22 months). Follow-up observations of those who did not develop osteonecrosis ranged from six to 76 months (average 24 months).

Table 6-4 shows the incidence of osteonecrosis in relation to dental status and extractions. The risk was significantly greater for patients whose teeth were extracted after radiation therapy than for those with extractions before radiation or no extractions at all. Of the 14 dentulous patients who had extractions and developed osteonecrosis, the necrosis was associated with dental extraction sites in only nine and was apparently spontaneous in the remaining five. All nine cases of necrosis associated with dental extractions occurred with postradiation extractions.

Conclusions. Certain facts emerge from this study:

1. Patients who were edentulous at the time of diagnosis of cancer had a relatively low risk of osteonecrosis.
2. Patients who were dentulous had a greater risk.
3. The increased risk in dentulous patients appeared to be associated with those who had tooth extractions after radiation therapy.
4. Dentulous patients with pretreatment extractions or no extractions appeared to have risks similar to those of the edentulous patients.

Table 6-2. REPORTED INCIDENCE OF OSTEONECROSIS IN PATIENTS IRRADIATED FOR HEAD AND NECK CANCER

Source, Year	Hospital	No. Patients	Years	Dosage (cGy)	Cases of Osteonecrosis
Beumer, 1972[39]	Univ. California (S.F.)	278	1961–69	5000– 7000	10 (4%)
Bedwinek, 1976[40]	M.D. Anderson (Tex.)	381	1966–71	6000– 7500	54 (14%)
Murray, 1980[41,42]	M.D. Anderson (Tex.)	397	1971–75	4000–>8000	77 (19%)
Morrish, 1981[38]	Univ. California (S.F.)	100	1971–77	5000– 7500	22 (22%)

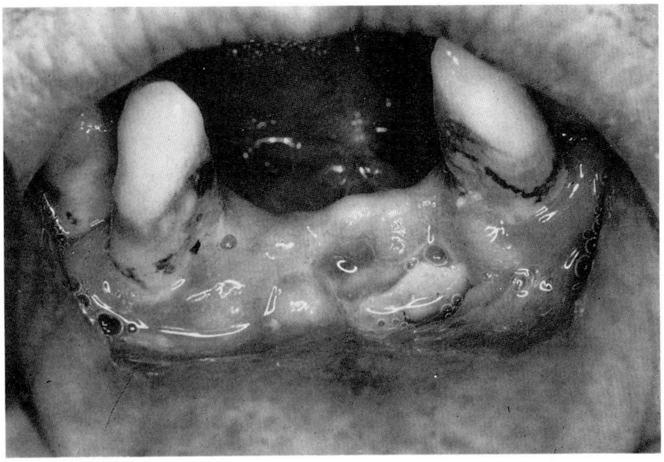

A

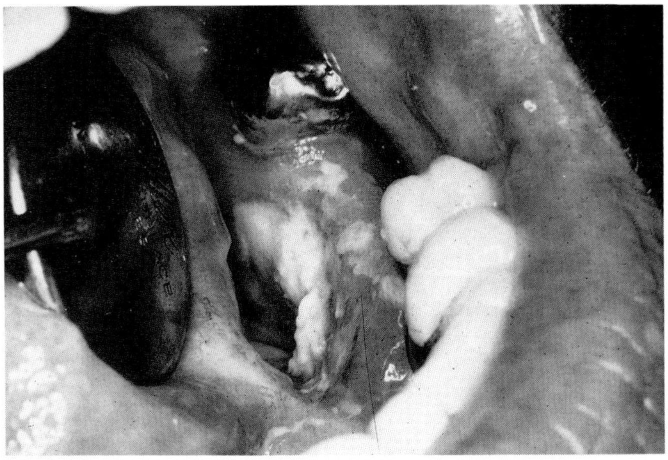

B

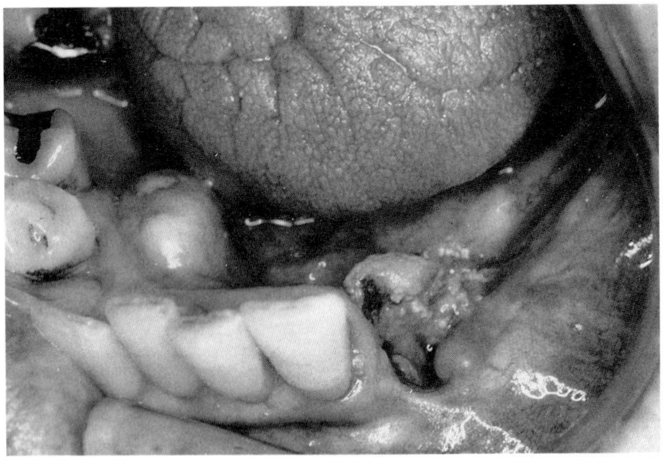

C

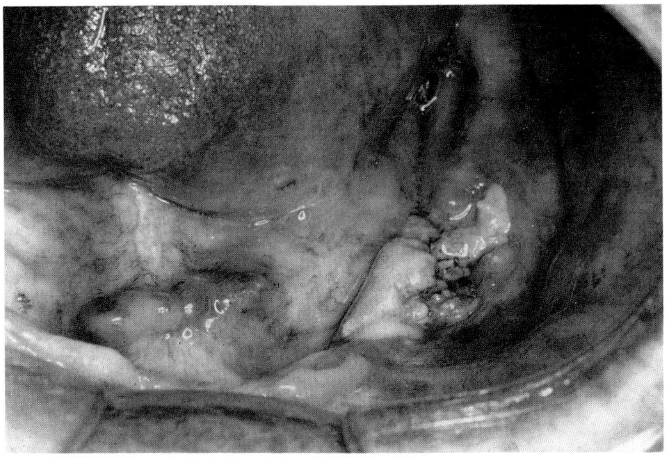

D

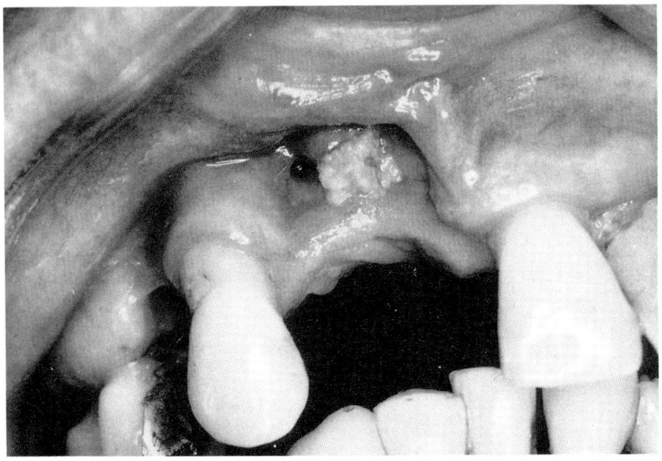

E

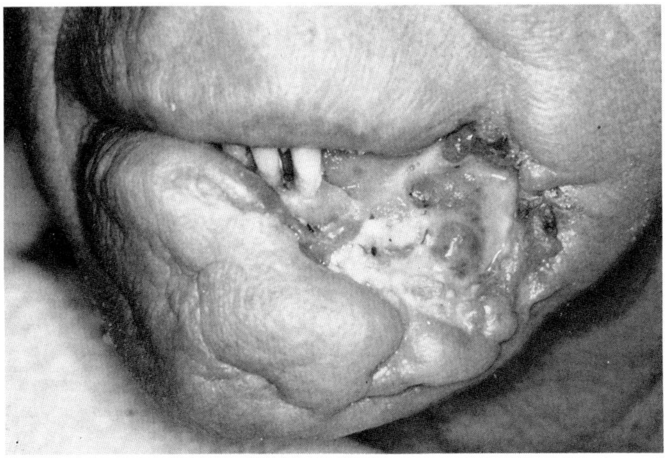

F

Fig. 6-5. Osteoradionecrosis after irradiation for head and neck cancer. This condition can occur spontaneously or after trauma. **A,** Spontaneous osteoradionecrosis of the mandible, which developed 3 years after treatment and responded to antibiotics. **B,** Osteoradionecrosis of the mandible appearing 6 months after treatment and developing after trauma. This did not respond to antibiotics and required mandibular resection. **C,** Osteoradionecrosis of the mandible developing 1 year after treatment, following extraction of the lower left cuspid. **D,** Osteoradionecrosis of the left mandible developing $1\frac{1}{2}$ years after treatment, even though lower denture was not worn. **E,** Osteoradionecrosis of the maxilla (an infrequent occurrence) developing 2 years after treatment. There had been no known trauma. **F,** Osteoradionecrosis of the mandible which was not controlled by antibiotics. Patient refused resection.

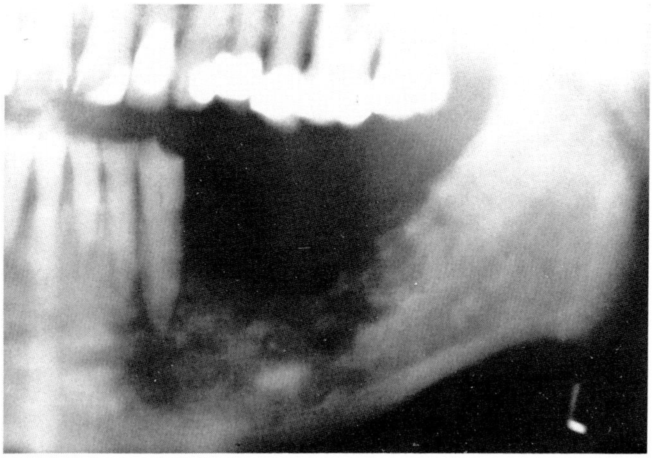

A

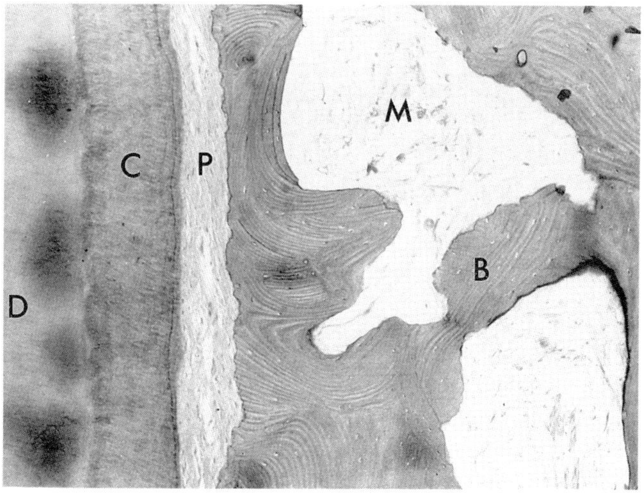

B

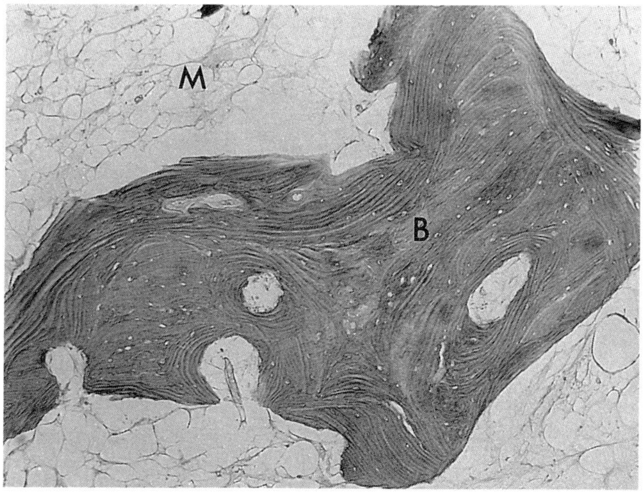

C

Fig. 6-6. Osteoradionecrosis. Histologic specimens showing devitalization of jawbone by radiation. **A,** Radiograph of advanced osteonecrosis that progressed to this stage four years after radiation (6800 cGy) for a squamous carcinoma of the mouth floor. There was exposed bone and severe pain. **B,** Dental socket area, including dentin (D), cementum (C), periodontal ligament (P), bone marrow (M), and alveolar bone (B). **C,** Higher-power view of an alveolar bone trabecula, showing bone (B) and marrow (M). Marrow is acellular and shows marked avascularity, lack of fibrous connective tissue, and some fatty degeneration. Note lack of osteocytes, osteoblasts, and osteoclasts.

Table 6-3. INCIDENCE OF OSTEONECROSIS ACCORDING TO RADIATION DOSE TO BONE*

Dose to Bone, cGy	Incidence of Osteonecrosis	
	Dentulous Patients	Edentulous Patients
<6500	0/36 (0%)	0/3 (0%)
6500–7500	8/29 (28%)	1/15 (7%)
>7500	11/13 (85%)	2/4 (50%)
Total	19/78 (24%)	3/22 (14%)

*Data from Morrish et al, 1981.[38]

Table 6-4. ASSOCIATION OF DENTAL EXTRACTIONS AND OSTEONECROSIS IN 78 IRRADIATED DENTULOUS PATIENTS*

Time of extraction	Radiation Dose (cGy)		Osteonecrosis	
	Range	Mean	Incidence	Mean Time of Onset After Treatment (mos)
No extractions	6940–9280	(7871)	5/41 (12%)	29
Before radiotherapy	7580–9610	(8500)	3/19 (16%)	41
After radiotherapy	6700–8100	(7346)	11/18 (61%)	20
Total	6700–9610	(7666)	19/78 (24%)	22

*Data from Morrish et al, 1981.[38]

†Radiation for dentulous patients without osteonecrosis ranged between 4950 and 9700 cGy (mean 6450 cGy).

5. Spontaneous osteoradionecrosis can occur.
6. The most important risk factor for the development of osteonecrosis appeared to be the radiation dose to the bone, particularly in the mandible.
7. Clinical changes in skin and/or mucosa indicating radiation damage was a risk indicator for osteonecrosis.
8. The risk for osteonecrosis continues indefinitely following radiation therapy.

Prior to 1977, osteoradionecrosis developed in less than 4% of patients irradiated for cancer of the oral cavity, oropharynx, and nasopharynx at the University of California, San Francisco.[39] During the period of this retrospective study,[38] an attempt to improve the cure rate in patients with head and neck cancer by means of aggressive radiation therapy may have led to an increase in complications. Osteonecrosis now seems to have been a significant problem in these individuals.

In our experience, the risk of osteonecrosis is negligible when the bone irradiation dose is less than 6500 cGy, but great when the dose exceeds 7500 cGy. Fortunately for patients' function and appearance, the risk for osteonecrosis related to denture-wearing is small (see Chapter 10).[40] Other investigators have found similar risk factors related to osteonecrosis.[34,41,42]

Treatment for Osteoradionecrosis

In the Morrish UCSF study,[38] 16 of the 22 patients with osteoradionecrosis were treated by conservative nonsurgical means. Four healed completely in three to 24 months, 10 had persistent but nonprogressive bone necrosis, and two refused surgical resection for progressive necrosis. Six of the 22 patients were resected and three had postsurgical recurrences of necrosis. Antibiotics are used to help control acute pain, swelling, and suppuration, and for prevention of these conditions if bone is exposed by accident or by treatment.

In Murray's study,[42] 47% of the 77 patients with osteoradionecrosis were controlled by conservative nonsurgical means. Since higher doses of radiation increase the risk of necroses, greater pain, and interference with function, the problem that eventually needs to be addressed is the balance between tumor cure rate and the morbidity associated with more aggressive radiation therapy.

SOFT TISSUE NECROSIS

Soft tissue necrosis may be defined as the occurrence of a mucosal ulcer in irradiated tissue that has no residual cancer (Fig. 6-7). The incidence of soft tissue necrosis is related to dose, time, and volume irradiated. The risk is far greater with interstital implantation and intraoral techniques because of the higher irradiation doses used.

In a University of California, San Francisco, study of 278 patients,[39] soft tissue necrosis occurred in 18 cases (6.5%). Eleven of these patients were treated by needle implantation or intraoral cone techniques. The average time of onset was within a year of therapy. Fifteen cases were self-limiting in time periods ranging from one to ten months (average three months), but three cases required surgical intervention.

Soft tissue necrosis is usually quite painful. Optimal hygiene is required and analgetics are usually helpful, but antibiotics are generally of little help in relieving pain and promoting healing. Since these ulcerations are often at the site of the primary tumor, periodic assessment for recurrence is essential until the necrosis heals.

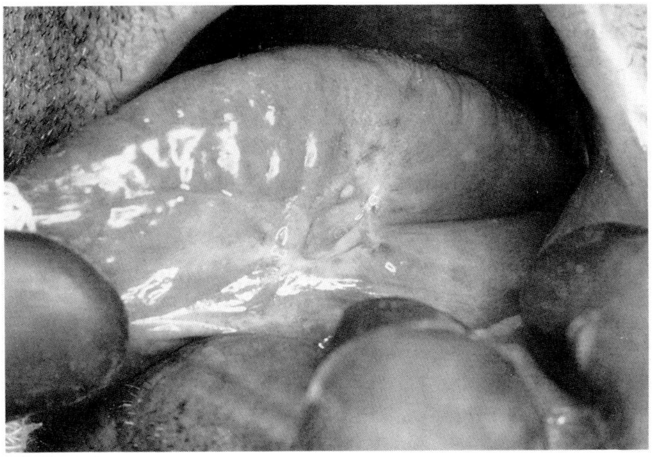

Fig. 6-7. Soft tissue necrosis. This painful ulcer appeared 6 months after radium needles were implanted for tongue carcinoma (calculated dose, 6800 cGy). Lesion healed in 4 months.

MANAGEMENT

In view of the risk that accompanies high-dose irradiation, special attention to preradiation dental planning appears critical. Factors important in the dental management of these patients include the following: (1) anticipated bone dose, (2) pretreatment dental status, dental hygiene, and retention of teeth that will be exposed to high-dose irradiation, (3) extraction techniques, (4) allowance of adequate healing time for teeth extracted before radiotherapy, and (5) patient motivation and capability of compliance to preventive measures.

Since many infections occur months or years after treatment, it is evident that the tissue changes induced by radiation persist for long periods of time and may be irreversible. Therefore, extreme care must be taken in evaluating the status of the teeth and periodontium before, during, and after treatment, and optimal oral and periodontal hygiene must be maintained because of the lowered biologic potential for healing in response to physical irritation, chemical agents, and microbial organisms.[44] Such attention is critical because of the potentially progressive nature of radiation osteonecrosis, which may involve large segments of bone and present a major therapeutic problem, possibly requiring extensive resection.

It is impossible to establish precise formulas for managing preradiation and postradiation dental problems. Extractions are considered primarily for teeth with a poor prognosis due to such conditions as advanced periodontal disease, extensive caries activity, and periapical lesions. Other considerations are sources of chronic soft-tissue irritation (trauma), and the degree of patient cooperation in preventive home care and dental office programs. The decision is modified further for each patient on the basis of the individual's prognosis, age, desires, economic aspects, and radiation delivery.

Reported studies and personal experience do not substantiate the advisability of extracting all teeth before treatment as a good preventive measure. When teeth are extracted before or after radiation, the alveolar bone must be evenly trimmed and carefully smoothed so that a primary tissue closure is possible. This is necessary because suppression of bone cell viability diminishes remodeling, and if a suitable alveolectomy is not performed, the resulting alveolar ridge will be irregular and may increase the risk of subsequent bone exposure and discomfort. A minimum of one week to ten days is arbitrarily allowed for initial healing before radiation is instituted. However, if the situation permits, more time is preferable, up to 14 or even 21 days.[34,45] Since dosages are fractionated, healing can usually continue before damaging levels of radiation are delivered to a surgical area. Obviously, teeth completely out of the treatment field are not affected similarly.

There is no evidence as to how many teeth should be extracted at one time. Therefore, whether before or after irradiation, all of the teeth indicated for removal are extracted as suits the needs of the surgeon and patient. The use of antibiotics during the healing period is important to minimize infection.

Whenever possible, an attempt is made to retain teeth to support tooth-borne appliances for the tentatively planned rehabilitation of these patients. It must be recalled that many teeth, either primarily or secondarily exposed to radiation, remain relatively free of disease and functional for long periods of time. This significantly facilitates rehabilitation. However, tissue-borne prostheses are not contraindicated (see Chapter 10).[41,43] In general, mucosa that appears fibrosed, telangiectatic, and atrophic is at greater risk.

The periodontium is maintained in optimal condition by periodic routine periodontal procedures. When areas exposed to radiation are treated, extreme care is exercised and antibiotics may be selectively administered. Fluoride applications (daily, in the form of mouth rinses or gels)[29] appear to aid in minimizing tooth decalcification and caries in these patients. There are no unusual contraindications for endodontic procedures.[46]

In conclusion, review of the literature and our own experience indicate that carefully controlled studies are necessary before more definitive guidelines can be formulated for managing dental structures which have been or are to be radiated. Until such information is available, each case must be managed individually, based on the patient's needs, the status of the tumor, and the risks known to exist for dental health in irradiated tissues. An overall "one-type" empirical approach for all patients is contraindicated.

REFERENCES

1. Hill M, Toto PD: Effects of human saliva on oral chemical carcinogenesis. *J Dent Res* 52:631, 1973.
2. Haselow RE, Nesbit M, Dehner LP et al: Second neoplasms following megavoltage radiation in a pediatric population. *Cancer* 42:1185, 1978.
3. Silverman JE, Weber CW, Silverman S Jr et al: Zinc supplementation and taste in head and neck cancer patients undergoing radiation therapy. *J Oral Med* 38:14, 1983.
4. Conger AD, Wells MA: Radiation and aging effects on taste structure and function. *Radiat Res* 37:31, 1969.
5. Mossman KL, Henkin RI: Radiation-induced changes in taste acuity in cancer patients. *Int J Radiat Oncol Biol Phys* 4:663, 1978.
6. Silverman S Jr, Thompson JS: Serum zinc and copper in oral/oropharyngeal carcinoma. *Oral Surg Oral Med Oral Pathol* 57:34, 1984.
7. Eneroth C, Henrickson CO, Jakobsson PA: Effect of fractionated radiotherapy on salivary gland function. *Cancer* 30:1147, 1972.
8. Bucher JA, Fleming TJ, Fuller LM et al: Preliminary observations on the effect of mantle field radiotherapy on salivary flow rates in patients with Hodgkin's disease. *J Dent Res* 67:518, 1988.
9. Fox PC: Systemic therapy of salivary gland hypofunction. *J Dent Res* 66:689, 1987.
10. Greenspan D, Daniels TE: Effectiveness of pilocarpine in postradiation xerostomia. *Cancer* 59:1123, 1987.
11. Nakamoto RY: Use of a saliva substitute in postradiation xerostomia. *J Prosthet Dent* 42:539, 1979.
12. Levine MJ, Aguirre A, Hatton MN et al: Artificial salivas: present and future. *J Dent Res* 66:693, 1987.
13. Shannon IL, Starcke EN, Wescott WB: Effect of radiotherapy on whole saliva flow. *J Dent Res* 56:693, 1977.
14. Dreizen S, Brown LR, Handler SH et al: Radiation-induced xerostomia in cancer patients. *Cancer* 38:273, 1976.
15. Makkonen TA, Tenovuo J, Vilja P et al: Changes in the protein composition of whole saliva during radiotherapy in patients with oral oropharyngeal cancer. *Oral Surg Oral Med Oral Pathol* 62:270, 1986.
16. Council on Dental Therapeutics: Concensus: Oral health effects of products that increase salivary flow rate. *J Am Dent Assn* 116:757, 1988.
17. Brown LR, Dreizen S, Handler SH et al: Effect of radiation-induced xerostomia on human oral microflora. *J Dent Res* 54:740, 1975.
18. Cowman RA, Baron SS, Glassman AH et al: Changes in protein composition of salivae from radiation-induced xerostomia patients and its effect on growth by oral streptococci. *J Dent Res* 61:336, 1983.
19. Keene HJ, Fleming TJ: Prevalence of caries-associated microflora after radiotherapy in patients with cancer of the head and neck. *Oral Surg Oral Med Oral Pathol* 64:421, 1987.
20. Schubert MM, Izutsu KT: Iatrogenic causes of salivary gland dysfunction. *J Dent Res* 66:680, 1987.
21. Frank RM, Herdly J, Philippe E: Acquired dental defects and salivary gland lesions after irradiation for carcinoma. *J Am Dent Assoc* 70:868, 1965.
22. Walker R: Direct effect of radiation on the solubility of human teeth in vitro. *J Dent Res* 54:901, 1975.
23. Shannon IL, Wescott WB, Starcke EN et al: Laboratory study of cobalt-60-irradiated human dental enamel. *J Oral Med* 33:23, 1978.
24. Shannon IL, Trodahl JN, Starcke EN: Remineralization of enamel by a saliva substitute designed for use by irradiated patients. *Cancer* 41:1746, 1978.
25. Hutton MF, Patterson SS, Mitchell DF et al: Laboratory study of cobalt-60 radiation on the dental pulps of monkeys. *Oral Surg Oral Med Oral Pathol* 38:279, 1974.
26. Nickens GE, Patterson SS, El-Kafrawy AH et al: Effect of cobalt-60 radiation on the pulp of restored teeth. *J Am Dent Assoc* 94:701, 1977.
27. Carl W, Schaaf NG, Chen TY: Oral care of patients irradiated for cancer of the head and neck. *Cancer* 30:448, 1972.

28. Dreizen S, Brown LR, Daly TE et al: Prevention of xerostomia-related dental caries in irradiated cancer patients. *J Dent Res* 56:99, 1977.
29. Wei SHY: Clinical uses of fluorides: A state-of-the-art conference on the uses of fluorides in clinical dentistry (Conference summary). *J Am Dent Assn* 109:472, 1984.
30. Jones GA, Purdy RB, Stoker HW et al: Use of dental x-rays on postirradiated patients with head and neck cancer. *J Am Dent Assn* 117:599, 1988.
31. Silverman S Jr, Luangjarmekorn L, Greenspan D: Occurrence of oral candida in irradiated head and neck cancer patients. *J Oral Med* 39:194, 1984.
32. Rossie KM, Taylor J, Beck FM et al: Influence of radiation therapy on oral *Candida albicans* colonization: A quantitative assessment. *Oral Surg Oral Med Oral Pathol* 64:698, 1987.
33. Rohrer MD, Kim Y, Fayos JV: The effect of cobalt-60 irradiation on monkey mandibles. *Oral Surg Oral Med Oral Pathol* 48:424, 1979.
34. Marx RE, Johnson RP: Studies in the radiobiology of osteoradionecrosis and their clinical significance. *Oral Surg Oral Med Oral Pathol* 64:379, 1987.
35. Hart GB, Mainous EG: The treatment of radiation necrosis with hyperbaric oxygen (OHP). *Cancer* 37:2580, 1976.
36. Marx RE, Johnson RP, Kline SN: Prevention of osteoradionecrosis: A randomized prospective clinical trial of hyperbaric oxygen versus penicillin. *J Am Dent Assn* 111:49, 1985.
37. Fattore LaD, Strauss RA: Hyperbaric oxygen in the treatment of osteoradionecrosis: A review of its use and efficacy. *Oral Surg Oral Med Oral Pathol* 63:280, 1987.
38. Morrish RB, Chan E, Silverman S Jr et al: Osteonecrosis in patients irradiated for head and neck carcinoma. *Cancer* 47:1980, 1981.
39. Beumer J III, Silverman S Jr, Benak SB: Hard and soft tissue necroses following radiation therapy for oral cancer. *J Prosthet Dent* 27:640, 1972.
40. Bedwinek JM, Shukovsky LJ, Fletcher GH et al: Osteonecrosis in patients treated with definitive radiotherapy for squamous cell carcinoma of the oral cavity and naso- and oropharynx. *Radiology* 119:665, 1976.
41. Murray CG, Herson J, Daly TE et al: Radiation necrosis of the mandible: A 10-year study. Part I. Factors influencing the onset of necrosis. *Int J Rad Oncol Biol Phys* 6:543, 1980.
42. Murray CG, Herson J, Daly TE et al: Radiation necrosis of the mandible: A 10-year study. Part II. Dental factors; onset, duration and management of necrosis. *Int J Rad Oncol Biol Phys* 6:549, 1980.
43. Beumer J III, Curtis TA, Morrish RB Jr: Radiation complications in edentulous patients. *J Prosthet Dent* 36:193, 1976.
44. Regezi JA, Courtney RM, Kerr DA: Dental management of patients irradiated for oral cancer. *Cancer* 38:994, 1976.
45. Starcke EN, Shannon IL: How critical is the interval between extractions and irradiation in patients with head and neck malignancy? *Oral Surg Oral Med Oral Pathol* 43:333, 1977.
46. Seto BG, Beumer J III, Kagawa T et al: Analysis of endodontic therapy in patients irradiated for head and neck cancer. *Oral Surg Oral Med Oral Pathol* 60:540, 1985.

7

Prognosis

KAREN FU
SOL SILVERMAN, JR.

The survival rates for oral cancer vary, depending upon several factors: the stage of the lesion (size of primary lesion, local extension, lymph node involvement, distant metastasis); the site of the primary tumor (in general, the more posterior the site, the more negative the prognosis); the adequacy of initial treatment; the Karnofsky performance status[1] (a patient's ability to cope); and the histological differentiation of the malignancy. The patient's general health, habits (especially tobacco and alcohol use), and predisposition toward multiple oral malignancies are important secondary factors.

STAGING AND REPORTING OF END RESULTS

Survival rates are reported in the following manner: the *observed rate,* which is based on the proportion of patients alive in a period of time after diagnosis, and the *relative rate,* which adjusts the cancer survival rates, taking into account deaths expected from other causes.

Classification

Staging of tumors (Table 7-1) takes into account the size of the primary tumor and evidence of spread. Staging is important because treatment modalities, prognosis, and accurate reporting depend on a uniform description of the malignancy, mucosa, alveolar ridge, floor of mouth, hard palate, anterior two-thirds of the tongue (oral tongue), retromolar trigone, and oropharynx (soft palate, uvula, tonsillar fossa and pillars), base of tongue, and glossoepiglottic and pharyngoepiglottic folds. Squamous carcinomas may also be graded according to Broder's classification as follows:

GX—Grade cannot be assessed,
G1—Well differentiated,
G2—Moderately well differentiated,
G3—Poorly differentiated,
G4—Undifferentiated.

However, the criteria for this cytologic assessment as well as therapeutic and prognostic significance creates many uncertainties.[2]

Table 7-1. CLASSIFICATION AND STAGING

TNM SYSTEM*

T	=	**primary tumor**
N	=	**lymph nodes regional**
M	=	**distant metastasis**
TX	=	primary tumor cannot be assessed
TIS	=	carcinoma in situ
T0	=	no evidence of primary tumor
T1	=	greatest diameter ≤ 2 cm
T2	=	greatest diameter > 2 cm but ≤ 4 cm
T3	=	greatest diameter > 4 cm
T4	=	massive tumor > 4 cm with deep invasion and/or invasion of adjacent structures
N0	=	no clinically positive nodes
N1	=	single clinically positive homolateral node ≤ 3 cm
N2	=	single clinically positive homolateral node > 3 but ≤ 6 cm (N2a) or multiple clinically positive nodes ≤ 6 cm (N2b) or bilateral nodes or contralateral nodes < 6 cm (N2c)
N3	=	metastasis in a lymph node > 6 cm
NX	=	regional lymph nodes cannot be assessed
M0	=	no evident metastasis
M1	=	distant metastasis present

STAGE GROUPING

Stage 0	=	TIS, N0, M0
Stage I	=	T1, N0, M0
Stage II	=	T2, N0, M0
Stage III	=	T3, N0, M0
		T1 or T2 or T3, N1, M0
Stage IV	=	T4, N0 or N1, M0
		Any T, N2 or N3, M0
		Any T, any N, M1

*From American Joint Committee for Cancer Staging and End Result Reporting, 1988.

Table 7-2. ORAL CANCER END RESULTS IN 1,570 CASES*
Percentage of 5-year survivals

Tumor Site	Stages: I	II	III	IV
Hard palate	93	40	6	8
Oral tongue	90	64	34	6
Soft palate	73	48	32	5
Buccal mucosa	72	61	42	0
Floor of mouth	68	70	50	9
Mandibular gingiva	64	49	37	10
Maxillary gingiva	62	64	36	29
Posterior tongue	50	44	26	1

*Data from American Joint Committee for Cancer Staging and End Result Reporting, 1968. (A more recent report has not been made.)

Table 7-3. ORAL CANCER: RELATIVE SURVIVAL RATES IN 11,375 CASES*

			Patient Survival (%)		
Site	**Stage†**	**No. Cases**	**1 yr**	**3 yr**	**5 yr**
Tongue:					
Base	Localized	81	92	64	50
	Spread	1449	63	30	22
Oral	Localized	787	93	76	67
	Spread	866	66	35	30
Oropharynx	Localized	736	87	68	53
	Spread	2841	68	38	30
Floor of mouth	Localized	324	92	77	68
	Spread	1669	75	49	41
Lip	Localized	1128	99	97	95
	Spread	288	96	85	78
Gingiva	Localized	70	94	72	55
	Spread	822	79	51	44
Buccal	Localized	58	98	84	78
	Spread	256	76	49	40

*Cases for which there was follow-up information. Source: National Cancer Institiute: Surveillance, Epidemiology and End Results Program (SEER), 1973–1984.[10]

†Localized (Stages I and II): 3184 (28%). Spread (Stages III and IV): 8191 (72%).

End Results

The size of an untreated tumor is usually directly related to the length of time it has been present. Therefore, both early detection and adequate treatment are extremely important to improve chances for survival.

Table 7-2 demonstrates the importance of detection at an early stage in reducing mortality. Other reports from large treatment centers confirm similar survival rates when Stage I and II lesions are compared with those that show metastases or are very extensive (Stage III and IV).[3-9] Survival data on 11,375 oral cancer patients which was obtained from nine cancer registries in the U.S. for the SEER program further document the improved survival for localized as compared with advanced disease (Table 7-3).[10] Table 7-4 compares the national SEER data to one of its 9 registry components, the San Francisco/Oakland Bay area. The overall survival is poor; less than half the patients survive their disease. Since most patients are treated for late-stage disease, delay in diagnosis appears to represent the most valid explanation for the dismal therapeutic results. This underscores the necessity for more effective public and professional education regarding signs, symptoms, and early diagnosis. In addition to stage and the primary tumor site, the patient's coping abilities (Karnofsky performance status) may have a significant influence on prognosis.[11]

CAUSE OF DEATH

As survival statistics indicate, more than half of the patients with oral cancer will die within five years from uncontrolled tumor. The most common cause of death is infection (septicemia or pneumonia). Infection results from two main sources: direct invasion by microorganisms entering through tumor-induced ulcerations; and "lowered resistance" due to anorexia or loss of masticatory function with resultant inability to consume adequate nutrients, causing anemia and weight loss (cachexia).[12] These problems may arise as a result of treatment or from mental depression and despair. Some patients die of hemorrhage evoked by tumor-induced erosion of blood vessel walls. In a study at M.D. Anderson Hospital in Houston, of 94 deaths due to head and neck cancer, 43 (46%) of the patients died of infection and 12 (13%) of hemorrhage.[13] Hypercalcemia is unusual in head and neck carcinomas. It occurs more frequently in advanced head and

Table 7-4. ORAL CANCER: EARLY DIAGNOSIS AND RELATIVE SURVIVAL*

	All Stages		Staging of All Lesions		5 yr. Survival	
	No. Cases	**Survival 5 yrs.**	**Localized (Stages I, II)**	**Spread (Stages III, IV)**	**Localized (Stages I, II)**	**Spread (Stages III, IV)**
SEER	12,792	45%	30%	70%	72%	34%
Bay Area	2,610	42%	23%	77%	66%	35%

*Includes nonspecified oral sites. Source: National Cancer Institute: Surveillance, Epidemiology and End Results Program (SEER), 1973–1984.[10]

neck cancers and indicates a poor prognosis as well as complicating management by causing gastrointestinal complaints, confusion, and dehydration.[14-16] Carcinomatosis is an infrequent cause of death, although distant spread probably occurs in over 10% of head and neck cancer patients.

A significant influence on survival is the extremely high risk for a second primary tumor in the respiratory and upper digestive tract in patients with mouth cancer (see Chapter 1). One study reported that 27% of 377 patients with treated floor-of-mouth carcinoma developed new primary cancers; two-thirds of these new cancers were of the respiratory and upper digestive tracts, the others were in the mouth.[17] These tumors were reported to have developed at a constant rate of 3.6% per year and led to an excess mortality of 5.2% per year.

REFERENCES

1. Mor V, Laliberte L, Morriss JN, et al: The Karnofsky Performance Status Scale: An examination of its reliability and validity in a research setting. *Cancer* 53:2002, 1984.
2. Anneroth G, Hansen LS, Silverman S Jr: Malignancy grading in oral squamous carcinoma. I. Squamous cell carcinoma of the tongue and floor of mouth: Histologic grading in the clinical evaluation. *J Oral Pathol* 15:162, 1986.
3. Kalnins IK, Leonard AG, Sako K et al: Correlation between prognosis and degree of lymph node involvement in carcinoma of the oral cavity. *Am J Surg* 134:450, 1977.
4. Shah JP, Shemen LJ, Strong EW: Buccal mucosa, alveolus, retromolar trigone, floor of mouth, hard palate, tongue tumors. In SE Thawley and WR Panje (eds), *Comprehensive Management of Head and Neck Tumors*. Philadelphia: WB Saunders Co., 1987, p.551.
5. Cummings BJ, Clark RM: Squamous cell carcinoma of the oral cavity. *J Otolaryngol* 11:359, 1982.
6. Fu KK, Lichter A, Galante M: Carcinoma of the floor of mouth: An analysis of treatment results and the sites and causes of failure. *Int J Radiat Oncol Biol Phys* 1:829, 1976.
7. Million RR, Cassisi NJ: Oral cavity. In RR Million and NJ Cassini (eds), *Management of Head and Neck Cancer. A Multidisciplinary Approach*. Philadelphia: JB Lippincott Co., 1984, p. 239.
8. Parsons JT, Million RR: Radiation therapy of tumors of the oral cavity. In SE Thawley and WR Panje (eds), *Comprehensive Management of Head and Neck Tumors*. Philadelphia: WB Saunders Co., 1987, p.516.
9. Wang CC: *Radiation Therapy for Head and Neck Neoplasms*. Boston: John Wright-PSG, 1983, p.73.
10. National Cancer Institute: Surveillance, Epidemiology and End Results Program (SEER), 1973-1984. Bethesda, MD (Computer Tape).
11. Pajak TF, Fazekas JT, Davis LW, Marcial VA: Analysis of radiation therapy oncology group head and neck database: Identification of prognostic factors and reevaluation of American joint committee staging system in head and neck cancer. In S Vogl (ed), *Head and Neck Cancer*. New York: Churchill Livingstone, 1988, p.41.
12. Costa G, Donaldson SS: Current concepts in cancer: Effects of cancer and cancer treatment on the nutrition of the host. *N Engl J Med* 300:1471, 1979.
13. Inagaki J, Rodriquez V, Bodey GP: Causes of death in cancer patients. *Cancer* 33:568, 1974.
14. Besarab A, Caro JF: Mechanisms of hypercalcemia in malignancy. *Cancer* 41:2276, 1978.
15. Won C, Decker DA, Drelichman A et al: Hypercalcemia in head and neck carcinoma. Incidence and prognosis. *Cancer* 52:2261, 1983.
16. Broaus AE, Mangin M, Ikeda K, et al: Humoral hypercalcemia of cancer. Identification of a novel parathyroid hormone-like peptide. *N Engl J Med* 319:556, 1988.
17. Tepperman BS, Fitzpatrick PJ: Second respiratory and upper digestive tract cancers after oral cancer. *Lancet* 2:547, 1981.

8

Leukemia and Lymphoma

SOL SILVERMAN, JR.
MARK SCHUBERT

Hematologic malignancies and malignant lymphomas make up a rather diverse group of diseases that can affect oral health care in a number of different ways. First, the initial signs and symptoms may appear in the mouth or neck. These oral manifestations may lead the patient to seek dental consultation, or they may be noticed on routine examination. Second, special precautions may be required during various oral procedures to minimize or avoid serious adverse reactions. Therefore, knowledge of these disorders—their general signs and symptoms, pathogenesis, treatment, complications, and prognosis—is extremely important for the providers of dental health care. Another important consideration is that the therapies used to treat these diseases are capable of having a profound effect both directly and indirectly on oral health which can result in significant morbidity or even fatal consequences.

MYELOPROLIFERATIVE AND LYMPHOPROLIFERATIVE DISEASES

Leukemias and lymphomas account for almost 78,000 new cases of cancer each year in the United States, about 8% of all malignancies. Oral and paraoral changes may be very early manifestations of disease and thus are important in establishing the diagnosis and prognosis. In addition, since patients with these conditions are immunosuppressed, oral infection must be minimized or avoided to decrease morbidity.

LEUKEMIAS

Leukemia, a neoplastic disorder of the blood-forming tissue, is characterized by proliferation of abnormal white cells. It occurs in all races and may develop at any age. Each year in the United States, approximately 27,000 new cases of leukemias are diagnosed. The etiology of leukemia remains unknown, but risks are increased by genetic and environmental factors including large doses of ionizing radiation and certain chemical compounds.[1,2] Although viral etiology is well established in many animal models, a link between virus and this disease in humans is less clear. A rare form of adult T-cell leukemia/lymphoma has been linked to exposure to a retrovirus known as human T-lymphotrophic virus (HTLV-1).[3] Although endemic to many areas of the world, it appears that only a small percentage of individuals exposed to this virus develop leukemia. Infection and hemorrhage are the chief causes of death. Of interest, blood banks now test for HTLV-1 in addition to HIV-1, hepatitis B, and syphilis.

The leukemias are customarily grouped into acute and chronic diseases, based on the degree of maturation of the cells and the survival time of patients. They are further subclassified according to the cell types involved, primarily lymphoblastic and myelogenous.

The proliferation of leukemic cells within the bone marrow does not occur at a much more rapid rate than normal myeloid cells, but the leukemic cells do have an added growth potential because of an inability to differentiate and mature. Normal erythroid, myeloid, and platelet production is decreased due to crowding and possibly by an inhibitory effect on normal cells by the leukemic cells. As the leukemia progresses, the peripheral blood shows increasing numbers of immature white cells or blasts (reflecting the ongoing leukocytosis), progressive anemia, reduction in platelets (thrombocytopenia), and reduction in polymorphonuclear leukocytes (neutropenia). In later stages of the disease, total marrow failure can occur.

Nearly half of the cases of leukemia seen in Western countries are acute leukemias, whereas approximately 30% are chronic lymphocytic leukemia (CLL) and 20% are chronic myelogenous leukemia (CML). Men are affected slightly more often than women.

In children between one and 14 years of age, malignancies are the leading disease-cause of death, and leukemia is the most common malignancy in this group. Acute lymphocytic leukemia (ALL) is the most common form in children.

ACUTE LEUKEMIA

Acute leukemias represent malignancies of blood-forming organs that result in a rapid and fulminant disease course which, if left untreated, can lead to death in a few weeks to

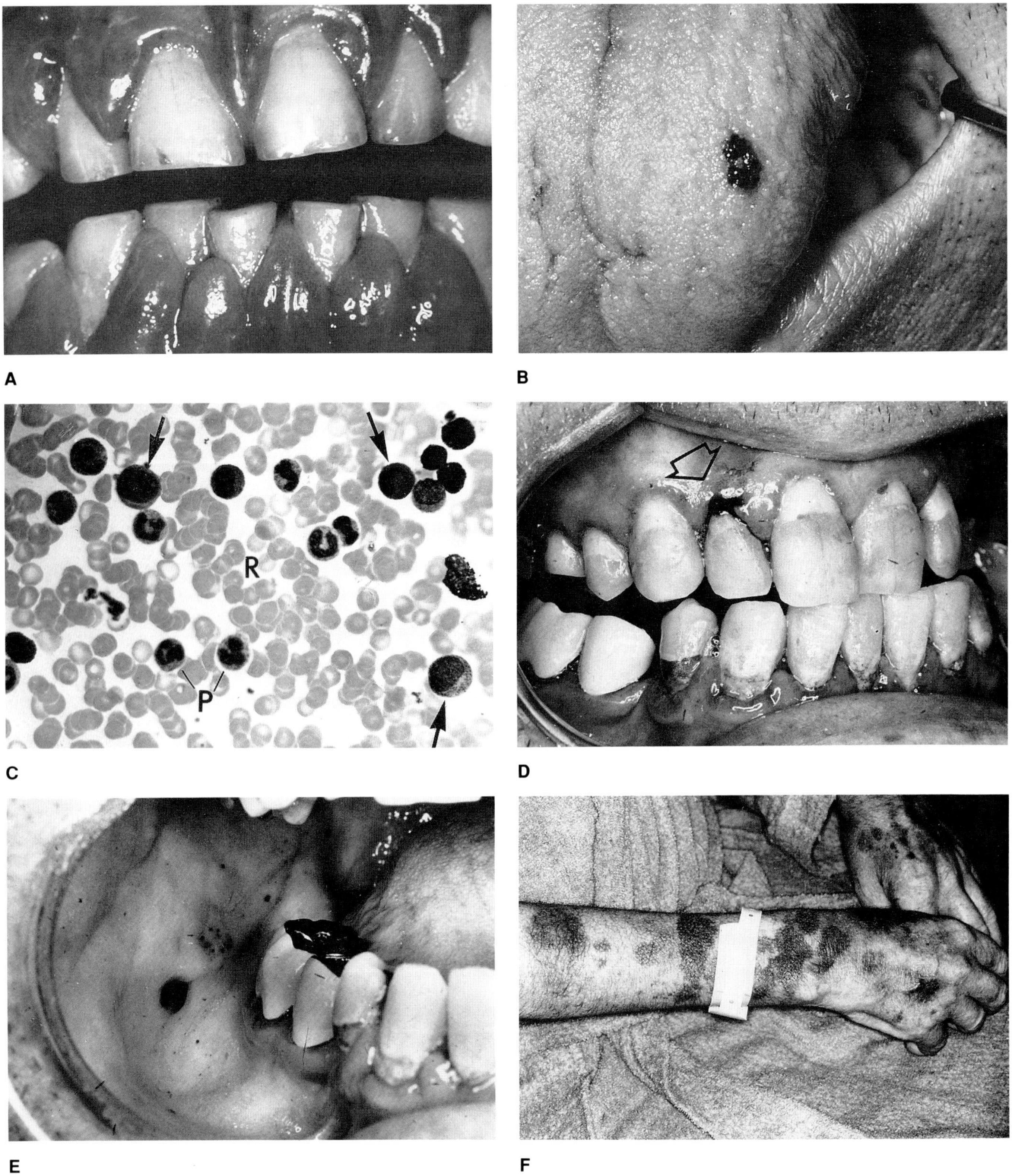

Fig. 8-1. Diagnostic signs of leukemia. **A,** Edematous, hyperplastic gingivae associated with pain, anorexia, and slight weight loss brought this 36-year-old man to the dental office. **B,** Examination of same patient revealed purpuric lesion on tongue, indicating a probable clotting abnormality. **C,** Differential smear showed an altered red/white blood cell ratio (usually 600:1) and numerous immature white blood cells, indicating the diagnosis of myelogenous leukemia. Note myeloblasts and myelocytes (arrows), a few normal polymorphonuclear leukocytes (P), and red blood cells (R). **D,** Subacute gingivitis and hemorrhage (arrow) in 50-year-old patient. **E,** Multiple buccal purpuric lesions in same patient. **F,** Multiple ecchymoses of the skin in same patient, further evidence of either capillary fragility or clotting defect or both. This patient had myelogenous leukemia.

months. Any of the myeloid cell lines can be involved. Presenting complaints are often general: weakness, malaise, pallor, anorexia, fever, purpura, and joint and bone pain. Lymphadenopathy may be present, as well as excessive bleeding or bruising after trauma.

The dentist is sometimes instrumental in the diagnosis of leukemia and lymphomas since unexplained necrotizing, ulcerative gingivitis, mucosal purpura, gingival edema with or without erythema and/or spontaneous bleeding, excessive bleeding after a surgical procedure, or cervical lymphadenopathy may be seen early in the course of the disease (Fig. 8-1).[4–7] The usual abnormally high peripheral white blood count can range from less than 10,000 to more than 100,000 per cubic millimeter. Anemia and thrombocytopenia also frequently occur early in the course of the disease. However, some patients are initially leukopenic. On the differential smear, immature and abnormal white cells are seen. There is a massive proliferation of primitive malignant cells in the bone marrow even when leukopenia exists.

It is estimated that the total burden of malignant cells when leukemia first presents clinically is approximately 10^{12} to 10^{13} cells. As the number of these cells is lowered by chemotherapeutic agents, signs and symptoms diminish and peripheral blood and marrow may temporarily appear normal. During the last 30 years, great progress has been made in the treatment of acute leukemias, especially ALL. In the early 1950s, nearly all patients diagnosed as having ALL died within three months; today nearly 50% of patients with ALL are long-term survivors after receiving cancer chemotherapy alone. While survival rates for other forms of acute leukemia are not as high as those for ALL, they have been increasing steadily. Multiple drug therapy attacks the leukemic cells in different phases of the mitotic cycle, however it is unknown what role the body's own immunologic defenses play in coping with residual disease.

Marrow transplantation is a therapy which involves the use of high-dose chemotherapy and total body irradiation followed by an infusion of marrow cells from an appropriate donor. It has become effective therapy for many patients, even an accepted treatment modality for certain individuals who have failed conventional chemotherapy.[8–10]

CHRONIC LEUKEMIA

Survival times are longer with chronic leukemia than with acute leukemias. Chronic myelogenous leukemia is characterized by a greatly elevated leukocyte count with all stages of granulocytic development in both peripheral blood and bone marrow. However, within a mean duration of three years after diagnosis, the relatively benign chronic phase may transform to a phase known as blast crisis. If untreated, it is inevitably fatal.

In contrast, chronic lymphocytic leukemia involves progressive accumulation of small B-lymphocytes that have lost the capacity to divide. The life span of these metabolically abnormal cells may be lengthened to several years, causing the total body lymphocyte mass to expand considerably. The cells, which originate in lymph nodes, aggregate chiefly in the lymph nodes, spleen, blood, and marrow. There is a subsequent progressive decline in levels of immunoglobulins. The onset of CLL is so insidious that often diagnosis is made accidently following blood studies performed as part of a routine medical examination. Adults with CLL may live for long periods of time and often show little clinical evidence of the disease. Whereas older patients have survival curves close to normal for their age group, the disease is more aggressive in younger patients, resulting in a shorter survival time (six to seven years).

The most common complaints of patients with chronic leukemia are those of fatigue, malaise, occasionally a fever or infection, lymphadenopathy, night sweats, and weight loss. Glandular swelling in the neck and gingival bleeding may be early signs that prompt a patient to the dental office before medical consultation is sought. Cellular and humoral immunity are both defective in CLL, and patients demonstrate lowered resistance to injuries and infections.

Currently CML management involves the use of several different chemotherapeutic strategies with or without splenectomy. However, once a patient progresses to blast crisis phase, these therapies are ineffective and survival times range from 2 to 10 months. The use of intensive (cellular lethal) chemoradiotherapy followed by marrow transplantation shows promising results in being able to clinically and cytogenetically induce complete remissions.[11] In contrast, therapy for CLL is usually not indicated until symptoms of anemia or thrombocytopenia, or both, are noted or if bulky lymphadenopathy develops.

Diagnostic Problems

From the characterization of the leukemias presented above, it is evident that most cases are diagnosed in the physician's office. However, the dentist should be suspicious of mucosal purpura, gingival bleeding, and lymphadenopathy, especially if these signs are also associated with complaints of weakness, malaise, intermittent fevers, anorexia, and pallor (Fig. 8-2). Furthermore, if a patient presents with gingival bleeding and/or infection and does not respond to routine therapy, a blood dyscrasia should be considered. It is important in these instances to correlate the oral signs and symptoms with any systemic signs and symptoms that may be present. When it is suspected that a patient may have leukemia, conservative empirical care should be prescribed while diagnostic blood work or appropriate referral is made to evaluate the possibility of a blood dyscrasia.

Temporary conservative management would include bland mouth rinses, antibiotics (if indicated), and analgetic agents. If leukemia is suspected in the differential diagnosis, aggressive dental procedures that could bring on a bleeding episode or induce bacteremia should be delayed until a definitive diagnosis is established.

Care of the Patient Diagnosed with Leukemia

The development of effective antileukemia therapy and advances in supportive care have resulted in dramatic changes in the treatment and prognosis of these disorders. Utilizing chemotherapy alone or chemoradiotherapy followed by marrow transplantation, the possibility of a cure or long-term disease-free response is a realistic goal.

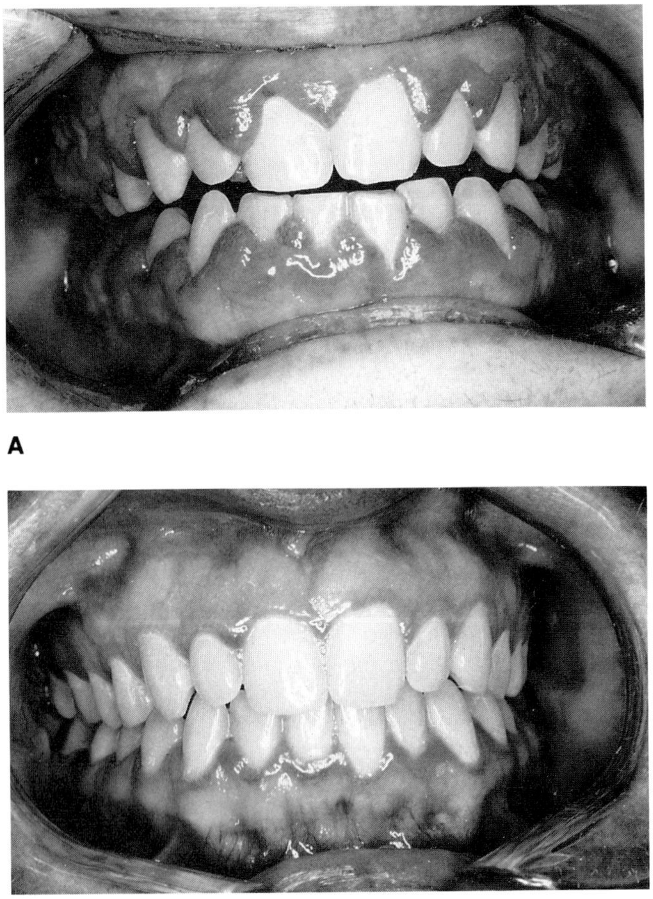

A

B

Fig. 8-2. Acute myelogenous leukemia first indicated by oral signs and symptoms of gingival swelling and pain in a 26-year-old woman. **A,** Gingival swelling and erythema accompanied by pain and slight bleeding had been noticed for 3 months. The patient also complained of malaise, fever, and slight weight loss. Laboratory findings included the following: white blood cells 80,000/mm^3, hemoglobin 9.2 g/100 ml, scarcity of platelets, and many immature cells in the monocyte series. **B,** Six months after chemotherapy and a bone marrow transplant (sister donor) the patient was without evidence of active leukemia and her gingiva appeared almost normal.

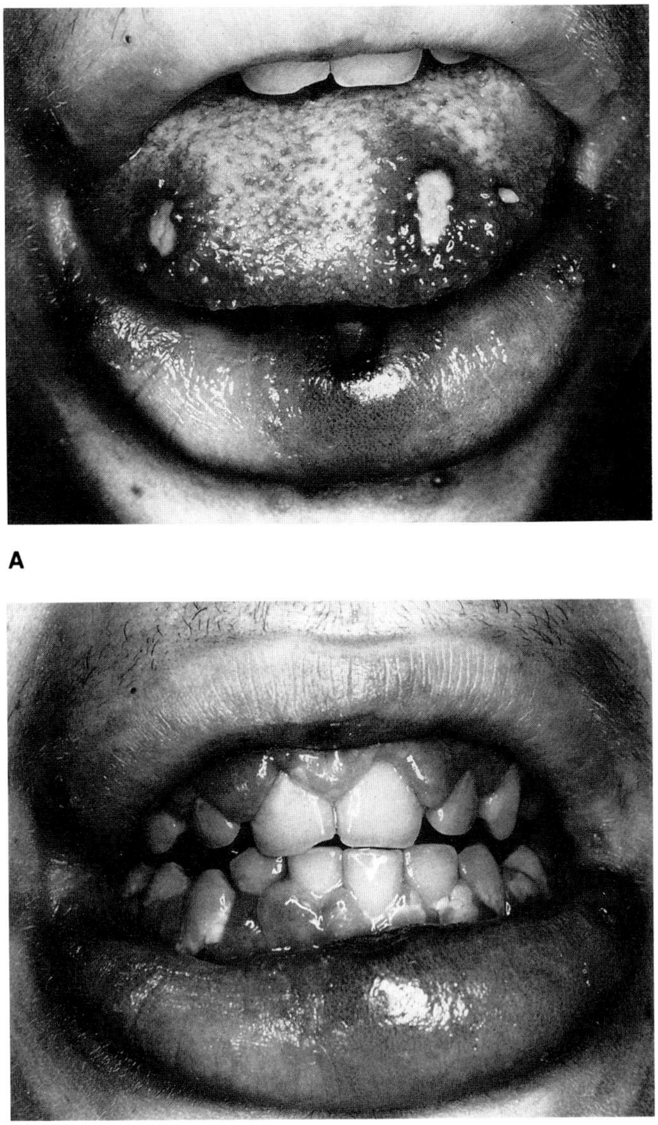

A

B

Fig. 8-3. Oral ulcerations and edema in a 16-year-old boy with leukemia being treated by chemotherapy. **A,** Ulcers on tongue and lip are manifestations of secondary infection, not leukemic infiltrates. **B,** Edema of gingiva and lip.

Once a diagnosis of leukemia has been made, it is extremely important to keep patients free from oral foci of infection and pain. In addition to the oral complications associated with the disease process, antileukemic therapy can also cause significant oral problems. The chemotherapeutic agents utilized to eradicate abnormal white-cell production also affect normal cells, particularly those that have relatively high turnover rates, such as those of the bone marrow and the gastrointestinal and oral epithelial tissues. The direct effect of therapy on the oral tissues can result in thinning and ulceration of the tissues, often referred to as mucositis (Fig. 8-3), as well as salivary gland[12,13] and taste dysfunction. The oral ulcerations may be due to direct cellular cytotoxicity from the chemotherapeutic agents, to increased susceptibility to microorganisms owing to neutropenia, to trauma, or to a combination of these factors.

It is important to realize that the ability of oral tissues to resist trauma and to repair themselves is significantly compromised, and even irritation from eating and talking can lead to mucosal breakdown. Therapy will further induce myelosuppression, leukopenia, and thrombocytopenia, and patients will become even more susceptible to infection and bleeding.[14–19]

The increased risk of infection is particularly important—not only can periodontal and dental infections have serious consequences, but the oral cavity can be the site of infections caused by viruses, fungi, and acquired bacterial pathogens. The reactivation of herpes-family viruses[20,21] such as herpes simplex I and *Varicella zoster*, can cause significant mucosal breakdown, pain, hemorrhage, and increase the risk of secondary infection. Fungal infections, caused by such organisms as Candida and Aspergillus species, in addition to producing local disease, can spread systemically and cause serious infections.[22–25] Bacterial infections can be caused by organisms normally found in the oral cavity, as well as by a number of opportunistic pathogens such as *Pseudomonas, Klebsiella, Serratia, Escherichia,* and other gram-negative bacteria.[26–28] Identification of the source of infection and appropriate selection of antimicrobial agent(s) are critical to effective management.

Marrow transplantation is associated with frequent and significant oral and head and neck complications.[29] High doses of chemotherapeutic agents, with or without total body irradiation and, occasionally, additional lymphoid irradiation, can result in severe oral and pharyngeal mucositis, pain, infections, and hemorrhage. An additional complication of marrow transplantation is graft-versus-host disease (GVHD) which results from the reaction of donor T-lymphocytes against host antigens.[30,31] The oral cavity can be the site of both acute and chronic GVHD.

Routine oral care plays an important role in maintaining oral health and preventing oral infections and bleeding. Efforts should be directed at effective and atraumatic plaque removal techniques, for example, frequent rinsing with chemotherapeutic mouth rinses (e.g. Peridex, Listerine) or with a normal saline solution, with or without sodium bicarbonate added (3/4 tsp. salt in one quart of water and 2 tsp. sodium bicarbonate, 8–16 oz. rinsed, gargled, then emptied out every 1 to 4 hrs. as needed). When oral pain increases, topical anesthetics (such as 2% viscous xylocaine) and rinsing with coating agents (such as aluminum hydroxide, milk of magnesia, kaolin suspension) can provide temporary help. Water rinses or sips, artificial salivas, and water-soluble lubricants (glycerol) provide temporary symptomatic relief of xerostomia in some patients.

Children who receive chemotherapy (and/or radiation therapy to the jaws) when permanent teeth are developing may suffer a number of abnormalities involving teeth and jaws: complete or partial dental agenesis, root malformation, and maldevelopment of jaws.[32]

LEUKOPENIA

Leukopenia, a deficiency in the number of white blood cells, may occur initially in certain forms of leukemia and lymphoma, and it commonly occurs in response to immunosuppressive drugs used for control of disease. Patients with leukopenia are less able to cope with infection and therefore require special precautions against infectious agents.[17,33,34]

Classification and Findings

The leukopenias may be classified in different ways. The relative or absolute reduction of polymorphonuclear leukocytes (neutrophils) is known as *neutropenia*. Suppression of all the granulocytes is known as *granulocytopenia* or *agranulocytosis*. In agranulocytosis, the lymphocytes and monocytes may also be slightly reduced. Marked suppression of all the white cells, along with red blood cells, is termed *pancytopenia*.

Depending on the cause of the leukopenia, the onset of clinical signs and symptoms can be variable. Most patients will complain of increasing weakness and malaise and demonstrate chills and fevers. These individuals are also susceptible to the spread of infection. Mouth and oropharyngeal ulcerations will frequently occur and be associated with pain (Fig. 8-4). The pathogenesis of these lesions is thought to be due to a poor response to trauma, allowing local and acquired bacterial flora to set up infections. This reaction can be further intensified in instances where patients are receiving cancer chemotherapeutic agents.

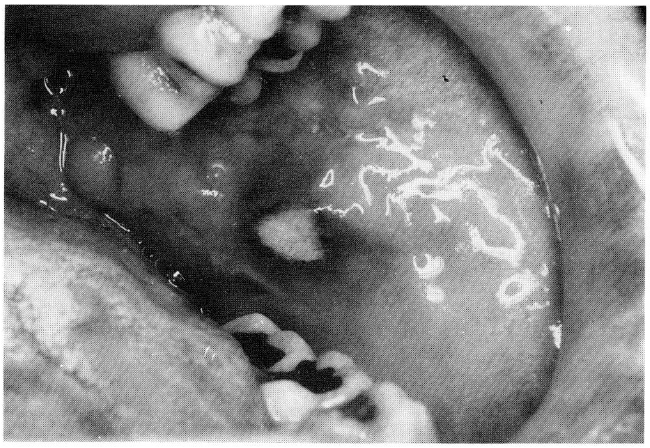

A

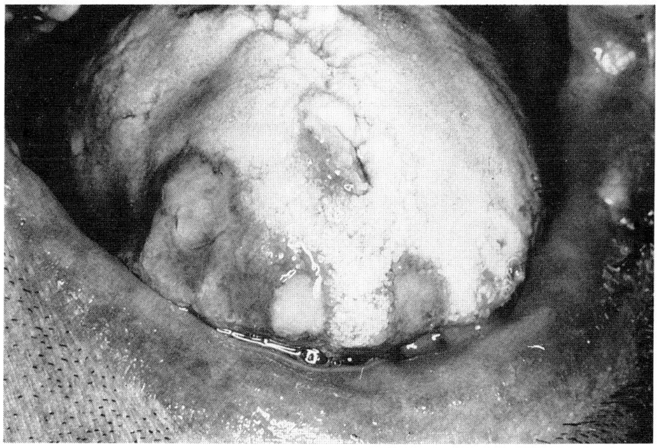

B

Fig. 8-4. Oral ulcerations in patients with leukopenia. Ulcers are due to epithelial breakdown and poor resistance to infection. **A,** Buccal ulcer in patient with lymphoma being treated with cytotoxic agents. Patient's white blood count was less than 500. **B,** Multiple tongue ulcers in leukemic patient whose white blood count was less than 1,000. Ulcers healed after blood transfusion raised white count to nearly 5,000.

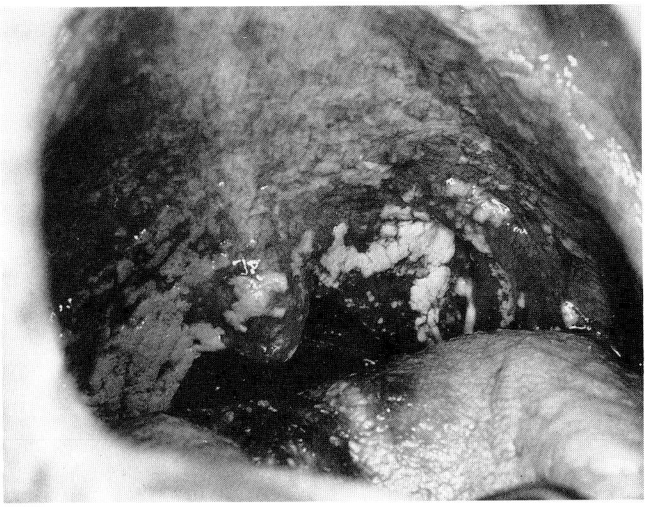

Fig. 8-5. Widespread oropharyngeal candidiasis in leukemic patient, secondary to partial xerostomia and immunosuppression caused by multiple drug therapy.

In view of the poor resistance in these patients, it is reasonable to expect a high risk of septicemia and a downhill course unless the leukopenia can be reversed. Persons with leukopenia are also prone to oral fungal (candidiasis, Fig. 8-5) and viral (herpes family, Fig. 8-6) infections which may further complicate their diagnosis and management. The viral infections could be in the form of herpes simplex gingivostomatitis, a cold sore, or varicella zoster (shingles).

Diagnosis and Prognosis

The diagnosis of leukopenia can be made from the complete blood count, based on the total number of white cells as well as the relative cell counts from the differential smear. Although the red cells are generally not affected, in drug-induced leukopenias the platelets are usually reduced or altered, resulting in bleeding problems. When there are associated infections, the sedimentation rates also rise. If causative factors can be corrected or, in the case of chemotherapy-induced leukopenia, once the drug is withdrawn, the subsequent recovery of the myeloid stem cells will lead to recovery and to a remission of clinical signs and symptoms. Most severe oral problems occur when the total white blood cell count drops below 2000 per mm^3 from normal values above 5000 mm^3.

The neutropenia and thrombocytopenia place these patients at risk for dental procedures, and consultation with the physician is recommended before performing any procedure. Often temporary withdrawal of the chemotherapeutic agent is required to increase the blood count. With or without this step, antibiotic coverage is recommended when a possible bacteremia is anticipated, and precautions should be taken against bleeding. It is important to realize that the least invasive means of managing a dental problem is usually indicated in these instances. Sometimes blood transfusions are indicated.

The patient's hematologic status often determines the extent of dental care that can be carried out. Some patients with leukemia in clinical remission (normal peripheral blood counts, clinically healthy) can receive comprehensive dental care with excellent tolerance; however, the recommended precautions should still be taken since the basic ability of these patients to cope with infection is still diminished. Patients in complete remission (normal marrow) are often considered and treated as normal.

Leukemic infiltrations may occur in the region of the head and neck and can be painful.[35] Appearances are variable and can resemble purpuric lesions, hemangiomas, and granulomas (Fig. 8-7). Chemotherapy will usually control these infiltrates, however resistant cases can be controlled with low-dose radiation therapy.

Oral candidal infections are relatively common in patients with leukemia. These infections are nurtured by antibiotic drugs, immunosuppression, and anemia. Often infections cannot be controlled until the patient's hematologic recovery (especially absolute neutrophils) is achieved. As the appropriate antifungal therapy is utilized and the drugs that increase the risk of fungal infections are discontinued, adequate nutrition and good oral hygiene can also be maintained.

The selection of an appropriate antifungal drug depends not only on the effectiveness of the agent against candidal infection, but also upon the mode of application and the patient's compliance with the agent. If an agent burns or stings or causes nausea and vomiting, it is less likely that the patient will continue the medication as prescribed. Patients who become immunosuppressed, especially when they also receive systemic antibiotics, will generally demonstrate a significant increase in oral colonization by candida. It has been demonstrated that it is not possible to prevent oral colonization completely in these patients by selective use of topical oral antifungals.[22,36,37] Topical antifungal forms include clotrimazole tablets and nystatin oral suspension, troches, or pastilles. Systemic therapy includes ketoconazole tablets to be swallowed or a solution used intravenously, and amphotericin B given intravenously. Hydrogen peroxide-saline mouth rinses (equal parts 3% hydrogen peroxide and normal saline) and chlorhexidine[38] can be effective against mild cases, although they can be irritating when mucositis is present. Patients must be monitored carefully for response to therapy because of variable agent effectiveness.

Viral infections are responsible for significant morbidity in patients who are immunosuppressed due to either underlying disease or chemotherapy (Fig. 8-6).[39–42] The reactivation of herpes simplex virus (HSV) when there is a deficiency in cellular immunity can result in severe oral lesions. The ulcerations can become very large, painful, and may persist for as long as the patient is immunocompromised or until appropriate therapy is instituted. Lesions caused by varicella zoster virus (VZV), cytomegalovirus (CMV), adenovirus, and coxsackieviruses are occasionally seen.

Acyclovir is used both prophylactically and therapeutically for HSV and VZV infections.[43–45] Either the oral capsules or the parenteral form has been used to prevent reactivation of HSV in patients previously demonstrated to be seropositive. True primary HSV infections in these patients is rare. In patients with mild lesions, treatment can often be supportive and palliative. However, in severely compromised patients or in patients with more extensive disease, the parenteral route or very high per oral dosages is preferred.

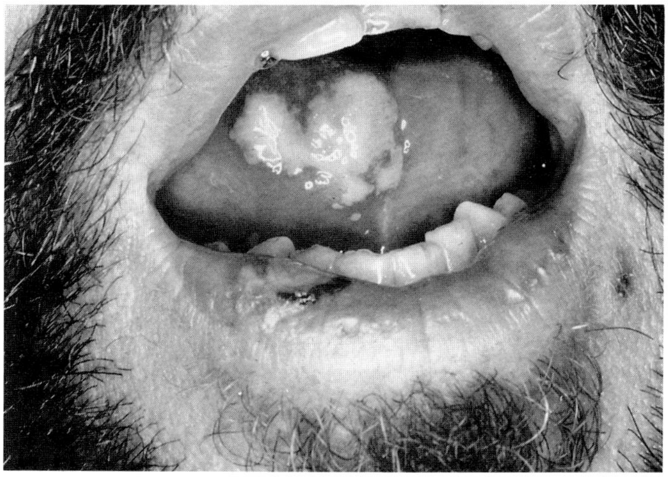

A

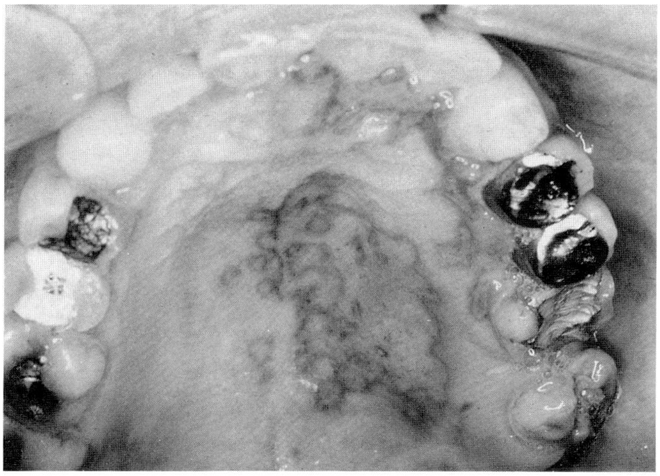

B

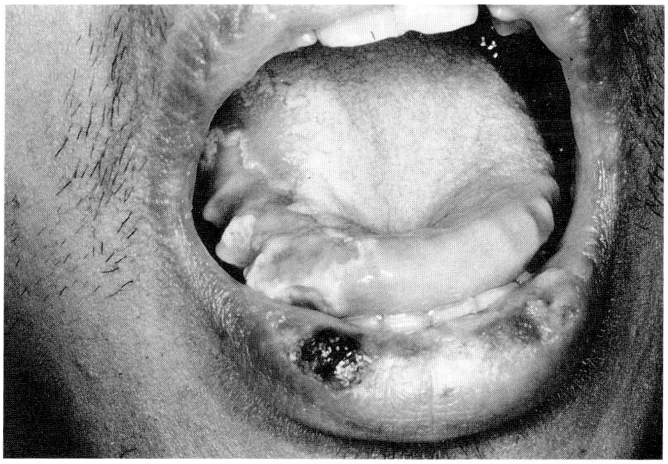

C

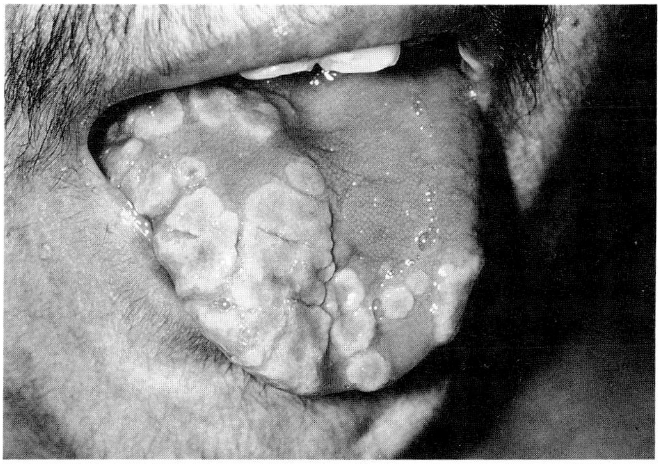

D

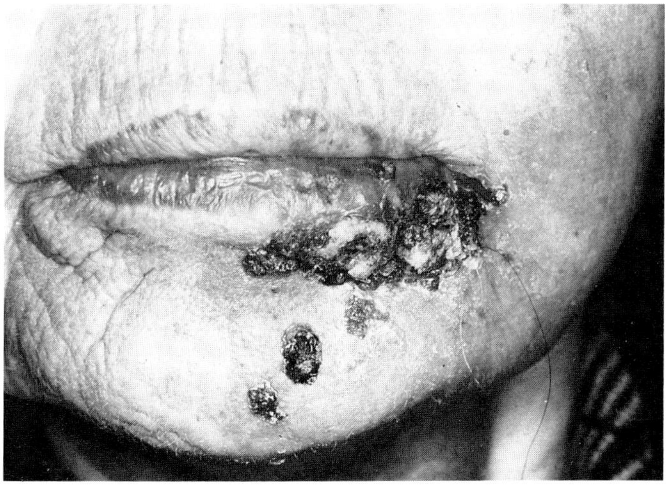

E

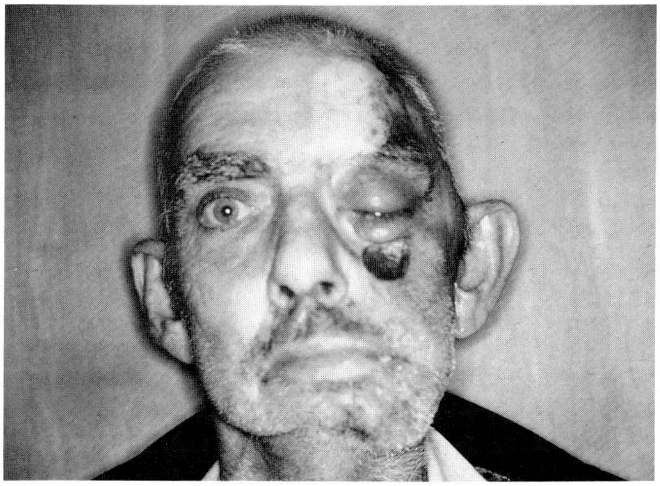

F

Fig 8-6. Herpes family virus infections in immunosuppressed patients. **A,** Recurrent herpes simplex infections of lip and tongue from reactivated virus. **B,** Recurrent herpes simplex infection of palate, fifth day. **C,** Primary herpetic gingivostomatitis in a leukemic patient being controlled with periodic chemotherapy, seventh day. **D,** Primary herpetic gingivostomatitis in an immunosuppressed kidney transplant patient, demonstrating the variety of clinical expressions. **E,** Varicella zoster (shingles) in an immunosuppressed lymphoma patient. Note unilateral distribution of the painful ulcerations. **F,** Severe varicella zoster in a leukemic patient undergoing induction therapy.

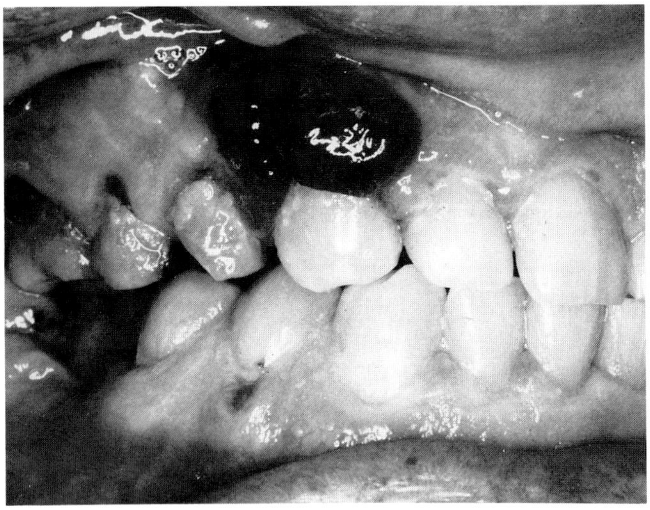

A

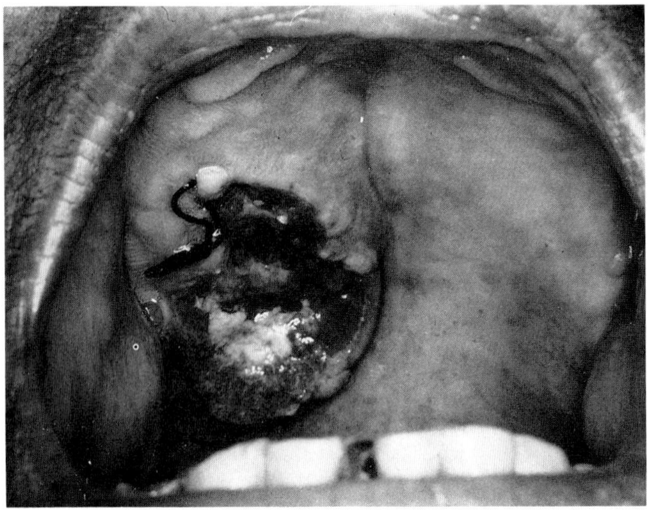

B

Fig. 8-7. Leukemic infiltrates in the mouth. These infiltrates are an accumulation of immature cells similar to those found in the marrow. **A,** Mildly symptomatic infiltrate of maxillary gingiva, which bled in response to mild irritation. **B,** Large leukemic infiltrate in the palate of patient with chronic lymphocytic leukemia. Lesion was controlled by a combination of chemotherapy and localized irradiation (600 cGy in two treatments).

MALIGNANT LYMPHOMAS

The term malignant lymphoma refers to a number of clinically related disorders caused by proliferation of the lymphoreticular system. Although these diseases usually present with lymphadenopathy or splenomegaly, extranodal sites, including the gingiva and other oral tissues, can be involved and cause clinical symptoms. The diseases to be considered here are Hodgkin's disease, non-Hodgkin's lymphomas, Burkitt's lymphoma, multiple myeloma, and mycosis fungoides.

HODGKIN'S DISEASE

Hodgkin's disease is a lymphoproliferative disorder.[46] The diagnosis is based on the histologic presence of the multinucleated Reed-Sternberg giant cells. At the present time there are no firm etiologic leads, and evidence of a genetic tendency is scant. There is a characteristic bimodal age-and-incidence curve with one peak in early adult life and a second sustained increase from the fifth decade. Hodgkin's disease is seen in all races. It afflicts about 7,400 Americans each year and kills approximately 1,500.

SIGNS AND SYMPTOMS

Complaints may include fever (temperatures greater than 38° C.), unexplained weight loss, excessive sweating, pruritus, and fatigue. However, the most important sign is lymph-node swelling, with most patients presenting with adenopathy in the supraclavicular or cervical area. While rare, oral and nasopharyngeal lesions have been reported.[47] The lymphadenopathy is in response to abnormal intranodal proliferation of lymphocytes, histiocytes, eosinophils, and the Reed-Sternberg giant cells (Fig. 8-8). Diagnosis is made by biopsy.

PATHOGENESIS, TREATMENT, AND SURVIVAL

Hodgkin's disease appears to start in regional lymph nodes and spreads in a somewhat unpredictable but orderly way as it progresses. Survival times vary enormously, from months to many, many years. The overall expected 5-year-survival rate is about 50 to 60%. Depending upon the staging, treatment ranges from minimal supportive care to intensive combinations of radiation and chemotherapy. Remissions and flares are not uncommon. The use of marrow transplantation to control otherwise incurable disease is meeting with increasing success.[48] There are complications with treatment, one of which is the risk of developing acute leukemia after combined-modality treatment. Patients receiving chemotherapy

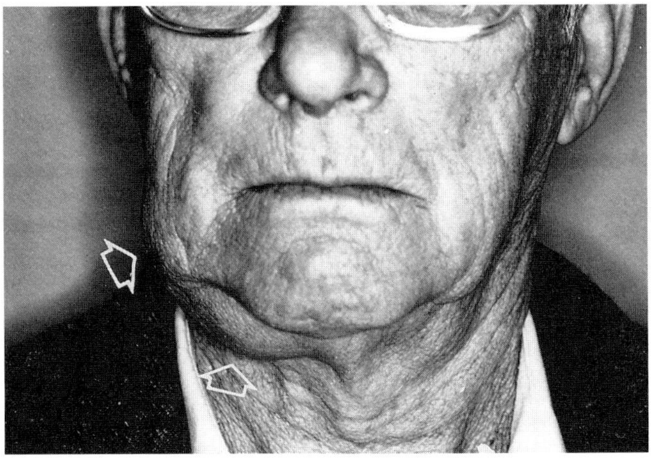

Fig. 8-8. Submandibular swelling (arrows) in patient with Hodgkin's disease. Evaluation showed the mass to be a tumor-filled lymph node that was the first clinical manifestation of widespread Hodgkin's lymphoma.

for Hodgkin's disease can demonstrate complications that are similar to those of patients receiving chemotherapy for leukemia, which include mucositis, severe infections, and inflammation.[49]

DENTAL IMPLICATIONS

The dentist becomes involved with Hodgkin's disease in two ways. First, the initial signs usually include cervical lymphadenopathy with associated symptoms. Because of the focal and orderly spread of this disease, the head and neck may be the only area involved early in the disease and possibly for a long time. Therefore, careful evaluation of persistent lymphadenopathy is important in the early recognition of this condition and in accelerating the proper staging and treatment.

Second, these patients have impaired immunity and thus require optimal oral health to keep their teeth and periodontal structures from acting as foci for infection. Bacteremias may be acute or chronic and greatly worsen a patient's condition, even to the point of threatening life. In addition, immunosuppression can be worsened by radiation or chemotherapeutic management. Therefore, the same precautions regarding anemia, thrombocytopenia, and neutropenia apply to patients with Hodgkin's disease that apply to patients with leukemia.

Those patients receiving head and neck radiotherapy to cervical lymph nodes usually will have radiation fields that include the salivary glands. The resulting xerostomia can lead to significant problems with dental caries and associated dental disease.[50]

NON-HODGKIN'S LYMPHOMA

Non-Hodgkin's lymphoma (NHL) represents a heterogeneous group of malignant disorders of lymphoid derivation that can range from diseases that are relatively indolent to some that are very aggressive. About 35,000 new cases of NHL are diagnosed each year in the United States. The etiology of these lymphomas remains unknown, although radiation and immune deficiencies have been implicated as associated factors. An increased incidence of NHL has been observed in survivors of Hiroshima, in organ transplant recipients undergoing immunosuppressive therapy, and in patients with immune deficiency syndromes. NHL is the second most common, as well as fastest increasing malignancy associated with AIDS-virus (HIV) infection.[51,52] Overall, the survival rate for persons with NHL is lower than that of Hodgkin's disease with a 5-year-survival rate of 30 to 40%. In HIV-infected patients it is invariably fatal.

CLINICAL FEATURES

NHL occurs in people of all races and in all age groups, arising in any lymphoid aggregate. Lymphadenopathy, often painful, is the usual initial finding and very frequently occurs in the head and neck area (Fig. 8-9). The early clinical signs and symptoms of NHL are similar to those in Hodgkin's disease, including malaise, fever, weight loss, and sweating. The diagnosis is made by biopsy.

Extranodal disease occurs in about 25% of patients with NHL. The two most common sites are the stomach and the head and neck region. In the head and neck region, intraoral NHL is uncommon, occurring most frequently in older persons.[53–56] When NHL occurs as localized extranodal involvement of the head and neck, nearly three-fourths involve Waldeyers's ring (nasopharynx) and one-fourth involve the paranasal sinuses. The most frequent oral sites are the soft and hard palate (Fig. 8-10). The involved lymphoid aggregate may be an extension from the nasopharynx or associated with lymphocytic infiltrates involving minor salivary glands.

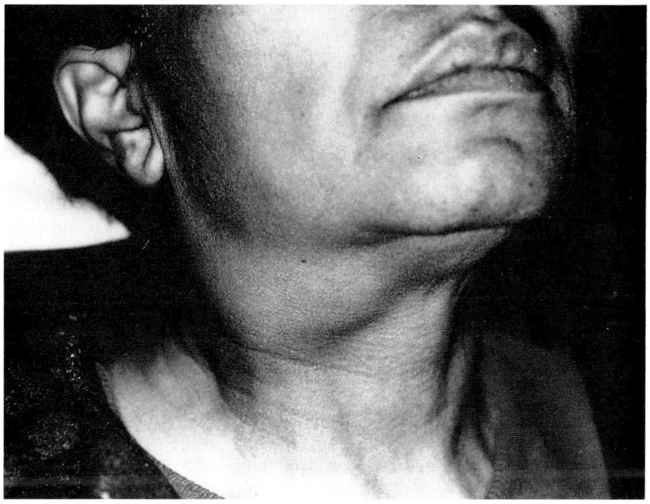

Fig. 8-9. Cervical lymphadenopathy caused by non-Hodgkin's lymphoma. Diagnosis was made by needle biopsy after dental disease was ruled out as the cause of the asymptomatic mass, which had been noticed for about 3 weeks. Lymphoma work-up revealed widespread disease.

CLASSIFICATION

Unlike Hodgkin's disease, the malignant lymphomas are usually multifocal, even from the beginning. Staging depends upon the cell morphology and extensiveness of disease. The classification of malignant lymphomas is complex, involving diffuse and nodular forms. In turn, these forms are characterized by the cell types: well-differentiated versus poorly differentiated lymphocytes and/or histiocytes, and the undifferentiated or stem cell.

TREATMENT

Treatment includes the use of radiation therapy and combinations of chemotherapeutic agents.[57] These tumors are usually radiosensitive. Surgery is often used in exploring the extent of disease, establishing a diagnosis, and reducing tumor mass to aid treatment or restore function. Marrow transplantation is utilized at times to treat patients with resistant disease.[9,58] Survival is variable, but overall control is poor because of the usually widespread nature of the malignant process.

Extranodal oropharyngeal lymphoproliferative disease appears to have a poor prognosis. Even solitary lesions designated as "benign lymphoproliferative disease" often have a tendency to demonstrate malignant behavior eventually (Fig. 8-11). Therefore, treatment should tend to be aggressive.

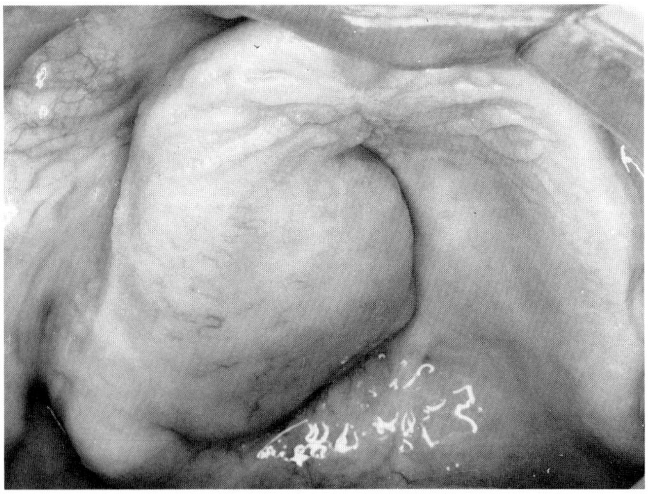

A

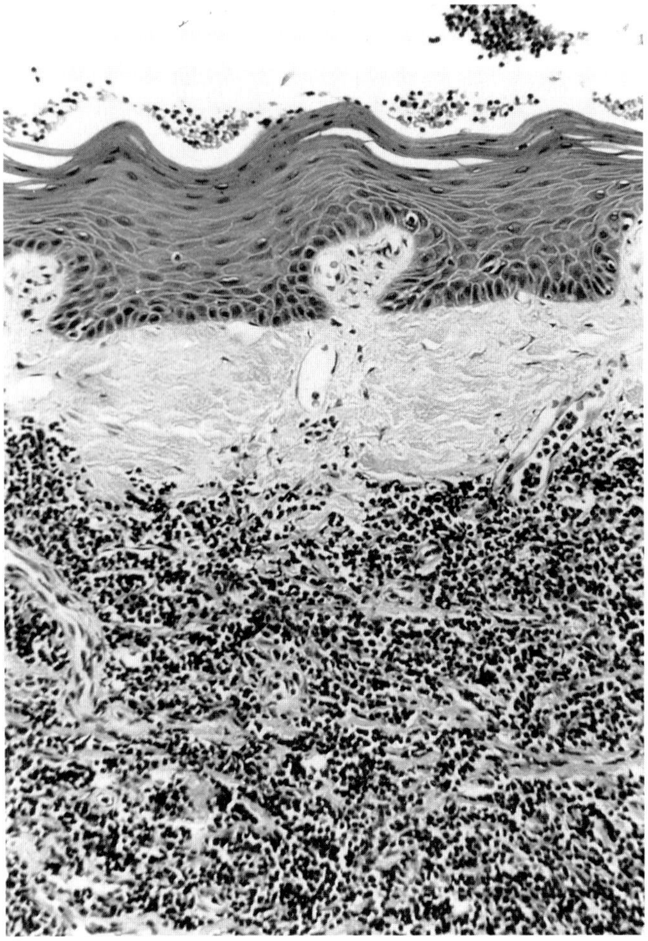

B

Fig. 8-10. Malignant lymphoma in the palate. Patient's only complaint was that this swelling of about 3 months' duration made her denture unstable. **A,** Rubbery, firm palatal swelling. **B,** Biopsy revealed malignant lymphocytic cellular infiltrate under normal-appearing epithelium.

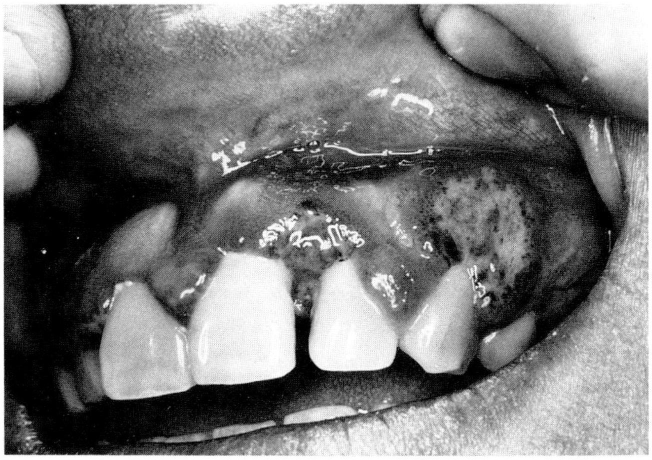

A

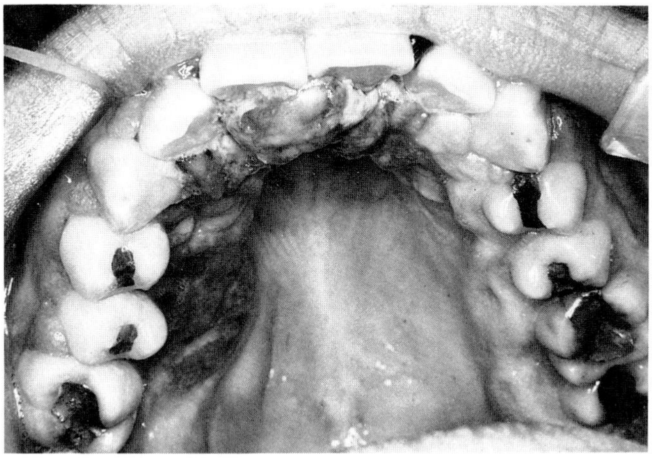

B

Fig. 8-11. Extranodal lymphoproliferative disease in the mouth. This 20-year-old woman had a 3-month history of progressive, painful, necrotic gingivitis involving the upper and lower gingiva. **A,** Buccal maxillary gingiva. **B,** Lingual maxillary gingiva. Biopsy revealed cellular infiltrate that was diagnosed as atypical lymphoreticular proliferation consistent with a variant of malignant lymphoma. Patient was successfully treated by local irradiation.

DENTAL MANAGEMENT

The dentist may be involved in the early diagnosis because of symptomatic or asymptomatic masses in the head and neck area.[59–64] Frequently the signs are not impressive and are thought to be benign because the masses may be slow-growing, small, and not bothersome to the patient. However, for any oral growth that does not resolve in a reasonable period of time, a biopsy should be considered. If a cervical mass persists and no oral cause can be found, the patient should be referred to a physician.

Since many NHL patients have had head and neck irradiation, chemotherapy, or both, precautions against oral sepsis and bleeding are critical. Because the radiation used rarely exceeds 6000 cGy, osteoradionecrosis is not a common complication. Xerostomia is somewhat more common and demands special attention to oral hygiene, saliva stimulants and substitutes, fluoride mouth rinses or applications, and diet. (See Chapter 6.) A burning sensation of the mouth (stomatopyrosis), if present, may be caused by drug toxicity, xerostomia, candidiasis, or anemia.

MULTIPLE MYELOMA

Multiple myeloma, a plasma-cell dyscrasia, occurs with equal frequency in men and women,[65,66] and it rarely occurs in patients under the age of 40 years. Currently in the United States there are almost 12,000 new cases each year. The average survival time from diagnosis is poor—approximately two years.

The plasma or myeloma cells, specialized for production of immunoglobulin, proliferate to an abnormally great degree in bone. This leads to marrow replacement, anemia, decalcification, and hypercalcemia. It can also lead to significant complications late in disease, including osteoporosis, multiple fractures, and diffuse pain. The inadequate production of blood cells and platelets lead to leukopenia and thrombocytopenia. In addition, normal immunoglobulin production is decreased, creating in these patients a susceptibility to infection which is exacerbated in those who have neutropenia.

The early signs and symptoms of myeloma include weakness, weight loss, recurrent infections, bone pain, and anemia. As marrow involvement progresses, pancytopenia can be noted with expected complications of immunodeficiency and hemorrhage. The dentist is very seldom involved with initial diagnosis.

Jaw lesions, when they do occur, are usually found in the mandible and tend to be asymptomatic. If they are found by the dentist they usually are chance findings.[67] Although extramedullary solitary plasmacytomas can occur in the oropharynx, these lesions are not related to generalized myeloma.[68]

Partial thromboplastin and prothrombin times may be prolonged and may cause oral purpuric lesions and gingival bleeding. When jaw bones are involved, the lesions can appear rounded, punched out, or mottled (Fig. 8-12). Cases where these lesions have mimicked periapical disease have been reported. In some cases amyloid protein will form in oral mucosa, primarily tongue or gingiva, causing swelling, induration, and pain.[69] Amyloid protein can be identified by biopsy and special stains.

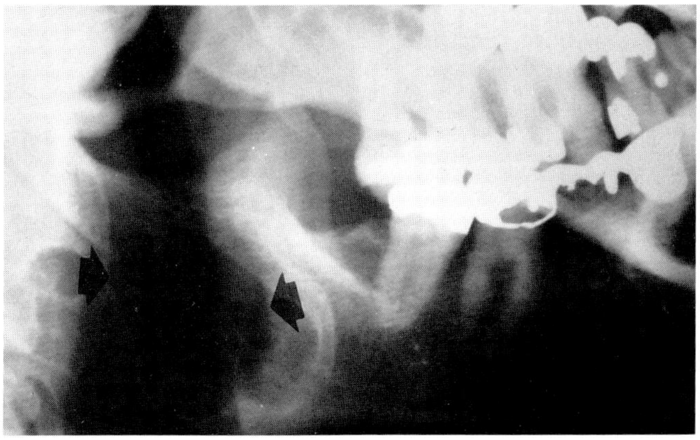

Fig. 8-12. Jawbone lesion in multiple myeloma. Patient with diagnosed multiple myeloma complained of mandibular pain. Radiograph revealed large "punched-out" (arrows) lesion of the right mandibular ramus that proved to be a myeloma infiltrate.

The diagnosis of multiple myeloma is made through assessing the clinical presentation of the patient, bone marrow morphologic findings, and measurements to detect excessive production of immunoglobulin molecules. The primary therapy for multiple myeloma is chemotherapy, with radiation therapy reserved for palliation of painful bony lesions. Results from marrow transplantation have not been encouraging to date.

There are a number of significant complications associated with the myeloma patient that can influence dental treatment. These include diminished resistance to infection, bleeding, anemia, hyperviscosity of blood, and chronic renal failure.[70] Since therapy induces temporary remission for about half of patients and long-term survivals are not common, dental treatment planning should be conservative.

BURKITT'S LYMPHOMA

An unusual type of cancer occurs in a narrow zone across Central Africa, Burkitt's lymphoma.[71] A characteristic feature is enlargement of jaw bones caused by proliferating tumor cells (Fig. 8-13). This disease was first thought to be

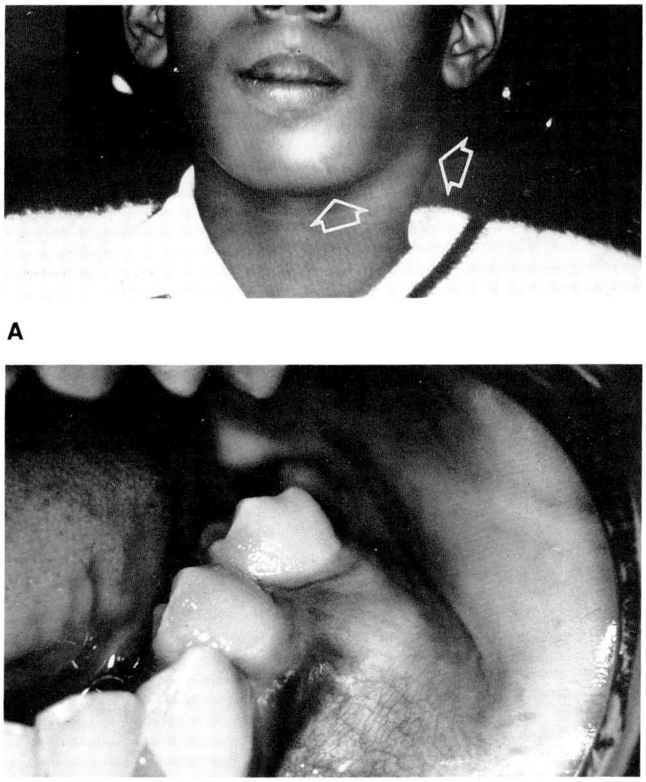

A

B

Fig. 8-13. Jawbone enlargement in Burkitt's lymphoma. Patient, a 13-year-old black boy born and raised in California, had pain and swelling in left jaw. **A,** Mandibular swelling and involved lymph node (arrows). **B,** Mandibular swelling displaced two bicuspids and caused moderate pain. Biopsy from the mass indicated Burkitt's lymphoma.

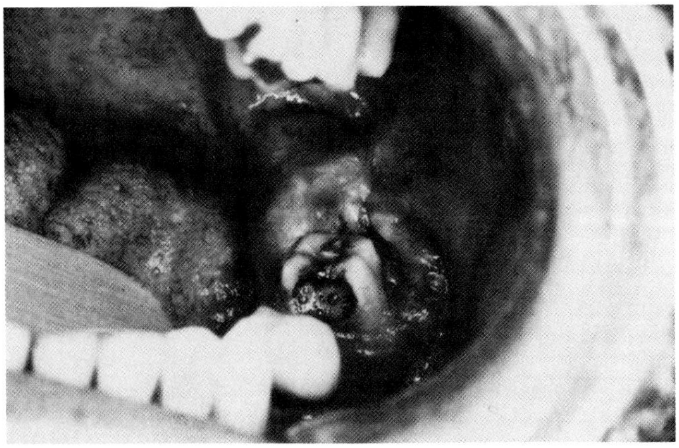

Fig. 8-14. Burkitt's lymphoma in a 26-year-old homosexual man. This retromolar swelling, extending to and involving the molar, was at first thought to be infection from an abscessed tooth. The patient died 4 months later from widespread lymphoma.

limited to African children, but subsequent reports have emphasized its worldwide distribution.[72–74]

Studies have identified Epstein-Barr virus (EBV) particles in cells cultured from Burkitt's tumor. In addition, high levels of antibodies to the EBV are found in all African children with Burkitt's lymphoma, but in only half of normal African children. American children with the disease also have demonstrated elevated levels of EBV antibody as compared with controls. Burkitt's lymphoma is routinely associated with cytogenetic abnormalities demonstrating several chromosome translocations.

Diagnosis is based on a characteristic microscopic pattern of B-cell lymphoid proliferation with a high mitotic count and a "starry-sky" pattern. Treatment consists of radiation and chemotherapy. The prognosis varies, depending upon stage and type of disease. The American type, which demonstrates more frequent initial involvement of lymph nodes and bone marrow, has a worse prognosis than the African form, which most frequently presents in the jaws. A Burkitt's-type lymphoma, which has become an increasing complication and cause of death in AIDS (Fig. 8-14), is thought to be associated with the interplay of the AIDS-related retrovirus and EBV.

MYCOSIS FUNGOIDES

Mycosis fungoides (MF), an uncommon malignant lymphoma, has the ability to undergo transition to other types of malignant lymphoma. MF appears to arise in the skin and eventually spreads into other organs.[75] The basic cause of MF is unknown, but the lesions are due to the proliferation of T-lymphocytes. Although MF may develop in young adults, most cases begin in the fifth decade of life. It is estimated that about 2,000 new cases develop each year in the United States. For unknown reasons, male victims outnumber female by about a 2:1 ratio. The disease occurs in all races. Its duration can be as short as one year or it may last for several decades, although the median survival from the time of diagnosis is less than five years.

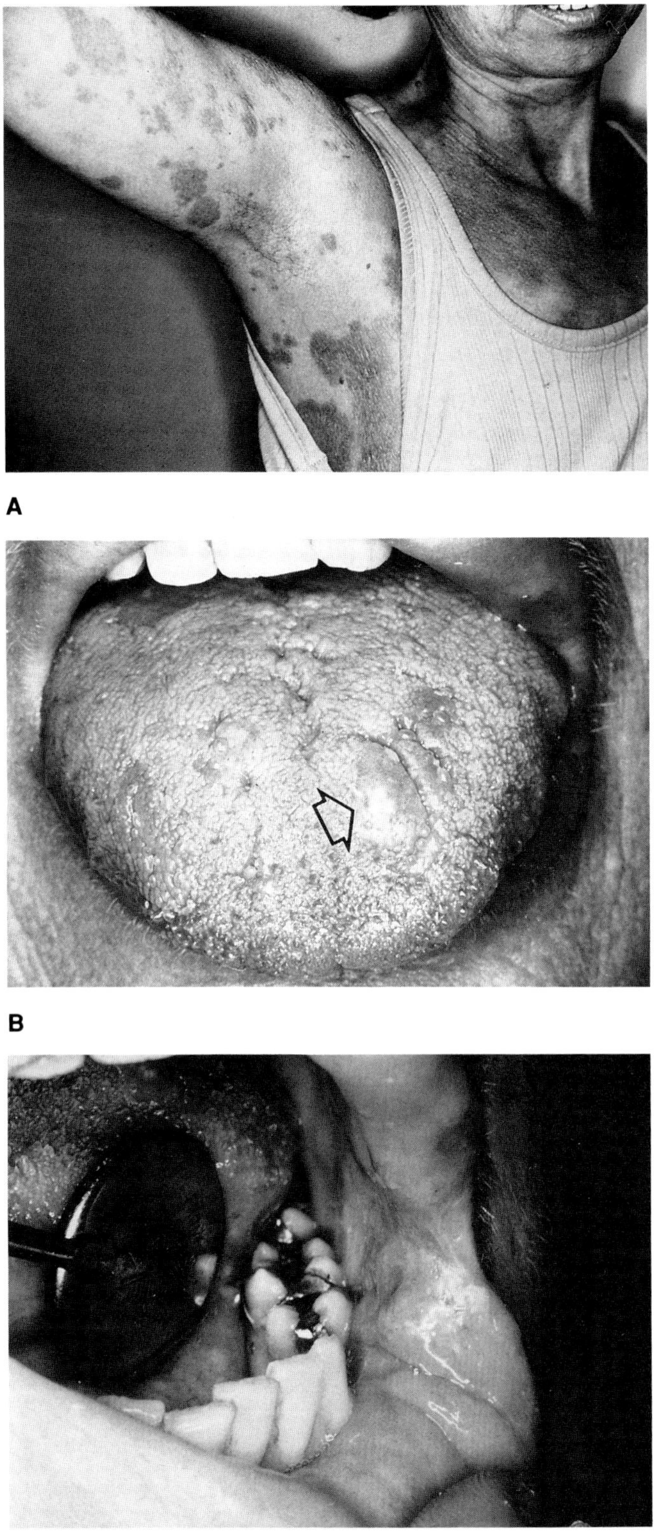

A

B

C

Fig. 8-15. Manifestations of mycosis fungoides. Patient was referred for evaluation of painful oral lesions. **A,** Widespread skin manifestations. **B,** Painful nodules on tongue (arrow) and **C,** Labial mucosa. Biopsy confirmed this was a lymphomatous infiltrate of mycosis fungoides, and the lesion was treated successfully by irradiation. Patient eventually died of her disease.

The initial skin manifestations of MF are somewhat nonspecific and are usually classified initially as benign dermatoses (Fig. 8-15). The lesions can appear as erythematous, eczematous, and psoriasiform lesions, usually associated with intense pruritus. Subsequently, MF progresses to infiltrated plaque and tumor phases.

Treatment is primarily by the use of radiation and chemotherapeutic agents. When the diagnosis is established in the early phases of the disease, survival time and chances for control are improved.[76] Pain, infection, cachexia, and despair often minimize the quality of life. Tumors of MF can occur in the mouth, and they are diagnosed by biopsy (Fig. 8-15).[77] While the oral manifestations can usually be controlled by radiation, other progressive aspects of the disease continue.

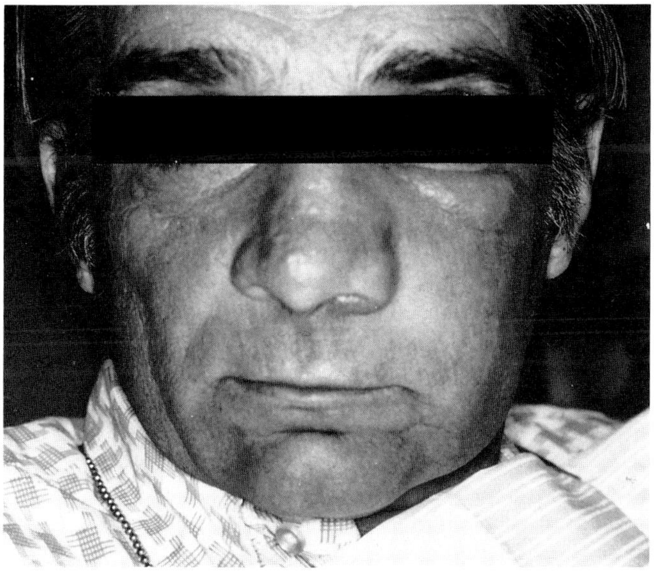

A

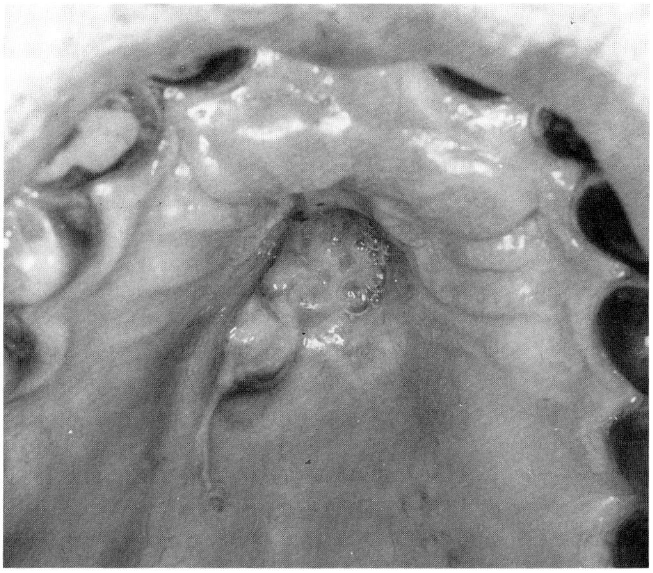

B

Fig. 8-16. Midline granuloma. This lesion occasionally transforms into or is associated with lymphoma. **A,** Left facial and nasal swelling in 48-year-old patient. **B,** Large, necrotic, foul-smelling ulcer observed in hard palate. Biopsy showed this to be consistent with a midline granuloma. Moderate-dose radiation controlled lesion.

MIDLINE "NONHEALING" GRANULOMA

The midline granuloma is considered under lymphoproliferative disorders because occasionally a lesion transforms into a lymphoma or is associated with a lymphomatous process.[78] This painful lesion of sudden onset is frequently manifested initially as a necrotic, progressive ulceration of the palatal or oropharyngeal mucosa (Fig. 8-16). Palatal bone and nasal cartilage are often involved. While this lesion mimics a malignancy or acute infection, biopsy specimens characteristically show nonspecific, benign inflammation and ulceration. These lesions are not self-limiting, and low-dose radiation is used for control. Clinically it is difficult to differentiate this disease from Wegener's granulomatosis, a more generalized disease that responds to chemotherapy.[79]

REFERENCES

1. Rinsky RA, Smith AB, Hornung R et al: Benzene and leukemia: An epidemiologic risk assessment. *N Engl J Med* 316:1044, 1987.
2. Miller KB, Rosenthal DS et al: Leukemia. In B. Cady (ed), *Cancer Manual*. Boston: American Cancer Society, 1986, p.318.
3. Gallo RC: The first human retrovirus. *Sci Am* 255:88, 1986.
4. Michaud M, Baehner RL, Bixler D et al: Oral manifestations of acute leukemia in children. *J Am Dent Assoc* 95:1145, 1977.
5. Stafford R, Sonis S, Lockhart P et al: Oral pathoses as diagnostic indicators in leukemia. *Oral Surg Oral Med Oral Pathol* 50:134, 1980.
6. Barrett AP: Oral changes as initial diagnostic indicators in acute leukemia. *J Oral Med* 41:234, 1986.
7. Epstein JB, Priddy RW, Sparling T et al: Oral manifestations in myelodysplastic syndrome. *Oral Surg Oral Med Oral Pathol* 61:466, 1986.
8. Doney KC, Buckner CD: Bone marrow transplantation: Overview. *Plasma Ther Transfusion Technol* 6:149, 1985.
9. Thomas ED: High-dose therapy and bone marrow transplantation. *Semin Oncol* 12:15, 1985.
10. Mayer RJ: Allogeneic transplantation versus intensive chemotherapy in first-remission acute leukemia: Is there a "best choice?" *J Clin Oncol* 6:1532, 1988.
11. Fefer A, Cliff RA, Thomas ED: Allogeneic marrow transplantation for chronic granulocytic leukemia. *J Natl Cancer Inst* 76:1295, 1986.
12. Schum CA, Izutsu KT, Molbo DM et al: Changes in salivary buffer capacity in patients undergoing cancer chemotherapy. *J Oral Med* 34:76, 1979.
13. Schubert MM, Izutsu KT: Iatrogenic causes of salivary gland dysfunction. *J Dent Res* 66:680, 1987.
14. Bodey GP, Rodriquez V, Chang HY et al: Fever and infection in leukemic patients. *Cancer* 41:1610, 1978.
15. Greenberg MS, Cohen SG, McKitrick JC et al: The oral flora as a source of septicemia in patients with acute leukemia. *Oral Surg Oral Med Oral Pathol* 52:32, 1982.
16. Dreizen S, Bodey GP, Valdivieso M: Chemotherapy-associated oral infections in adults with solid tumors. *Oral Surg Oral Med Oral Pathol* 55:113, 1983.

17. DePaola LG, Peterson DE, Overholser CD et al: Dental care for patients receiving chemotherapy. *J Am Dent Assoc* 112:198, 1986.
18. Dreizen S, McCredie KB, Bodie GP, Keating MJ: Quantitative analysis of the oral complications of antileukemia chemotherapy. *Oral Surg Oral Med Oral Pathol* 62:650, 1986.
19. Barrett AP: Clinical characteristics and mechanisms involved in chemotherapy-induced oral ulceration. *Oral Surg Oral Med Oral Pathol* 63:424, 1987.
20. Rand KH, Kramer B, Johnson AC: Cancer chemotherapy-associated symptomatic stomatitis: Role of herpes simplex virus (HSV). *Cancer* 50:1262, 1982.
21. Lam MT, Pazin GJ, Armstrong JA et al: Herpes simplex infection in acute myelogenous leukemia and other hematologic malignancies. *Cancer* 48:2168, 1981.
22. Rodu B, Carpenter JT, Jones MR: The pathogenesis and clinical significance of cytologically detectable oral Candida in acute leukemia. *Cancer* 62:2042, 1988.
23. Barrett AP: Recognition and management of invasive pharyngeal candidiasis in acute leukemia. *Oral Surg Oral Med Oral Pathol* 67:275, 1989.
24. Dreizen S, Bodey GP, McCredie KB, Keating MJ: Orofacial aspergillosis in acute leukemia. *Oral Surg Oral Med Oral Pathol* 59:499, 1985.
25. Schubert MM, Peterson DE, Meyers J, Truelove EL: Head and neck aspergillosis in patients undergoing bone marrow transplantation. *Cancer* 57:1092, 1986.
26. Dreizen S, Brown LR: Oral microbial changes and infections during cancer chemotherapy. In DE Peterson and ST Sonis (eds), *Oral Complications of Cancer Chemotherapy*. The Hague, Boston: Martinus Nijhoff, 1983, p.41.
27. Minah GE, Rednor JL, Peterson DE et al: Oral succession of gram-negative bacilli in myelosuppressed cancer patients. *J Clin Microbiol* 26:2105, 1988.
28. Bergmann OJ: Oral infections and septicemia in immunocompromised patients with hematologic malignancies. *J Clin Microbiol* 26:2105, 1988.
29. Kolbison DA, Schubert MM, Flournoy N, Truelove EL: Early oral changes following bone marrow transplantation. *Oral Surg Oral Med Oral Pathol* 66:130, 1988.
30. Sale GE, Shulman HM, Schubert MM et al: Oral and ophthalmic pathology of graft-versus-host disease in man: Predictive value of the lip biopsy. *Hum Pathol* 12:1022, 1981.
31. Schubert MM, Sullivan KM, Morton TH et al: Oral manifestations of chronic graft-versus-host disease. *Arch Intern Med* 144:1591, 1984.
32. Rosenberg SW, Kolodney H, Wong GY et al: Altered dental root development in long-term survivors of pediatric acute lymphoblastic leukemia. *Cancer* 59:1640, 1987.
33. Nachman JB, Honig GR: Fever and neutropenia in children with neoplastic disease. *Cancer* 45:407, 1980.
34. Lockhart PB, Sonis ST: Relationship of oral complications to peripheral blood leukocyte and platelet counts in patients receiving cancer chemotherapy. *Oral Surg Oral Med Oral Pathol* 48:21, 1979.
35. Dreizen S, McCredie KB, Keating MJ et al: Malignant gingival and kin "infiltrates" in adult leukemia. *Oral Surg Oral Med Oral Pathol* 55:572, 1983.
36. DeGregorio MW, Lee WM, Ries CA: Candida infections in patients with acute leukemia: Ineffectiveness of nystatin prophylaxis and relationship between oropharyngeal and systemic candidiasis. *Cancer* 50:2780, 1982.
37. Barrett AP: Evaluation of nystatin in prevention and elimination of oropharyngeal Candida in immunosuppressed patients. *Oral Surg Oral Med Oral Pathol* 58:148, 1984.
38. Ferretti GA, Ash RC, Brown AT: Chlorhexidine for prophylaxis against oral infections and associated complications in patients receiving bone marrow transplants. *J Am Dent Assoc* 114:461, 1987.
39. Cohen SG, Greenberg MS: Chronic oral herpes simplex virus infection in immunocompromised patients. *Oral Surg Oral Med Oral Pathol* 59:465, 1985.
40. Montgomery MT, Redding SW, LeMaistre CF: The incidence of oral herpes simplex virus infection in patients undergoing cancer chemotherapy. *Oral Surg Oral Med Oral Pathol* 61:238, 1986.
41. Barrett AP: A long-term prospective clinical study of oral complications during conventional chemotherapy for acute leukemia. *Oral Surg Oral Med Oral Pathol* 63:313, 1987.
42. Greenberg MS, Cohen SG, Boosz B et al: Oral herpes simplex infections in patients with leukemia. *J Am Dent Assoc* 114:483, 1987.
43. Wade JC, Newton B, Flournoy N et al: Oral acyclovir for prevention of herpes simplex virus reactivation after marrow transplantation. *Ann Int Med* 100:823, 1984.
44. Lundgren G et al: Acyclovir prophylaxis in bone marrow transplant patients. *Scand J Infec Dis (Suppl)* 47:137, 1985.
45. Gold D, Corey L: Acyclovir prophylaxis for herpes simplex virus infection. *Antimicrob Agents Chemother* 31:361, 1987.
46. Desforges JF, Rutherford CJ, Pira A: Hodgkin's disease. *N Engl J Med* 301:1212, 1979.
47. Baden E, Al Saati T, Caverivière P et al: Hodgkin's lymphoma of the oropharyngeal region: Report of four cases and diagnostic value of monoclonal antibodies in detecting antigens associated with Reed-Sternberg cells. *Oral Surg Oral Med Oral Pathol* 64:88, 1987.
48. Sullivan KM, Appelbaum FR, Horning SJ et al: Selection of patients with Hodgkin's disease and non-Hodgkin's lymphoma for bone marrow transplantation. *Int J Cell Cloning* 4(Suppl 1): 94, 1986.
49. Reboul F, Donaldson SS, Kaplan HS: Herpes zoster and varicella infections in children with Hodgkin's disease. *Cancer* 41:95, 1978.
50. Kaplan P: Mantle irradiation of the major salivary glands. *J Prosthet Dent* 54:681, 1985.
51. Levine AM: Non-Hodgkin's lymphomas and other malignancies in the acquired immune deficiency syndrome. *Semin Oncol* 14:34, 1987.
52. Loureiro C, Gill PS, Meyer PR et al: Autopsy findings in AIDS-related lymphoma. *Cancer* 62:735, 1988.
53. Reddy S., Pellettiere E, Saxena V et al: Extranodal non-Hodgkin's lymphoma. *Cancer* 46:1925, 1980.
54. Eisenbud L, Sciubba J, Mir R et al: Oral presentations in non-Hodgkin's lymphoma: A review of thirty-one cases. Part I. Data analysis. *Oral Surg Oral Med Oral Pathol* 56:151, 1983.
55. Eisenbud L, Sciubba J, Mir R et al: Oral presentations in non-Hodgkin's lymphoma: A review of thirty-one cases. Part II. Fourteen cases arising in bone. *Oral Surg Oral Med Oral Pathol* 57:272, 1984.
56. Eisenbud L, Mir R, Sciubba J: Oral presentations in non-Hodgkin's lymphoma: A review of thirty-one cases. Part III. Six cases in children. *Oral Surg Oral Med Oral Pathol* 59:44, 1985.
57. Mill WB, Lee FA, Franssila KO: Radiation therapy treatment of stage I and II extranodal non-Hodgkin's lymphoma of the head and neck. *Cancer* 45:653, 1980.
58. Appelbaum FR, Thomas ED: Review of the use of marrow transplantation in the treatment of non-Hodgkin's lymphoma. *J Clin Oncol* 1:440, 1983.

59. Lehrer S, Roswit B, Federman O: The presentation of malignant lymphoma in the oral cavity and pharynx. *Oral Surg Oral Med Oral Pathol* 41:441, 1976.
60. Mittleman D, Kahan LB: Recurrent "non-Hodgkin's lymphoma" presenting with gingival enlargement. *Oral Surg Oral Med Oral Pathol* 42:792, 1976.
61. Tomich CE, Shafer WG: Lymphoproliferative disease of the hard palate: a clinicopathologic entity. *Oral Surg Oral Med Oral Pathol* 39:754, 1975.
62. Howell RE, Handlers JP, Abrams AM et al: Extranodal oral lymphoma. Part II. Relationships between clinical features and the Lukes-Collins classification of 34 cases. *Oral Surg Oral Med Oral Pathol* 64:597, 1987.
63. Fukuda Y, Ishida T, Fujimoto M et al: Malignant lymphoma of the oral cavity: Clinicopathologic analysis of 20 cases. *J Oral Pathol* 16:8, 1987.
64. Griffin TJ, Hurst PS, Swanson J: Non-Hodgkin's lymphoma: a case involving four third-molar extraction sites. *Oral Surg Oral Med Oral Pathol* 65:671, 1988.
65. McIntyre OR: Current concepts in cancer. Multiple myeloma. *N Engl J Med* 301:193, 1979.
66. Blattner WA, Blair A, Mason TJ: Multiple myeloma in the United States, 1950–1975. *Cancer* 48:2547, 1981.
67. Lambertenghi-Deilelers G, Bruno E, Corelezzi A et al: Incidence of jaw lesions in 193 patients with multiple myeloma. *Oral Surg Oral Med Oral Pathol* 65:533, 1988.
68. Glover GR, Nesbitt JA, North AF: Maxillary plasmacytoma/plasma cell myeloma. *Oral Surg Oral Med Oral Pathol* 64:680, 1987.
69. Raubenheimer EJ, Dauth J, de Coning JP: Multiple myeloma presenting with extensive oral and perioral amyloidosis. *Oral Surg Oral Med Oral Pathol* 61:492, 1986.
70. Barrett AP, Buckley DJ: Oral complications of high-dose melphalan in multiple myeloma. *Oral Surg Oral Med Oral Pathol* 64:264, 1987.
71. Burkitt DP: The discovery of Burkitt's lymphoma. *Cancer* 51:1777, 1983.
72. Sariban E, Donahue A, Magrath IT: Jaw involvement in American Burkitt's lymphoma. *Cancer* 53:1777, 1984.
73. Levine PH, Kamaraju LS, Connelly RR et al: The American Burkitt's Lymphoma Registry: Eight years' experience. *Cancer* 49:1016, 1982.
74. Anaissie E, Geha S, Allam C et al: Burkitt's lymphoma in the Middle East. *Cancer* 56:2539, 1985.
75. Cohen SR, Stenn KS, Braverman IM et al: Mycosis fungoides: Clinicopathologic relationships, survival, and therapy in 59 patients with observations on occupation as a new prognostic factor. *Cancer* 46:2654, 1980.
76. Merlo CJ, Hoppe RT, Abel E et al: Extracutaneous mycosis fungoides. *Cancer* 60:397, 1987.
77. Wright JM, Balciunas BA, Muus JH: Mycosis fungoides with oral manifestations. Report of a case and review of the literature. *Oral Surg Oral Med Oral Pathol* 51:24, 1981.
78. Ishii Y, Yamanaka N, Ogawa K et al: Nasal T-cell lymphoma as a type of so-called "lethal midline granuloma." *Cancer* 50:2336, 1982.
79. Batsakis JG: Wegener's granulomatosis and midline (nonhealing) "granuloma." *Head Neck Surg* 1:213, 1979.

9

Other Head and Neck Cancers

SOL SILVERMAN, JR.
ROGER BOLES • Salivary Gland Tumors
HERBERT H. DEDO • Laryngeal Carcinomas
KAREN FU • Nasopharyngeal Carcinomas

Cancers of the salivary glands, jaw bones, larynx, nasopharynx, skin, and lips, as well as oral malignant melanomas and AIDS-related tumors, are discussed in this chapter since they must be considered in the differential diagnosis of numerous benign conditions. With the exception of skin cancer, these malignancies occur infrequently. Nevertheless, an understanding of the signs and symptoms, diagnostic approaches, and treatment implications is important in differentiating malignant from nonmalignant oral diseases as well as in caring for patients with these conditions.

MALIGNANT SALIVARY GLAND TUMORS

Salivary gland cancers account for about 0.5% of all malignancies (approximately 5000 new cases each year in the U.S.). Most of these cancers occur in the major salivary glands (the paired parotid, submandibular, and sublingual) as opposed to the minor salivary glands, which are distributed throughout the oral mucosa.

The initial sign is usually a lump, which may be painful. These lumps may resemble benign growths, cysts, inflammations, or infections, making the differential diagnosis difficult.[1] Enlargement of salivary glands caused by systemic disease is seldom mistaken for tumor.

An extremely important difference in the approach to salivary gland diagnosis is that early or even immediate biopsy of minor salivary gland lesions is in order, whereas biopsy of major salivary gland lesions should be avoided in favor of less invasive diagnostic approaches. This is because a biopsy of the major glands prior to definitive treatment tends to spill tumor cells into adjacent tissues as well as to cause scar formation, both of which complicate surgical resection and diminish the effectiveness of radiation. Fine needle aspiration biopsy (FNA) is accurate and has become an acceptable diagnostic modality in distinguishing neoplasia from infections or inflammatory disease before conventional or open biopsy.[2] Equipment for FNA consists of a 22-gauge needle and special syringe holder that provides a good vacuum in a 10- or 20-ml syringe. The aspirated contents are prepared by cytologic technique methods. Magnetic resonance imaging (MRI) has also proved to be extremely helpful in assessing type and extent of salivary gland disease. Therefore, accurate noninvasive diagnostic techniques are available and indicated where biopsy is considered to establish the diagnosis. (See Chapter 3.)

MAJOR SALIVARY GLANDS

By far the most frequently involved major salivary gland is the parotid. It accounts for about 85% of all major salivary gland tumors, and about one fourth of all parotid tumors are malignant. The relative incidence of tumors in the three types of major salivary glands and the percentage of these tumors that are malignant are shown in Table 9-1.

More than 80% of these tumors occur in patients over 35 years of age, and they are infrequent in individuals under 21 years.[3,4] There is essentially no difference in occurrence between men and women or by race. Mucoepidermoid cancers and adenocarcinomas are the most frequent histologic types.[5] Squamous carcinomas and malignant mixed tumors develop from preexisting benign mixed tumors.[6,7] Primary lymphomas arising in salivary glands are very uncommon (see Chapter 8).[8]

Table 9-1. MAJOR SALIVARY GLAND TUMORS

Gland	Approximate Distribution of Tumors (%)	Approximate Malignant Tumors (%)
Parotid	85–90	25
Submaxillary	10–15	50
Sublingual	1	75

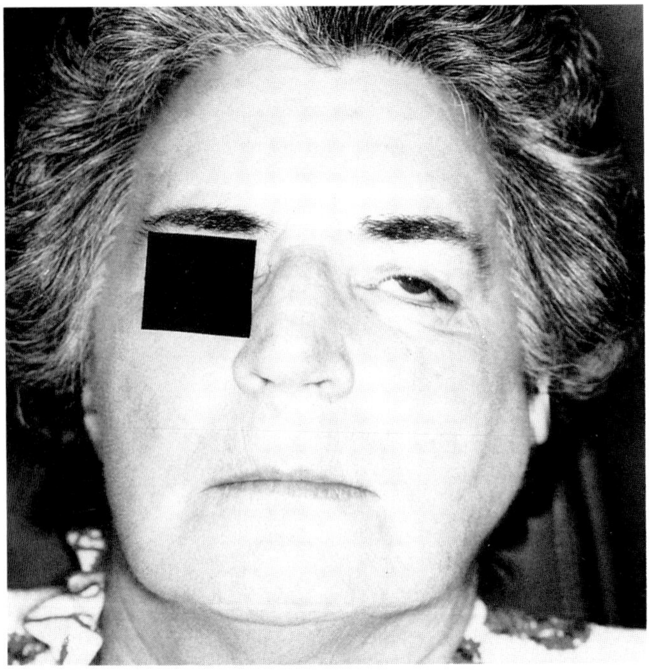

A

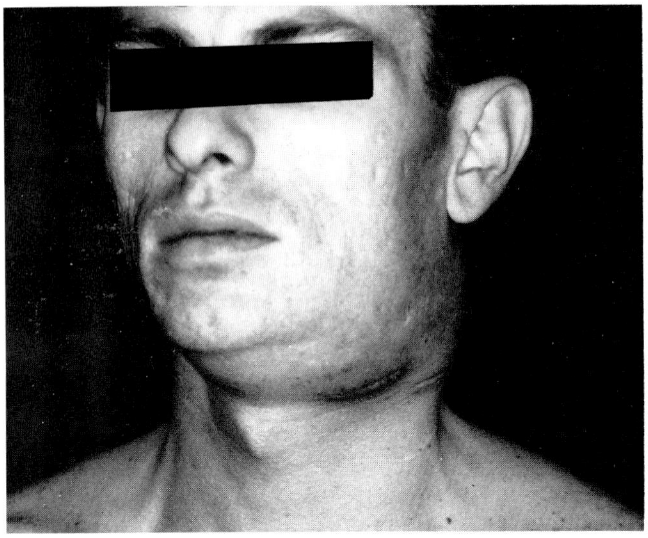

B

Fig. 9-1. Diagnosis of major salivary gland tumors. **A,** Painful left facial swelling of 1 month's duration. There was no evidence of dental disease, and the patient did not respond to empirical treatment. Needle biopsy confirmed an adenocarcinoma (parotid). Note the inability to blink the left eye, indicating nerve involvement. **B,** Cervical swelling of less than 2 weeks' duration, thought to be an acute infection of dental origin. No dental disease could be found, and incision and drainage did not reveal any suppurative material. Biopsy showed this to be a squamous carcinoma of parotid gland origin.

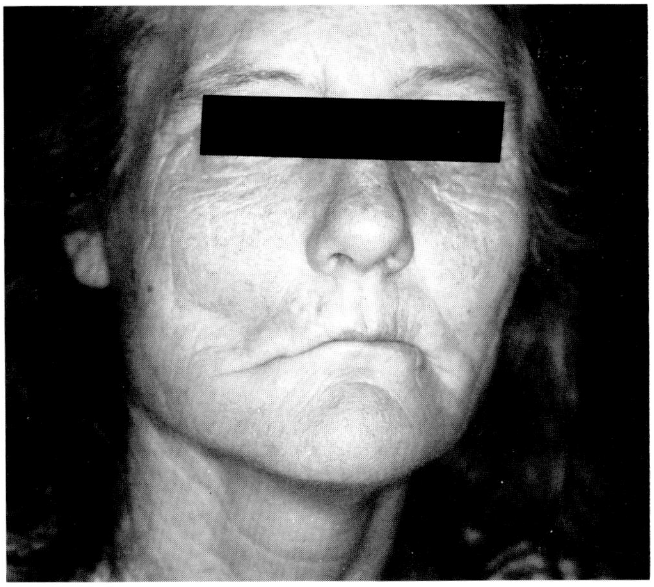

Fig. 9-2. Right facial paralysis (Bell's palsy) of 3 months' duration. Radiograph revealed a destructive lesion in the posterior mandible which was diagnosed as an extension of a parotid mucoepidermoid carcinoma. Lip drooping and inability to close the eyelid (loss of blink reflex) are characteristic of facial nerve involvement.

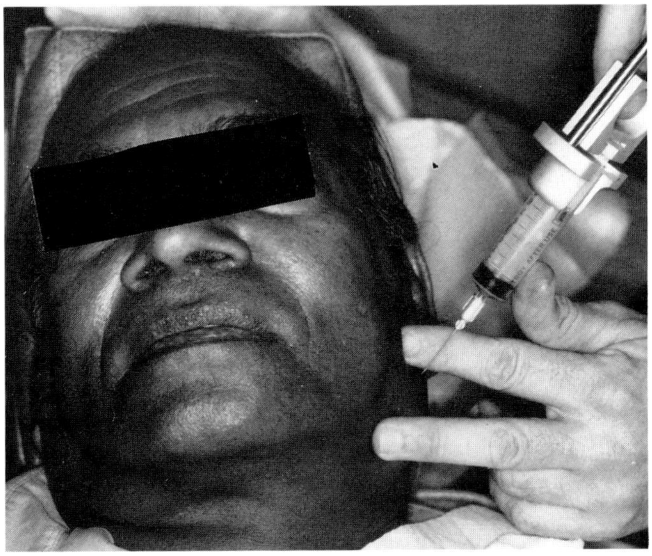

Fig. 9-3. Parotid swelling of 4 months' duration that did not respond to antibiotics. Needle biopsy indicated Warthin's tumor, later confirmed by limited resection of this benign growth.

The most common first sign of malignant tumor is swelling (Fig. 9-1). Growth is often moderately rapid, and usually there is associated pain. However, sometimes enlargement is slow, which diminishes patient concern and delays diagnosis. Facial paralysis may be an early sign, resulting from involvement of the seventh nerve (Fig. 9-2). The differential diagnosis must include conditions such as infections, stones, adenomas, or inflammatory/autoimmune enlargement. Sialography, radiographic imaging, and response to heat and antibiotics are helpful in selected cases, both in management and as diagnostic approaches before biopsy. If a lesion persists, the diagnosis of a malignancy can be determined only by tissue analysis. Fine needle aspiration biopsy has been extremely useful in differentiating benign and malignant tumors, and often in classifying lesions (Fig. 9-3). Treatment is usually surgical, often accompanied by radiation therapy.

An incisional biopsy should be performed by the tumor therapist. This is best done at the time of surgery. Radiation is used when surgery is contraindicated, for tumors at high risk for local recurrence or spread, or for tumors that are large, aggressive, or have spread to regional lymph nodes.[9,10] Chemotherapy for recurrent and widespread salivary gland malignancy remains relatively ineffective.[11]

Most cancers of salivary gland origin have a good prognosis if they are diagnosed early and treated adequately (Table 9-2). Fortunately, most salivary gland tumors are localized and the poorer prognoses and outcomes are due to the tumor types and their biologic behavior. Classified by histologic type, treatment results appear to be best for low-grade mucoepidermoid carcinoma[12] and worst for adenoid cystic carcinomas.[13,14] Data on 349 Caucasian women with malignancies of salivary glands indicated a twofold risk for subsequent breast cancer.[15] Malignant tumors of major salivary glands occasionally can represent metastases from other primary sites. In these cases the diagnostic approaches and treatments are variable and the prognosis poor.

Table 9-2. LOCALIZATION AND RELATIVE SURVIVAL RATES OF 923 PATIENTS WITH SALIVARY GLAND MALIGNANCIES, 1973–1984*

Stage	n	Patient Distribution (%)	5-Year Survival (%)
Localized	487	52.8	91
Regional Spread	337	36.5	56
Distant Metastasis	99	10.7	25

*Source: Data from National Cancer Institute: Surveillance, Epidemiology and End Results Program (SEER), 1973–1984[28]

MINOR SALIVARY GLANDS

Minor salivary gland carcinomas occur infrequently and usually after age 30. They show great diversity in histologic appearance, anatomic site, and clinical course (Fig. 9-4).[16–19]

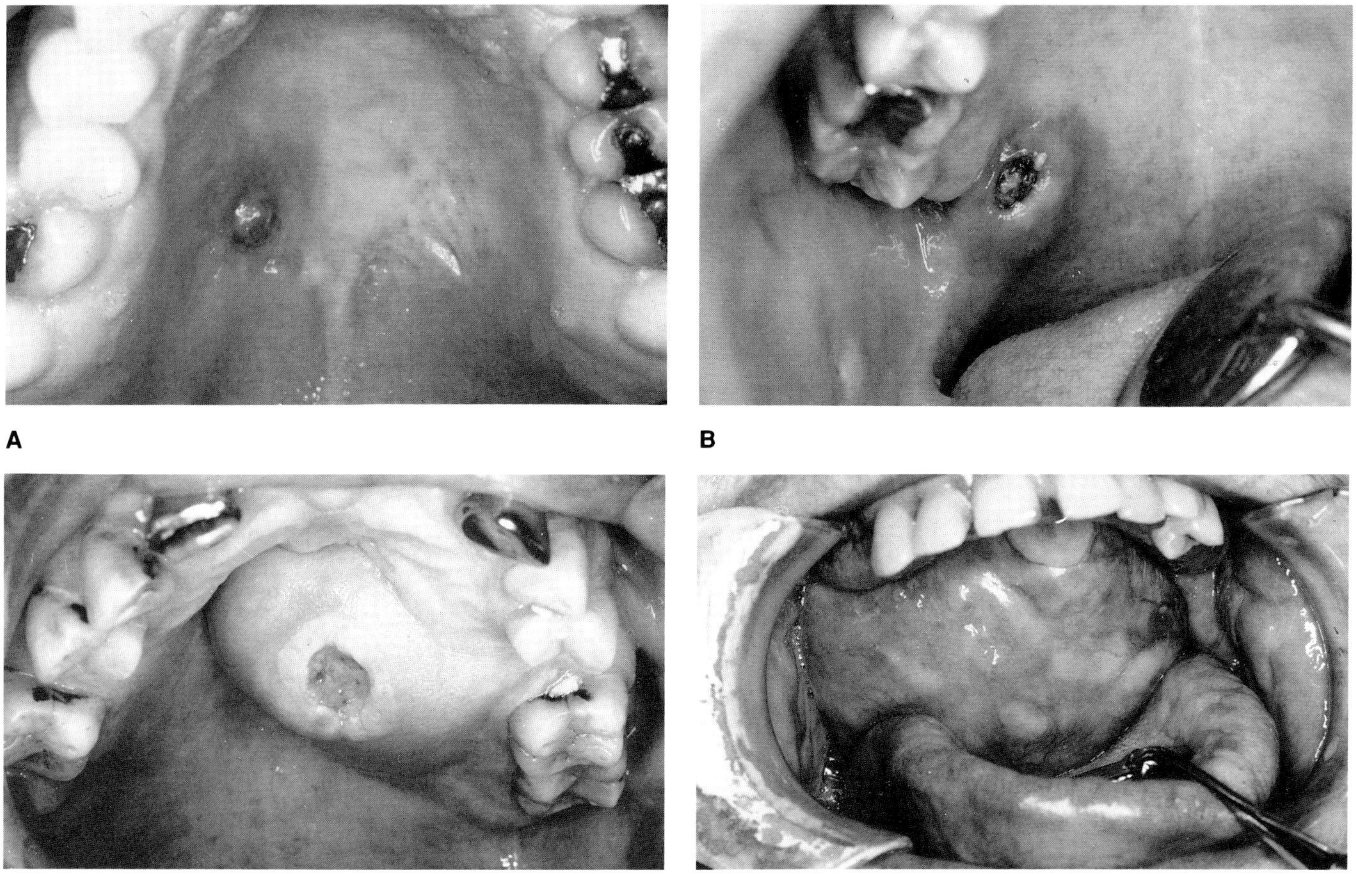

Fig. 9-4. Variable appearances of malignant minor salivary gland tumors. **A,** Mucoepidermoid carcinoma, noticed by patient for about 1 month and first thought to be a mucocele. **B,** Adenocarcinoma of minor salivary gland origin in a 15-year-old schoolboy, who had noticed small lump in right posterior palate for about 1 month. Ulceration indicates area where incision and drainage was attempted. **C,** Malignant mixed tumor, noticed by patient for more than 3 months. Lesion had been covered with intact, normal-appearing epithelium before biopsy induced an ulcer. **D,** This large, relatively painless mass had been noticed by patient for more than 6 months and caused partial obstruction of airway and difficulty in breathing. Biopsy showed it to be an adenocarcinoma of minor salivary gland origin.

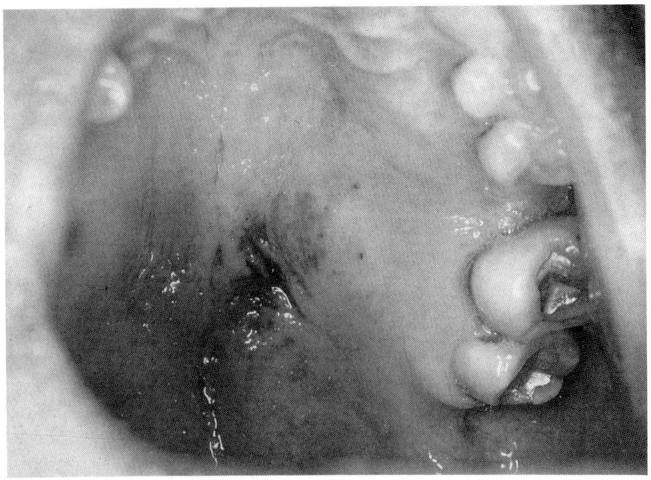

A

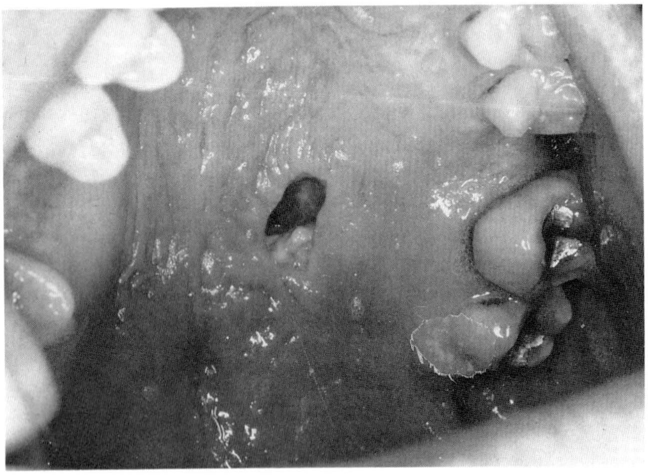

B

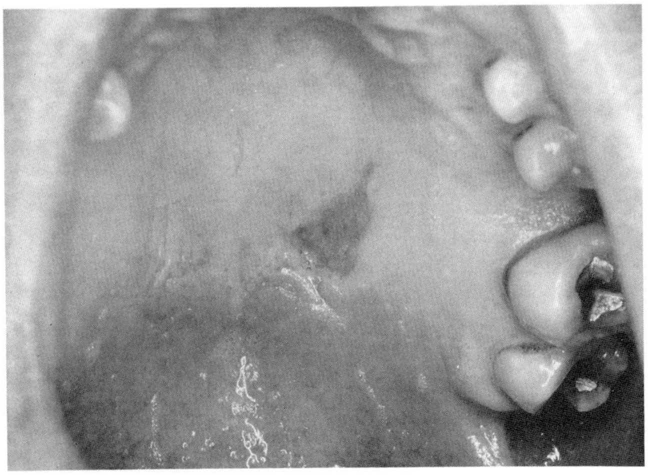

C

Fig. 9-5. Necrotizing sialometaplasia. This condition can be mistaken for malignancy. **A,** Painful, erythematous, mildly erosive palatal lesion of 2 weeks' duration, confirmed by biopsy to be necrotizing sialometaplasia. **B,** Typical punched-out appearance of maturing lesion. Defect is not due to biopsy. **C,** Lesion spontaneously healed 6 weeks after initial signs and symptoms appeared.

Their usual location is the palate, followed by lip and buccal mucosae. However, they can even occur in the tongue.[20] A painless lump, often resembling a cyst, a fibroma, or even a vascular growth, is the most common first complaint.

Necrotizing sialometaplasia, a nonneoplastic, inflammatory disease of minor salivary glands,[21] most commonly occurs as a sudden progressive ulceration of the palate (Fig. 9-5). It can be confused with a malignant process both clinically and microscopically. The cause is unknown and the disease is self-limiting, usually lasting four to six weeks. It occurs most frequently in individuals over 40 years of age, another reason for including malignancy in the differential diagnosis.

Tumors of minor oral salivary glands probably account for about 15% of all salivary gland neoplasms; about half of them are malignant. The most common histologic type appears to be mucoepidermoid carcinoma.[18] Benign mixed tumors (pleomorphic adenomas) are the most common of benign and minor salivary gland tumors. However, they have a tendency toward aggressive local spread and recurrence and thus can mimic malignant behavior.

Minor salivary gland malignancies are usually treated by surgical excision, followed by radiation therapy for high-grade tumors and/or large tumors with questionable margins (Chapter 5, Fig. 5-5). Sometimes in critical or surgically inaccessible areas, these malignant tumors are treated by irradiation alone. Local recurrence and metastasis are common. In a clinicopathologic study of 492 cases, the five-year survival was 42%.[16] Experience at the University of California, San Francisco, has been that major and minor salivary gland malignancies have similar survival times.[10] However, since with minor salivary gland malignancies 5-year survival does not indicate cure, many patients eventually die of their disease more than five years after diagnosis.

MALIGNANCIES INVOLVING THE JAWBONES

CARCINOMA

A primary intraoral carcinoma may invade the mandible or maxilla by local extension (see Chapter 4). These are advanced lesions, since the periosteum is usually a moderately resistant barrier. Dental radiographs will reflect advanced osseous destruction, but early microscopic invasion is usually not visible in an x-ray film. On rare occasions, epithelium lining odontogenic cysts can transform into carcinoma.[22]

SARCOMA

Primary sarcomas in the jawbones are rare. They are usually manifested by rapid expansion and pain and have a poor prognosis.

Osteogenic sarcoma[23] is the most common primary malignant lesion of bone (Fig. 9-6). This tumor is found in the jawbones at an incidence rate of less than one case per million population. It occurs in all age groups, in both sexes, and in the mandible and maxilla. Osteogenic sarcoma is a highly malignant tumor; about one third of cases show metastases, primarily to the lung. Combination therapeutic approaches using surgery, radiation, and chemotherapy have helped increase survival rates (see Chapter 5, Fig. 5-1).

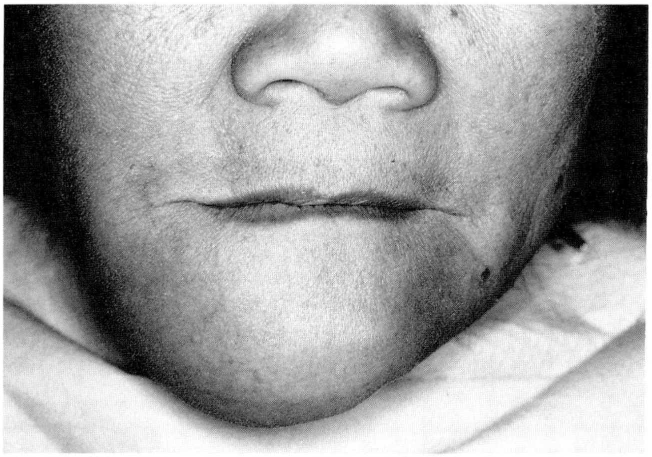

A

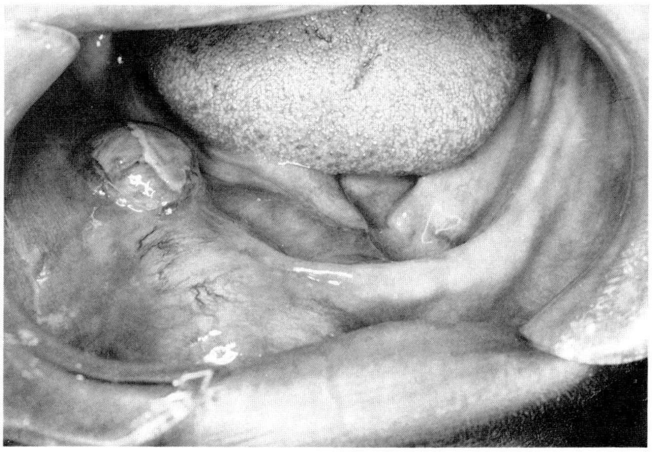

B

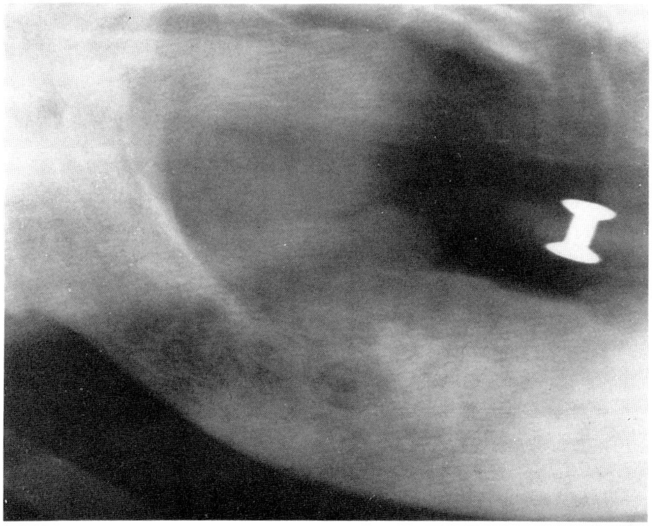

C

Fig. 9-6. Osteogenic sarcoma. **A,** Patient noticed mandibular growth and change in appearance over a 9-month period. **B,** Intraoral swelling. Biopsy of bone revealed osteogenic sarcoma. **C,** Radiograph shows altered trabeculation, frayed alveolar crest margin, and overall expansion in diseased area.

MAXILLARY SINUS CANCER

Early signs and symptoms of maxillary sinus cancer often consist of palatal swelling, pain, or loose maxillary teeth (Fig. 9-7). These signs and symptoms may be mistaken for denture injury or dental infection. Radiographs will show bone destruction and/or a dense obliteration of part or all of the sinus. Computed tomography (CT scan) has been extremely useful in identifying the extent of tumor involvement (see Chapter 3). Even with combined radiation and surgical therapy, cure rates are poor, primarily because most lesions are diagnosed in advanced stages.

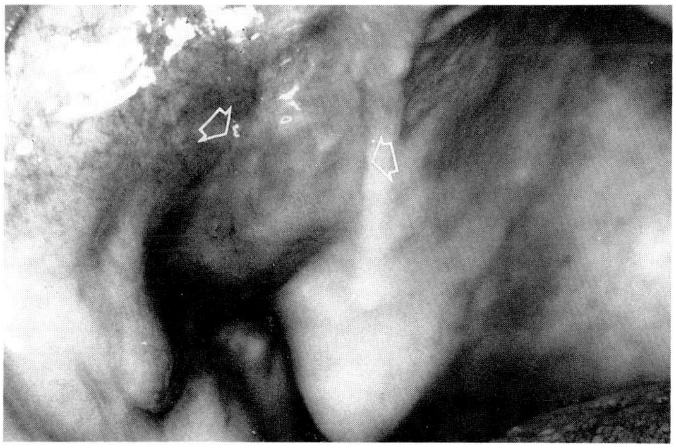

A

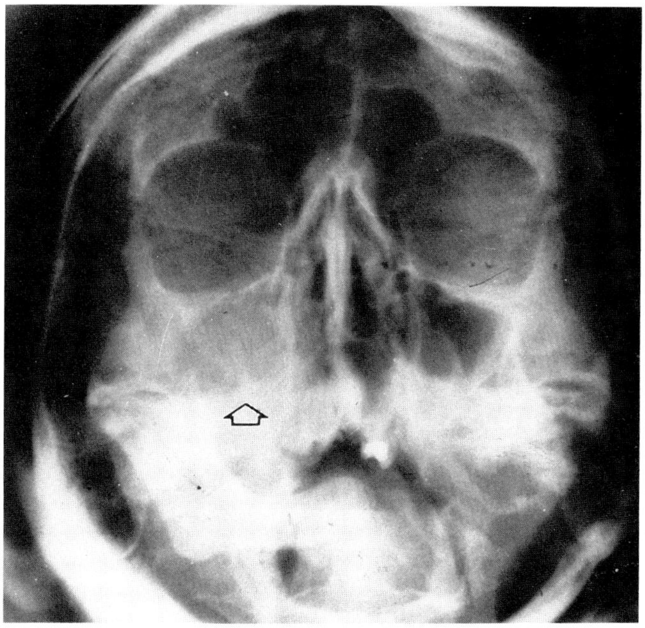

B

Fig. 9-7. Maxillary sinus cancer. **A,** Mass (arrows) in right maxillary reflex dislodged patient's denture. Patient complained of nasal stuffiness and sinusitis. **B,** Radiograph of anteroposterior head revealed opacity of right maxillary sinus (arrow), which was obliterated by tumor. Reflex mass was an extension of tumor, a low-grade adenocarcinoma, which had eroded sinus walls and invaded adjacent tissues.

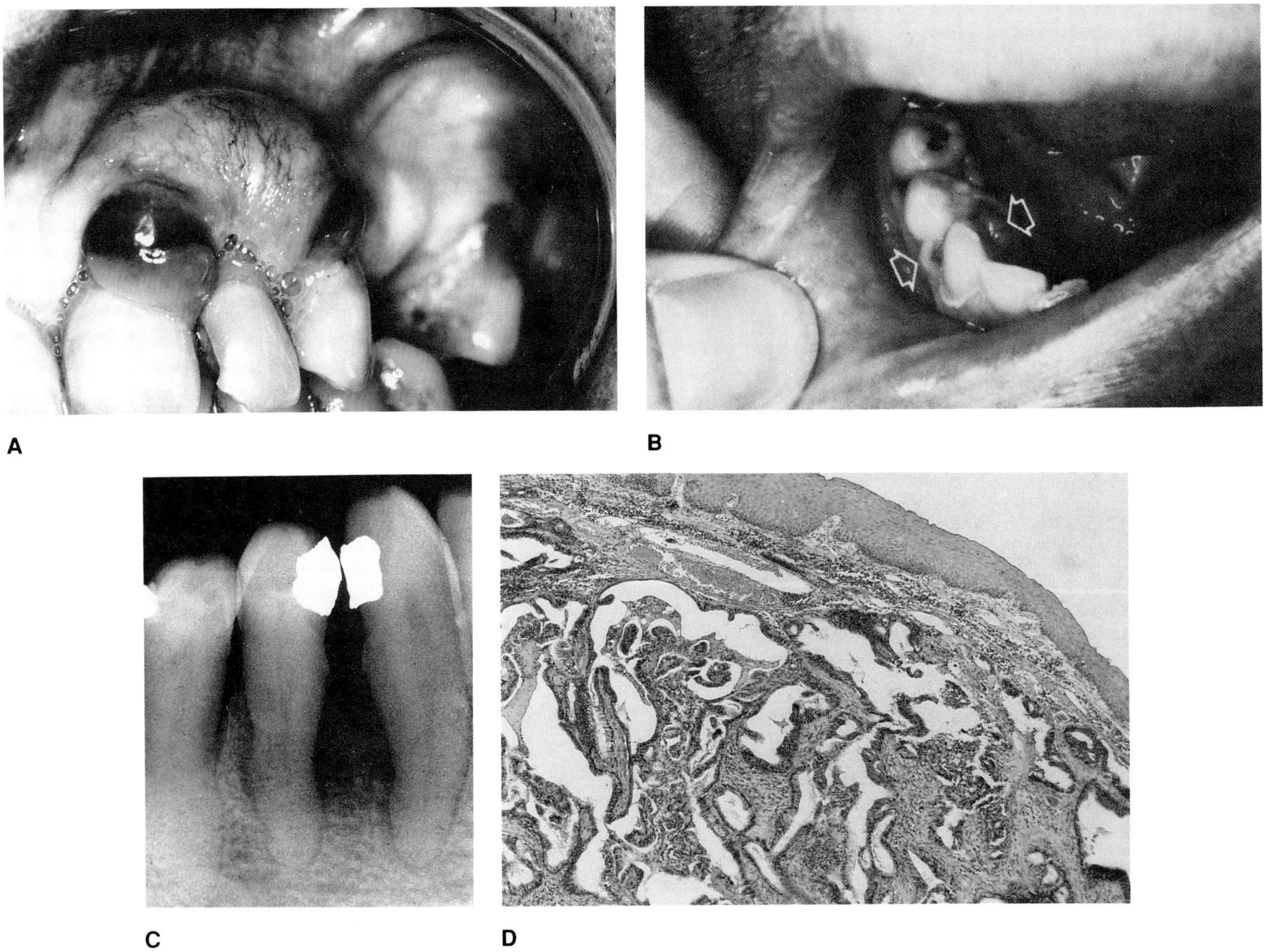

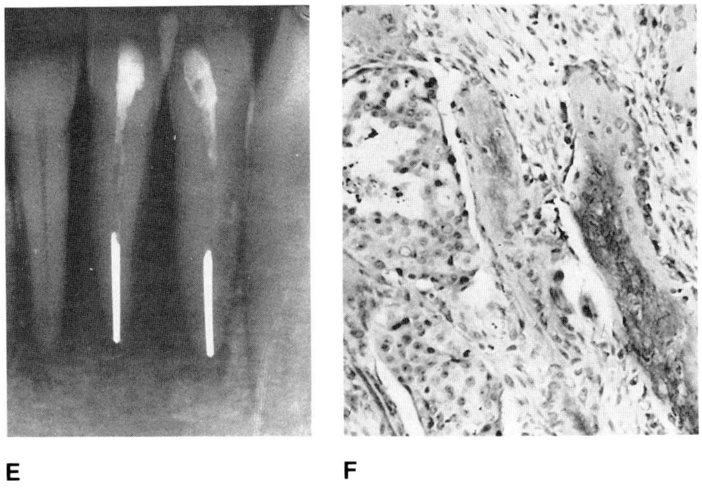

Fig. 9-8. Metastatic lesions to the jawbones. **A,** Adenocarcinoma metastatic from the breast. **B,** Metastasis to mandible from testicular carcinoma (arrows). **C,** Patient undergoing treatment for cancer of uterine cervix was seen because of denture pain. Radiograph showed marked bone loss between cuspid and bicuspid. **D,** Biopsy from same patient revealed metastatic adenocarcinoma. **E,** Patient being treated for lung cancer experienced pain in anterior mandible. Radiograph showed radiolucency involving lower anterior teeth. Endodontic treatment was unsuccessful in relieving pain. **F,** Biopsy from this patient indicated metastatic adenocarcinoma.

METASTASES

Metastatic lesions to the jawbones occur infrequently and are evidence of advanced and generalized tumor spread (Figs. 9-8, 9-9). Most often they stem from multiple myeloma or from adenocarcinoma of the breast. They are usually symptomatic and may be mistaken for either dental disease of local infective origin or sometimes for a neuralgic syndrome.

Neuroblastoma, a highly malignant tumor originating in the sympathetic nervous tissue, is the second most common malignancy of children, preceded only by leukemia. One study indicated that the jawbones were affected in approximately 25% of the patients.[24]

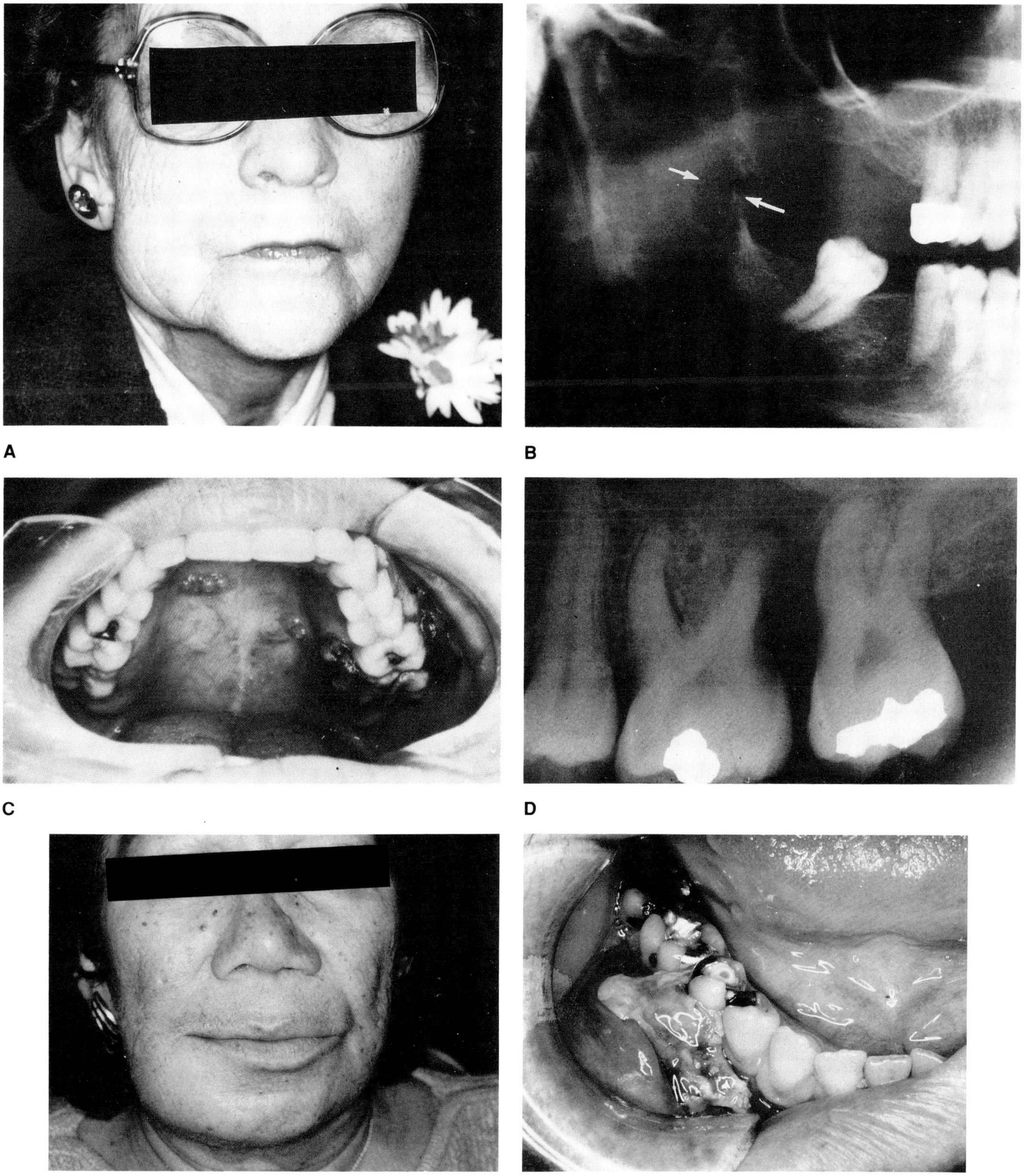

Fig. 9-9. Malignant tumors metastatic to jawbones. **A,** Patient, 70 years old, experienced painful swelling of right mandible and face for 5 weeks. **B,** Radiograph showed radiolucency and fracture of mandible (arrows). Biopsy revealed adenocarcinoma of bowel origin. **C,** Patient, 26 years old, with apparently controlled breast carcinoma noticed a painful gingival swelling of 2 months' duration in left maxilla. **D,** Radiograph revealed a destructive bone lesion between first and second molars. Biopsy showed metastatic breast cancer. **E,** While undergoing radiation therapy for a recurrent carcinoma of the lung, patient had an acute, painful swelling of the right mandible. **F,** Oral examination revealed a buccogingival mass primarily involving the bicuspid area. Biopsy proved this to be metastatic carcinoma from the lung.

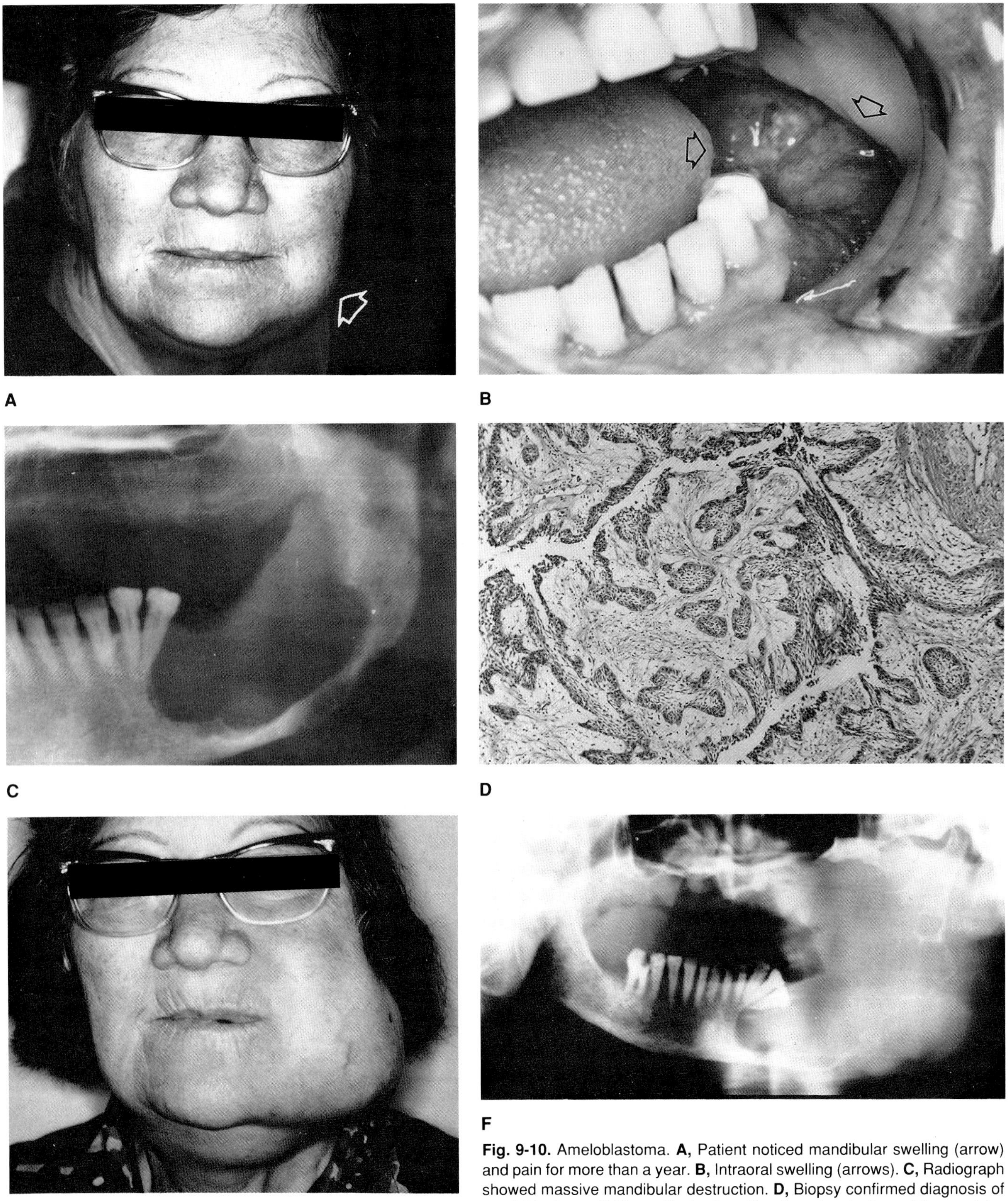

Fig. 9-10. Ameloblastoma. **A,** Patient noticed mandibular swelling (arrow) and pain for more than a year. **B,** Intraoral swelling (arrows). **C,** Radiograph showed massive mandibular destruction. **D,** Biopsy confirmed diagnosis of ameloblastoma. **E,** The patient refused treatment and returned 2 years later because of marked pain and inability to chew and swallow. **F,** Radiograph reflects massive local extension of the tumor, which did not respond to an attempt at control by radiation therapy.

AMELOBLASTOMA

Ameloblastomas (adamantinomas) have a very low malignant potential (Fig. 9-10).[25] Usually they tend toward local aggressive spread and recurrence. It has been substantiated that the true ameloblastoma can metastasize, although very few cases have been unequivocally documented.[26] While management is primarily surgical, radiation has been a useful adjunct in some extensive cases.[27]

GIANT CELL TUMORS

Giant cell tumors occurring in the jawbones are extremely rare (Fig. 9-11). Malignant transformation is almost nonexistent. However, the tumors can be locally destructive and painful, and malignancy must be carefully ruled out. Giant cell tumors usually can be easily differentiated from giant cell granulomas and giant cell lesions (osteitis fibrosa cystica, "brown" tumor) associated with hyperparathyroidism.

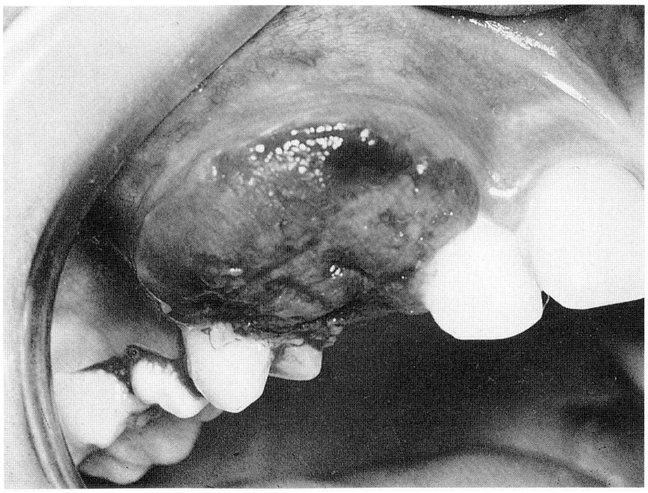

Fig. 9-11. Giant cell tumor. A 13-year-old boy experienced painful swelling of right maxillary gingiva for 3 weeks. Biopsy revealed numerous giant cells and active-appearing connective tissue stroma consistent with giant cell tumor. The underlying cuspid was impacted and there was evident alveolar bone destruction.

LARYNGEAL CARCINOMA

Carcinoma of the larynx accounts for about 1.4% of all cancers in the United States each year (more than 14,000 new cases). About 80% of cases occur in men. Early signs and symptoms include a chronic sore throat, hoarseness, change in voice, and blood spotting in saliva. These complaints should alert the clinician to suspect tumor.

Early diagnosis and treatment greatly improve survival and curability. Recent SEER program data covering the years 1979–1984 and 5,458 cases showed an overall 5-year patient survival rate of 65%.[28] However, 52% of the lesions were localized and the 5-year survival rate for patients in this group was 80%. Radiation therapy has been very effective by itself or in combination with surgery in extending survival, increasing curability, and decreasing morbidity (by avoiding some laryngectomies, thus saving speech). These tumors can usually be seen well by indirect laryngoscopy, and diagnosis is confirmed by biopsy.

As with oral cancer patients, most laryngeal cancer victims are heavy users of tobacco and alcohol, and leukoplakia is a common precancerous lesion of the larynx.

Pretreatment dental planning and posttreatment care are important. Since the radiation field is often extended to major salivary gland tissue (to include regional lymph nodes), alterations in saliva and subsequent radiation caries may become rehabilitation problems (see Chapter 6).

NASOPHARYNGEAL CARCINOMA

Cancers of the nasopharynx account for about 0.2% of all malignancies, approximately 2,000 cases in the United States each year. The main histologic type is squamous carcinoma. Chinese people are known to have a genetic predisposition to this disease; their risk is up to 30 times greater (depending on the population used for comparison) than that of persons in other ethnic groups. Nasopharyngeal carcinoma is one of the most common malignancies in Southeast Asia. The risk increases with age and is twice as great for men as for women. Smoking, working in poor ventilation, use of nasal balms or oils, the consumption of salted fish, herbal drugs, and a high Epstein-Barr antibody titer (specifically anti-IgA VCA) have all been statistically associated as predisposing risk factors.[29–34]

Dental clinicians may become involved in either diagnosis or management. Often the initial signs are enlarged cervical lymph nodes, nasopharyngeal pain, and nasal stuffiness or bleeding. Early diagnosis and aggressive treatment help to increase survival.

Because therapy requires aggressive irradiation (including the major salivary glands, the oropharynx, and the neck), xerostomia, dental caries, and osteonecrosis are major problems (see Chapter 6). Pretreatment dental planning is extremely important. Furthermore, although mortality from nasopharyngeal carcinoma exceeds 50%, the survival time is often prolonged, and most patients require preventive and therapeutic oral care during and after treatment as well as before (Table 9-3). Chinese patients with nasopharyngeal carcinoma treated in China have shown similarly poor long-term survival.[35]

Table 9-3. LOCALIZATION AND RELATIVE SURVIVAL RATES OF 739 PATIENTS WITH NASOPHARYNGEAL CARCINOMA, 1973–1984*

Stage	Distribution (%)	5-Year Survival (%)
Localized	19	57
Regional Spread	46	47
Distant Metastasis	22	26
Unknown	13	38
	100	43

*Source: Data from National Cancer Institute: Surveillance, Epidemiology and End Results Program (SEER), 1973–1984.[28]

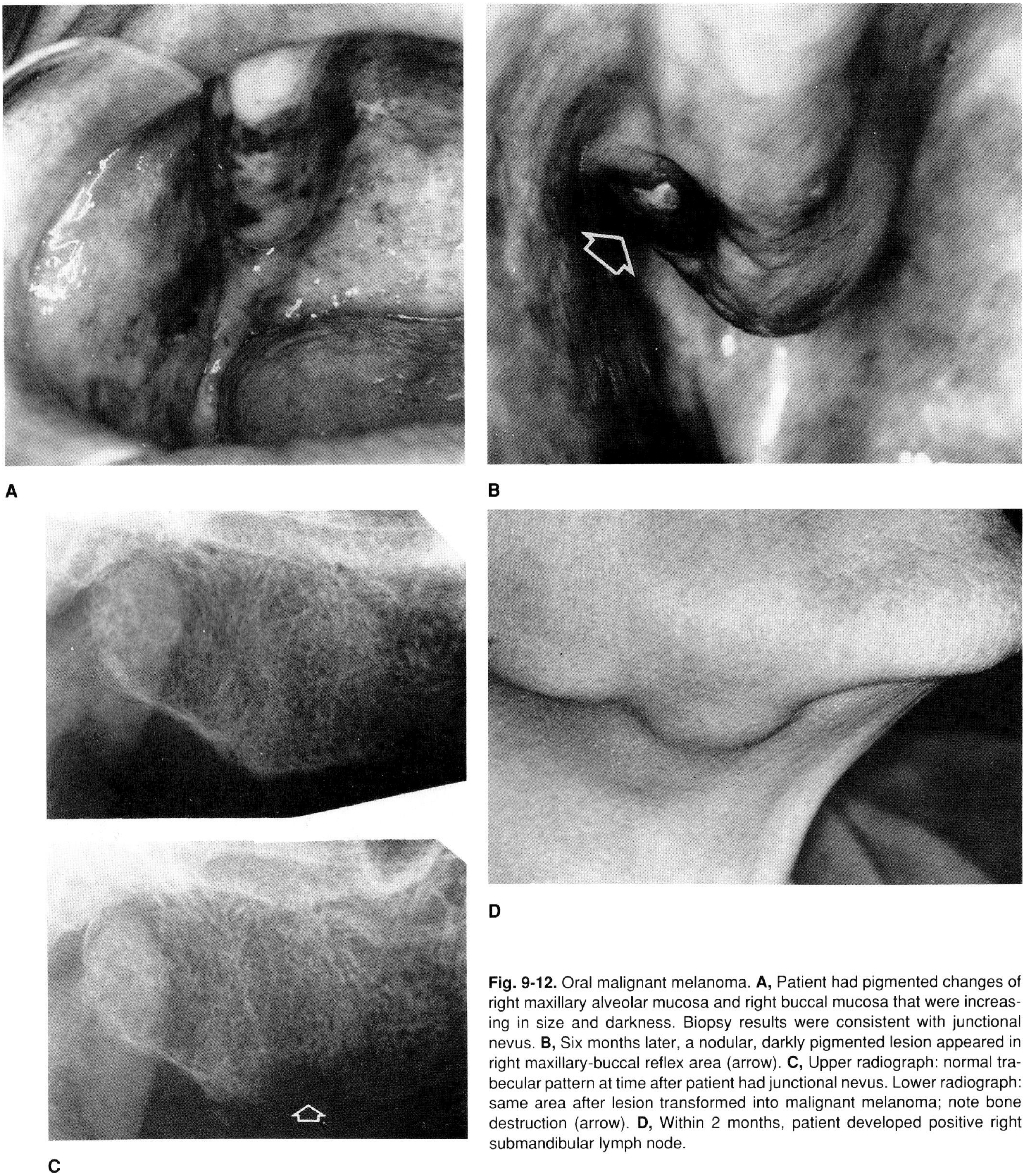

Fig. 9-12. Oral malignant melanoma. **A,** Patient had pigmented changes of right maxillary alveolar mucosa and right buccal mucosa that were increasing in size and darkness. Biopsy results were consistent with junctional nevus. **B,** Six months later, a nodular, darkly pigmented lesion appeared in right maxillary-buccal reflex area (arrow). **C,** Upper radiograph: normal trabecular pattern at time after patient had junctional nevus. Lower radiograph: same area after lesion transformed into malignant melanoma; note bone destruction (arrow). **D,** Within 2 months, patient developed positive right submandibular lymph node.

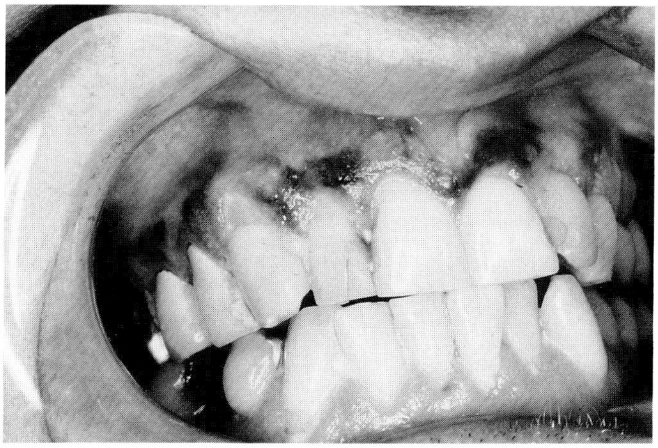

A

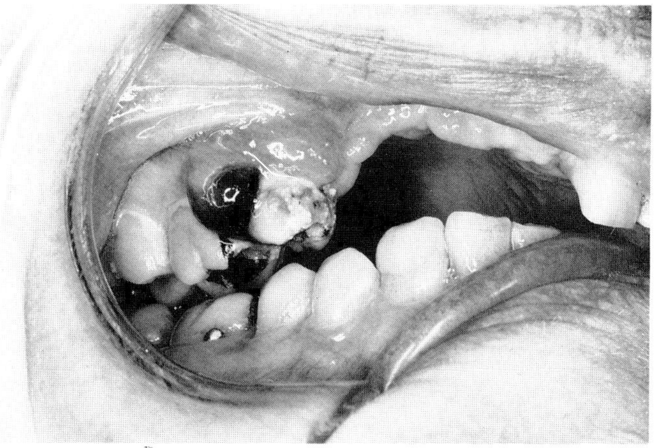

B

Fig. 9-13. Malignant melanomas of the gingiva. **A,** These flat, pigmented lesions were at first thought to be a benign melanosis. **B,** This sessile pigmented mass was the first sign of malignant melanoma which also involved underlying bone and maxillary sinus.

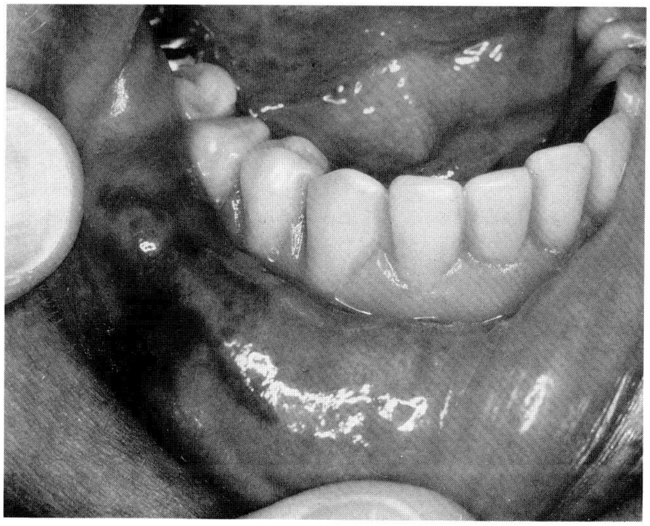

A

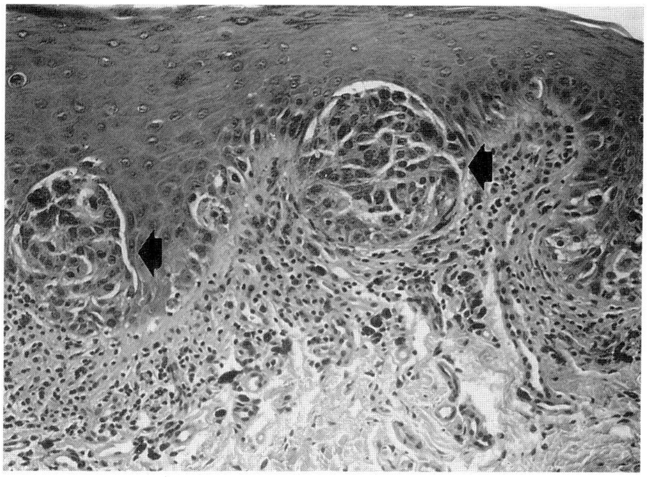

B

Fig. 9-14. Junctional nevus. **A,** Asymptomatic, spreading, darkly pigmented lesion of lower lip. **B,** Biopsy indicated junctional nevus, without evidence of malignancy. Note nests of nevus cells (arrows).

MALIGNANT MELANOMA

Pigmented lesions of the oral cavity often present a diagnostic problem. The discoloration may be due to melanin deposition (e.g., nevi, melanosis, systemic disorders, racial origin), amalgam particles,[36-38] or precipitation products from other metals and drugs. However, the most important possibility to consider in the differential diagnosis of a pigmented lesion is malignant melanoma. Oral malignant melanomas are extremely rare (Figs. 9-12, 9-13).

Nevi of the oral mucosa are also important considerations because they can transform into malignancies (Fig. 9-14).[39] However, so few cases with adequate follow-up have been reported that the risk of malignant transformation cannot be ascertained.[37]

Some sizable studies of intraoral malignant melanoma have been reported.[40-43] In these reviews it was found that the average age of the patients was approximately 50 years with about 80% of cases being in patients over 40 years old. Males were affected more often than females. Most cases occurred in the maxillary mucosa (palate and gingiva). The average time between onset of symptoms and diagnosis was approximately 16 months. In about one third of the cases, the tumor was preceded by pigmentation which was present for periods ranging from several months to several years. Ulceration and bleeding were most often the signs that brought attention to the tumor. The lesions usually were not indurated, and the margins often were flat and not rolled. Bone involvement with loosening and exfoliation of teeth was a common finding in the later stages of the disease. Regional metastasis was observed in about 50% of the cases, and generalized metastasis occurred in about 20%. Follow-up of these cases revealed that the prognosis was poor with 5-year survival varying from 3 to 20%.

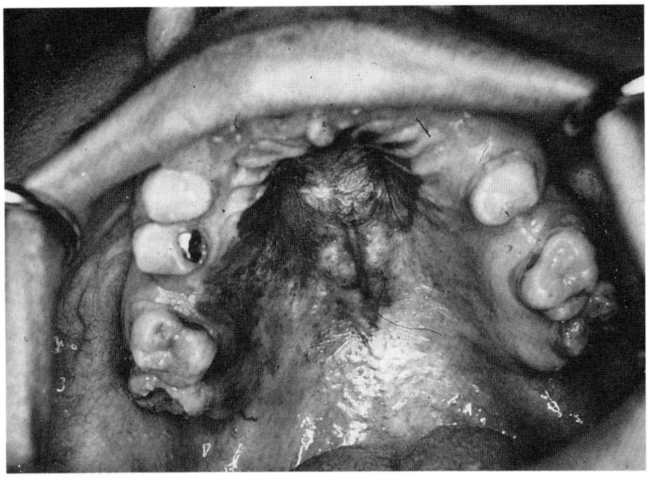

A

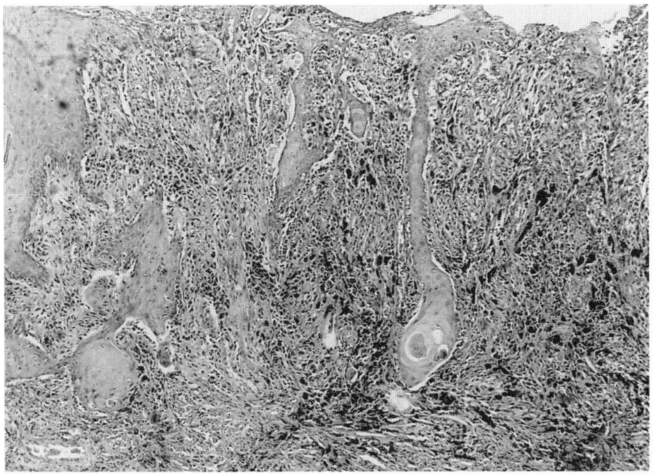

B

Fig. 9-15. Malignant melanoma. **A,** Mildly symptomatic, spreading, pigmented lesion of palate. **B,** Incisional biopsy confirmed malignant melanoma diagnosis. Note malignant proliferation of epithelium and numerous melanin-producing cells (dark reaction) in connective tissue.

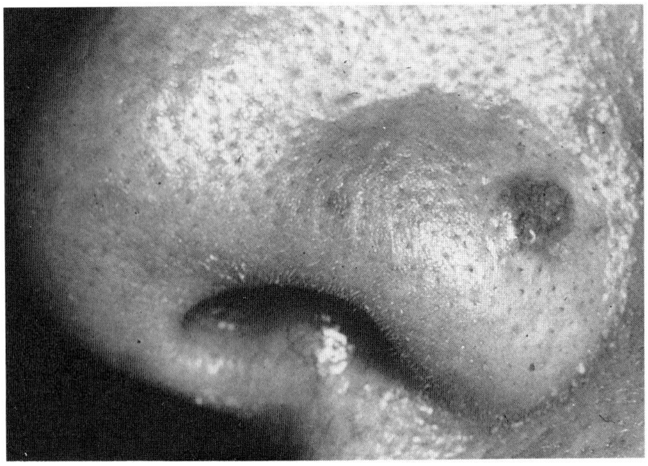

A

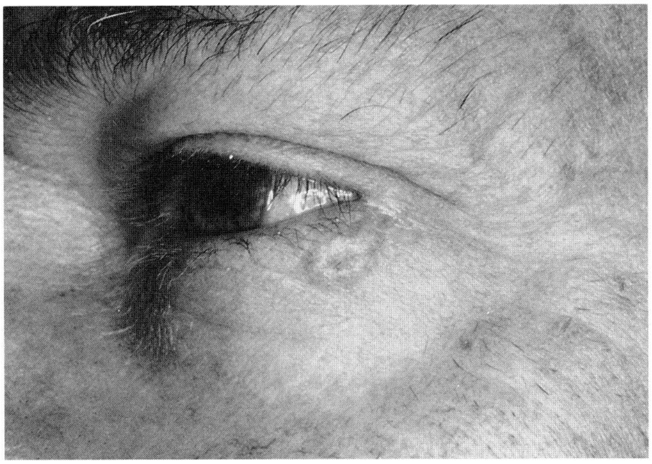

B

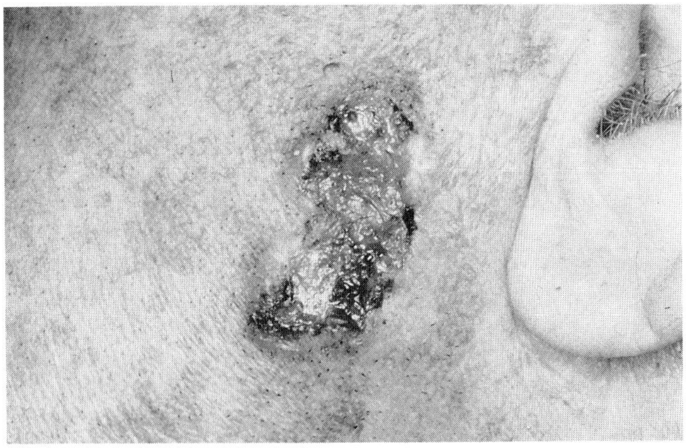

C

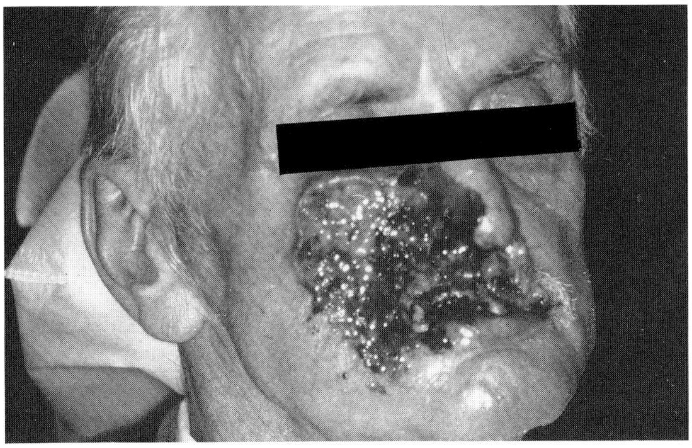

D

Fig. 9-16. Basal cell carcinoma. **A,** Early basal cell carcinoma of nose which had been noticed for 5 months but showed little change. **B,** Early basal cell carcinoma at the outer canthus of the eye. **C,** Moderately advanced basal cell carcinoma of the cheek anterior to the tragus of the ear. The lesion had been ignored for 3 years. **D,** Advanced basal cell carcinoma, neglected for many years. Though locally destructive, these lesions rarely metastasize.

Tissue analysis is required for diagnosis (Fig. 9-15). Excisional biopsy is preferred, theoretically, but the size and extent of the lesion often make this procedure impractical. Even though incisional biopsy could possibly disseminate tumor cells, the paramount consideration is to establish the diagnosis. Furthermore, there is no study which indicates that incisional biopsy gives a less favorable prognosis in patients with oral malignant melanoma.[44,45]

The only adequate treatment has been surgical, although occasionally radiation and chemotherapy have been used as adjunctive measures. Prognosis of malignant melanoma of the oral cavity is very poor as compared with that of cutaneous melanomas. Absolute 5-year survival rates for all patients with cutaneous melanoma range from 35 to 45%. When the diagnosis is made early and the lesions are thin (superficial), long-term survival rates approach 75%.[45,46] For patients with malignant melanoma of the mouth, survival appears to be less than 15%. This difference between cutaneous and mucosal tumor cure rates may be due to paucity of symptoms, delayed diagnosis, or difficulty in obtaining good surgical margins in and about the oral cavity.

SKIN AND LIP CANCERS

Skin cancer is important to the dentist because it is by far the most common cancer of man and its most frequent site is the head and neck. Yearly, new cases in the U.S. probably exceed a half million. Predisposing factors include light complexion, exposure to actinic rays, and age. Fortunately, these cancers seldom metastasize and respond well to treatment. Five-year cure rates are in excess of 95%. Initial signs may not arouse the patient's concern for many months, or even years, because these malignancies are usually slow-growing and are not painful.

Basal cell carcinoma is the most prevalent skin cancer. The early lesion may appear as a small ulcer, scab, or waxy pearl-like formation (Fig. 9-16). It may be mistaken for a benign skin condition.

The nevoid basal cell carcinoma syndrome is a rare condition that involves oral care because multiple jaw cysts are often found (Fig. 9-17).[47] This syndrome includes multiple nevi and basal cell carcinomas of the skin, rib anomalies, epidermal pits of the hands and feet, and a variety of other defects. The prognosis is good, but constant examination and continual treatment are required.

Lip cancer is often preceded by a premalignant change of cheilitis or keratosis (Fig. 9-18A). Chronic out-of-door exposure and pipe smoking appear to be causally related. Protective or therapeutic ointments should be initiated in an attempt to reverse these changes. In case of persistence and clinical suspicion, diagnosis should be made by biopsy. Cytology in this area is usually not representative and is difficult to interpret because of the high degree of squamous cell differentiation and cornification.

The lower vermilion border is by far the most common site, and squamous carcinoma is the most common type (Fig. 9-18B-D). Since most of these lesions remain localized, cure rates are extremely good. This is the only oral cancer that is decreasing in incidence.

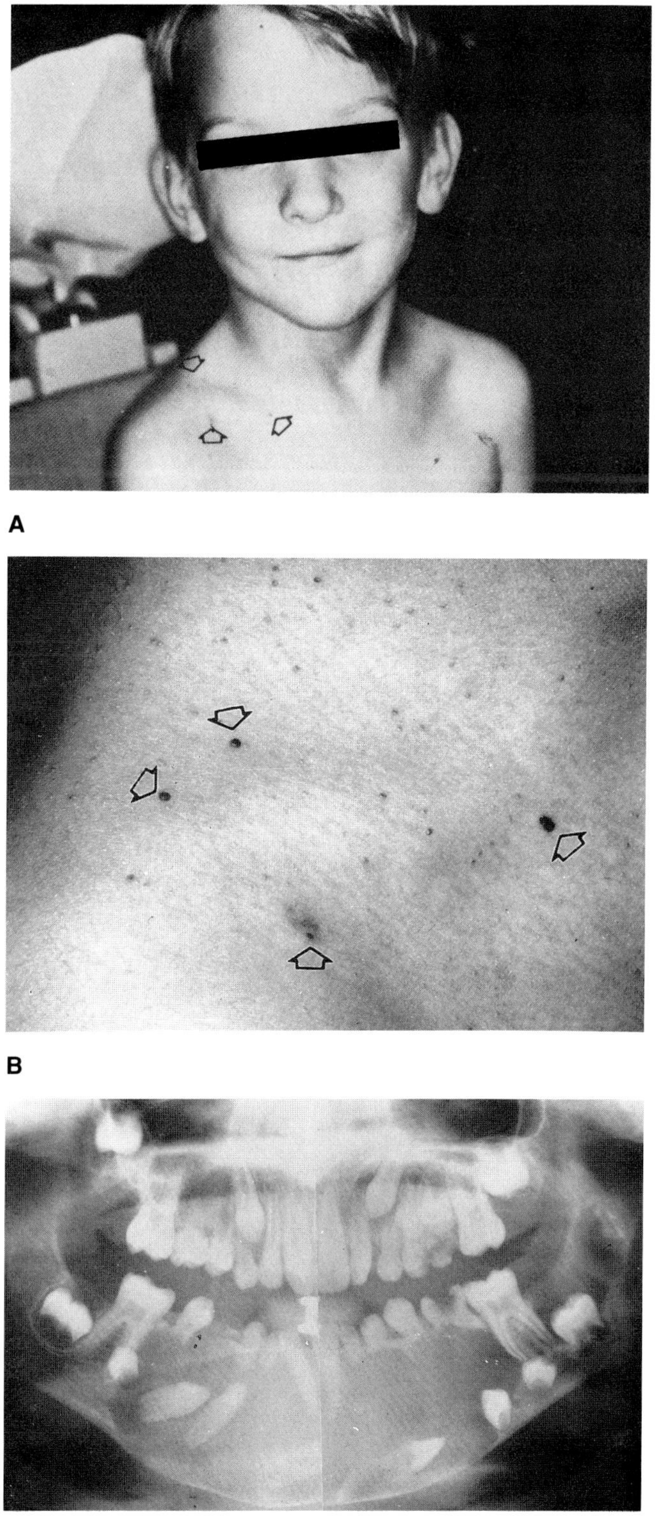

Fig. 9-17. Basal cell nevoid syndrome. **A,** Patient was normal except for multiple jawbone and skin lesions (arrows). **B,** Closer view of pigmented lesions. On histologic examination, many clinical lesions showed basal cell carcinoma (arrows). **C,** Panoramic radiograph of mandible shows multiple cysts and dislocated teeth, an occasional manifestation of this condition.

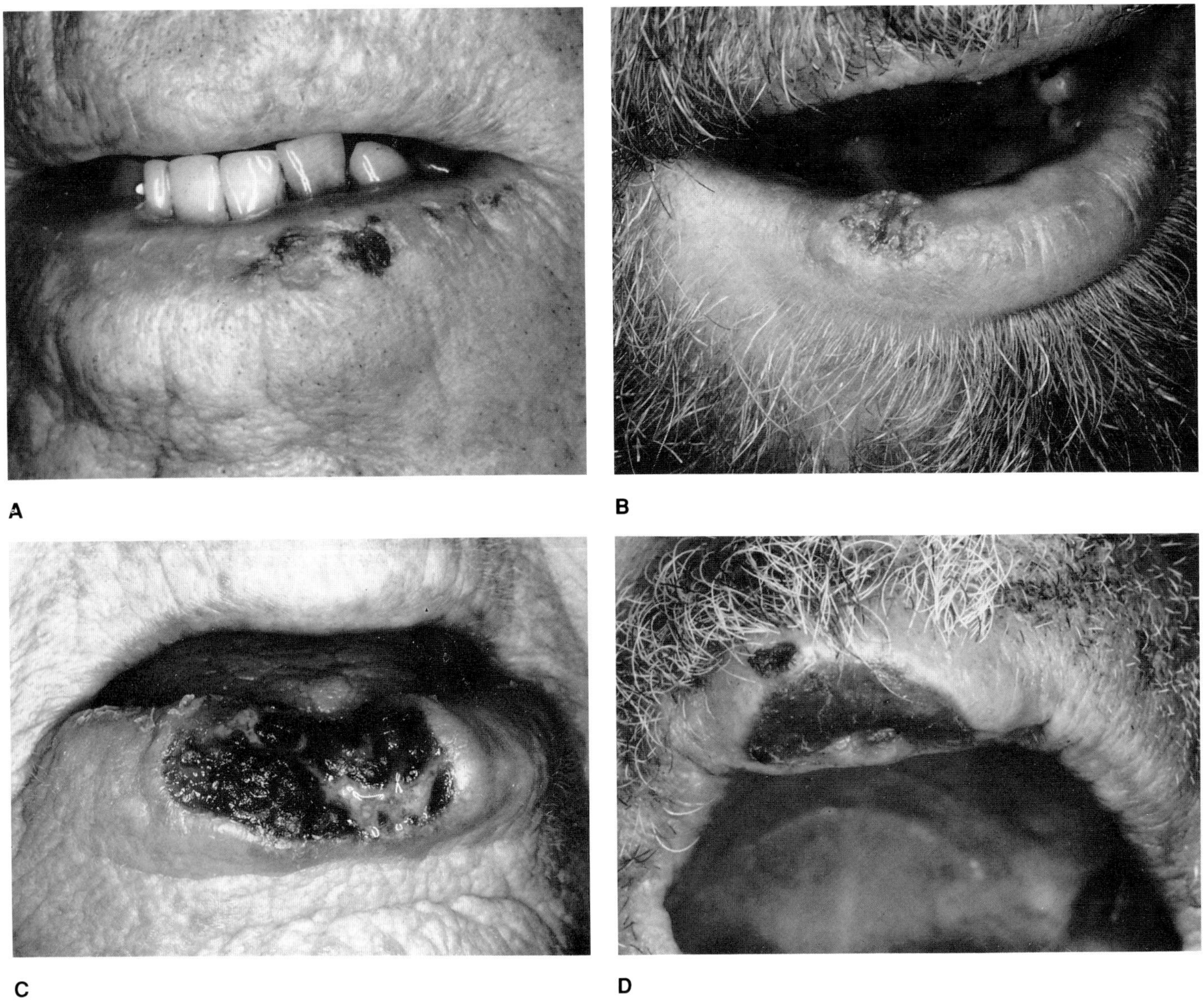

Fig. 9-18. Cancer of the lip. **A,** Solar cheilitis, a common precancerous change. **B,** Early squamous cell carcinoma of lower lip. **C,** Moderately advanced squamous cell carcinoma of lower lip; there was no evidence of regional spread. **D,** Squamous cell carcinoma of upper lip, an infrequent site.

ACQUIRED IMMUNODEFICIENCY SYNDROME (AIDS)

The AIDS pandemic has implications for the field of oral oncology. More than 15% of AIDS patients develop Kaposi's sarcoma (KS), a malignant tumor of fibrous and vascular connective tissue proliferation. It appears that the tumors represent multifocal lesions caused by a growth factor released by AIDS-virus-infected lymphocytes. While most of these patients die of opportunistic infections, in some cases KS is the primary cause. While KS is primarily a tumor involving the skin, many of these individuals, perhaps more than half of them, have KS lesions in the oral mucosa. The palate has been the most common intraoral site (Fig. 9-19). In a study of 134 patients with KS at the University of California, San Francisco, oral KS was the first site afflicted in 22% of the cases and, in many patients, led to the diagnosis of AIDS.[48]

In its early stages, oral KS is flat and asymptomatic, but it usually progresses into the nodular and symptomatic forms. The diagnosis is confirmed by biopsy. Treatment is palliative and primarily accomplished with low-dose radiation or chemotherapy.

Squamous carcinomas, primarily of the tongue, have occurred at a higher-than-expected frequency in AIDS patients, as have malignant, non-Hodgkin's lymphomas (Chapter 8, Fig. 8-14).

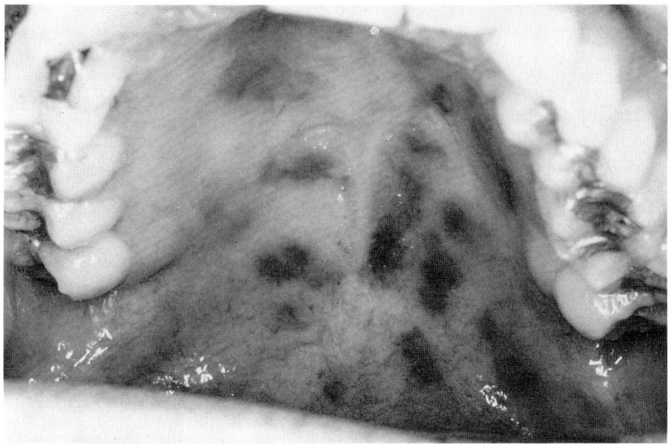

A

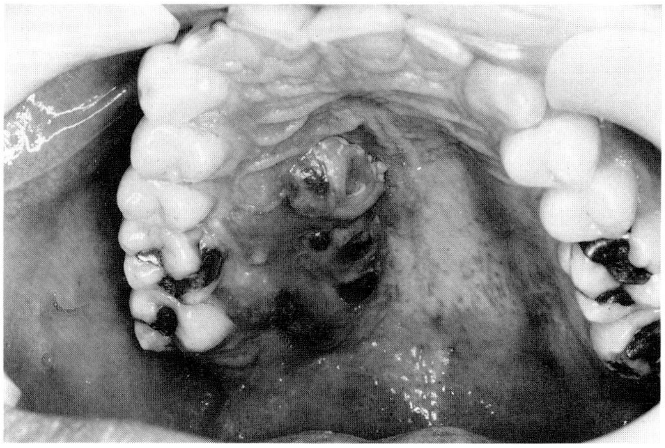

B

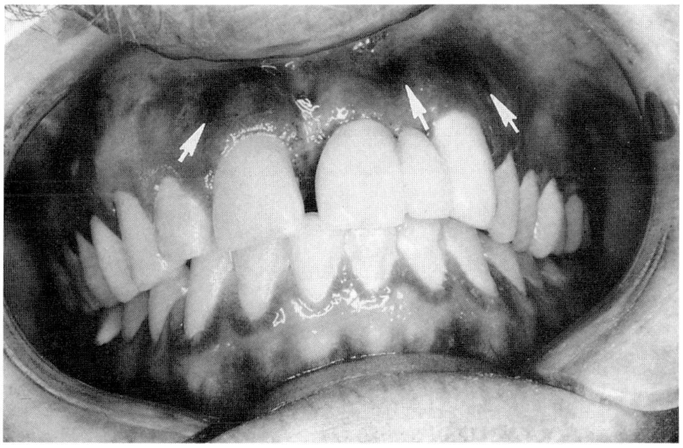

C

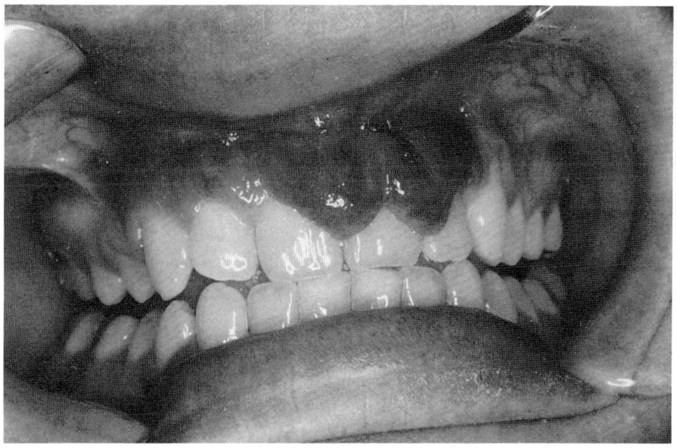

D

Fig. 9-19. Kaposi's sarcoma (KS). **A,** Flat KS lesions of palate which were asymptomatic. **B,** Nodular form of KS causing discomfort. **C,** Flat KS lesions of gingiva (arrows). **D,** Nodular KS of gingiva causing pain, bleeding, interference with hygiene and concern regarding appearance. **E,** Vascular-appearing skin lesions of KS. Esthetics are the usual complaints regarding skin lesions.

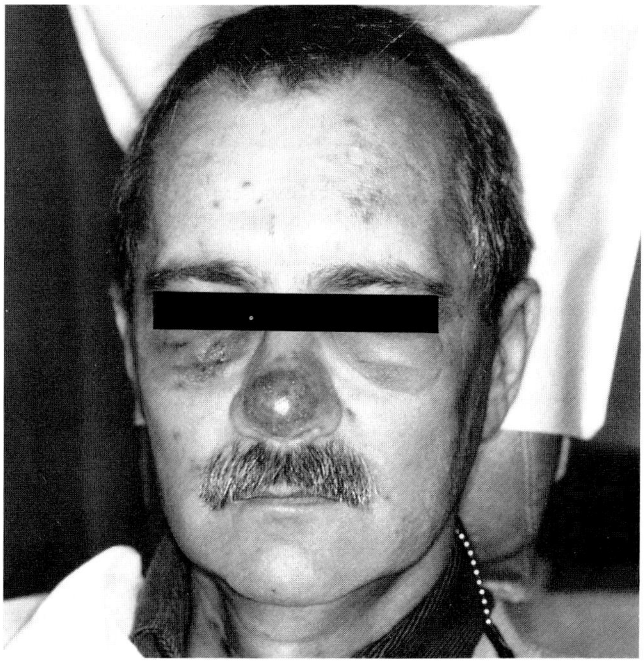

E

REFERENCES

1. Blitzer A: Inflammatory and obstructive disorders of salivary glands. *J Dent Res* 66 (Spec Iss): 675, 1987.
2. O'Dwyer P, Farrar WB, James AG et al: Needle aspiration biopsy of major salivary gland tumors: Its value. *Cancer* 57:554, 1986.
3. Krolls SO, Trodahl JN, Boyers RC: Salivary gland lesions in children. A survey of 430 cases. *Cancer* 30:459, 1972.
4. Baker SR, Malone B: Salivary gland malignancies in children. *Cancer* 55:1730, 1985.
5. Levitt SH, McHugh RB, Gomez-Marin O et al: Clinical staging system for cancer of the salivary gland: A retrospective study. *Cancer* 47:2712, 1981.
6. Krolls SO, Boyers RC: Mixed tumors of salivary glands. Long-term follow-up. *Cancer* 30:276, 1972.
7. Spiro RH, Huvos AG, Strong EW: Malignant mixed tumor of salivary origin. A clinicopathologic study of 146 cases. *Cancer* 39:388, 1977.
8. Gleeson MJ, Bennett MH, Cawson RA: Lymphomas of salivary glands. *Cancer* 58:699, 1986.
9. Shidnia H, Hornback NB, Hamaker R et al: Carcinoma of major salivary glands. *Cancer* 45:693, 1980.
10. Fu KK, Leibel SA, Levine ML et al: Carcinoma of the major and minor salivary glands. Analysis of treatment results and sites and causes of failure. *Cancer* 40:2882, 1977.
11. Rentschler R, Burgess MA, Byers R: Chemotherapy of malignant major salivary gland neoplasms. A 25-year review of M.D. Anderson Hospital experience. *Cancer* 40:619, 1977.
12. Spiro RH, Huvos AG, Berk R et al: Mucoepidermoid carcinoma of salivary gland origin: A clinicopathologic study of 367 cases. *Am J Surg* 136:461, 1978.
13. Spiro RH, Huvos AG, Strong EW: Adenoid cystic carcinoma: Factors influencing survival. *Am J Surg* 138:579, 1979.
14. Matsuba HM, Spector GJ, Thawley SE et al: Adenoid cystic salivary gland carcinoma. A histopathologic review of treatment failure patterns. *Cancer* 57:519, 1986.
15. Dunn JE, Bragg KU, Sautter C et al: Breast cancer risk following a major salivary gland carcinoma. *Cancer* 29:1343, 1972.
16. Spiro RH, Koss LG, Hajdu SI et al: Tumors of minor salivary gland origin. A clinicopathologic study of 492 cases. *Cancer* 31:117, 1973.
17. Chaudry AP, Labay GR, Yamane GM et al: Clinicopathologic and histogenetic study of 189 intraoral minor salivary gland tumors. *J Oral Med* 39:58, 1984.
18. Waldron CA, El-Mofty SK, Gnepp DR: Tumors of the intraoral minor salivary glands: A demographic and histologic study of 426 cases. *Oral Surg Oral Med Oral Pathol* 66:323, 1988.
19. Neville BW, Damm DD, Weir JC et al: Labial salivary gland tumors. *Cancer* 61:2113, 1988.
20. Goldblatt LI, Ellis GL: Salivary gland tumors of the tongue. Analysis of 55 new cases and review of the literature. *Cancer* 60:74, 1987.
21. Lynch DP, Crago CA,. Martinez MG: Necrotizing sialometaplasia. A review of the literature and report of two additional cases. *Oral Surg Oral Med Oral Pathol* 47:63, 1979.
22. Eversole LR, Sabes WR, Rovin S: Aggressive growth and neoplastic potential of odontogenic cysts. With special reference to central epidermoid and mucoepidermoid carcinomas. *Cancer* 35:270, 1975.
23. Clark JL, Unni KK, Dahlin DC et al: Osteosarcoma of the jaw. *Cancer* 51:2311, 1983.
24. Stern MH, Turner JE, Coburn TP: Oral involvement in neuroblastoma. *J Am Dent Assoc* 88:346, 1974.
25. Sehdev MK, Huvos AG, Strong EW et al: Ameloblastoma of maxilla and mandible. *Cancer* 33:324, 1974.
26. Laughlin EH: Metastasizing ameloblastoma. *Cancer* 64:776, 1989.
27. Atkinson CH, Harwood AR, Cummings BJ: Ameloblastoma of the jaw. A reappraisal of the role of megavoltage irradiation. *Cancer* 53:869, 1984.
28. National Cancer Institute: Surveillance, Epidemiology and End Results Program (SEER), 1973–1984. Bethesda, MD (computer tape).
29. Lin TM, Yang CS, Tu SM et al: Interaction of factors associated with cancer of the nasopharynx. *Cancer* 44:1419, 1979.
30. Armstrong RW, Armstrong MJ, Yu MC et al: Salted fish and inhalants as risk factors for nasopharyngeal carcinoma in Malaysian Chinese. *Cancer* Res 43:2967, 1983.
31. Pearson GR, Weiland LH, Neel HB III et al: Application of Epstein-Barr virus (EBV) serology to the diagnosis of North American nasopharyngeal carcinoma. *Cancer* 51:260, 1983.
32. Zeng Y: Seroepidemiological studies on nasopharyngeal carcinoma in China. *Advances in Cancer Research* 44:121, 1985.
33. Mabuchi K, Bross DS, Kessler II: Cigarette smoking and nasopharyngeal carcinoma. *Cancer* 55:2874, 1985.
34. Yu MC, Ho JHC, Lai SH et al: Cantonese-style salted fish as a cause of nasopharyngeal carcinoma: Report of a case-control study in Hong Kong. *Cancer Res* 46:956, 1986.
35. Wang DC, Cai WM, Hu YH et al: Long-term survival of 1035 cases of nasopharyngeal carcinoma. *Cancer* 61:2338, 1988.
36. Buchner A, Hansen LS: Amalgam pigmentation (amalgam tattoo) of the oral mucosa. A clinicopathologic study of 268 cases. *Oral Surg Oral Med Oral Pathol* 49:139, 1980.
37. Buchner A, Hansen LS: Pigmented nevi of the oral mucosa: A clinicopathologic study of 36 new cases and review of 155 cases from the literature. Part II. Analysis of 191 cases. *Oral Surg Oral Med Oral Pathol* 63:676, 1987.
38. Whitt JC, Jennings DR, Arendt DM et al: Rapidly expanding pigmented lesion of the buccal mucosa. *J Am Dent Assoc* 117:620, 1988.
39. Hansen L, Silverman S Jr, Beumer J III: Primary malignant melanoma of the oral cavity. *Oral Surg Oral Med Oral Pathol* 26:352, 1968.
40. Chaudry AP, Hampel A, Gorlin RJ: Primary malignant melanoma of the oral cavity: A review of 105 cases. *Cancer* 11:923, 1958.
41. Takagi M, Ishikawa G, Mori W: Primary malignant melanoma of the oral cavity in Japan: With special reference to mucosal melanosis. *Cancer* 34:358, 1974.
42. Liversedge RL: Oral malignant melanoma. *Br J Oral Surg* 13:40, 1975.
43. Rapini RP, Golitz LE, Greer RO et al: Primary malignant melanoma of the oral cavity. A review of 177 cases. *Cancer* 55:1543, 1985.
44. Paslin DA: The effects of biopsy on the incidence of metastases in hamsters bearing malignant melanoma. *J Invest Dermatol* 61:33, 1973.
45. Epstein E, Bragg K: Curability of melanoma: A 25-year retrospective study. *Cancer* 46:818, 1980.
46. Balch CM, Soong SJ, Milton GW et al: Changing trends in cutaneous melanoma over a quarter century in Alabama, USA and New South Wales, Australia. *Cancer* 52:1748, 1983.
47. Southwick GJ, Schwarz RA: The basal cell nevus syndrome. Disasters occurring among a series of 36 patients. *Cancer* 44:2294, 1979.
48. Ficarra G, Berson AM, Silverman S Jr. et al: Kaposi's sarcoma of the oral cavity: A study of 134 patients with a review of the pathogenesis, epidemiology, clincal aspects, and treatment. *Oral Surg Oral Med Oral Pathol* 66:543, 1988.

10

Rehabilitation

JOHN BEUMER III
IAN ZLOTOLOW
THOMAS A. CURTIS

The care of patients with head and neck cancer does not cease with elimination of the tumor. Rehabilitation, an essential phase of cancer care, should be considered from the time of diagnosis. Surgical resections often create large defects accompanied by dysfunction and disfigurement, and radiation therapy produces significant morbidities and unique tissue management problems. Speech, swallowing, control of saliva, and mastication can be adversely affected. If these cosmetic and functional impairments are not corrected or minimized, the patient may be unable to resume a normal working and social life.

TREATMENT OBJECTIVES

The primary objective of rehabilitation is the restoration of appearance and function. How successfully this is accomplished depends upon the judgment and skill of the therapist and the posttreatment anatomic, physiologic, and psychological makeup of the patient. In the rehabilitation of head and neck cancer patients, certain basic considerations apply:

1. The process of rehabilitation begins at the time of diagnosis. For example, if surgery is to be employed, the configuration of the surgical defect can have great impact on the design and effectiveness of the prosthetic restoration. These issues should be discussed before surgery if the level of rehabilitation is to be maximized.
2. The teeth should be preserved if possible. Teeth that might be considered inadequate for conventional prosthodontic purposes may prove valuable in patients with large oral defects.
3. Treatment plans should be carefully developed using basic prosthodontic principles with the aid of mounted diagnostic casts and appropriate radiographs. The prostheses are designed to be as simple and lightweight as possible.
4. Further surgery to improve existing anatomic configurations may be required. The successful use of a prosthesis may directly depend upon secondary surgical procedures—creating a sulcus, freeing a restricted tongue, or restoring mandibular continuity.
5. Ideally, comprehensive care of the cancer patient recognizes that this disease has both physical and psychological components and demands teamwork by health-care professionals with expertise in these areas. Surgeons, radiotherapists, and dentists are responsible for the physical management of the patient's disease, but psychological intervention is equally important if recovery is to be as complete as possible. After primary treatment, many patients with cancer of the head and neck fail to return to work, become socially isolated, and experience feelings of shame, worthlessness, and dejection—even when they have been fitted with adequate prostheses.[1] Therefore, a support system should be initiated at the patient's entry into the health care system and should continue throughout the course of treatment. A physically restored patient who withdraws from a usual pattern of social interaction represents a failure of the health-care team.

THE TEAM APPROACH TO REHABILITATION

Rehabilitation of the head and neck cancer patient requires the team approach, employing specialists outside the medical and dental professions who are available at a large medical center complex.

Two important members of a maxillofacial rehabilitation team are the *clinical social worker* and the *vocational rehabilitation counselor*. Since severe emotional distress accompanies the diagnosis and treatment of head and neck cancer, the patient's emotional resources can be strained, sometimes beyond endurance. The patient's family, which is called upon to provide support and comfort, often does not know just how to help.

The clinical social worker sees the patient at the time of diagnosis (whenever possible), during primary cancer treatment, and during the long period of rehabilitation. The primary function of this team member is to help the patient understand the process of treatment and to mobilize his or her resources to cope with the situation. The social worker also serves as the patient's advocate in the large medical center and with government agencies, as well as dealing with the myriad of other problems that patients and their families must face. When specific problems arise in the patient's relationship with his work, a vocational rehabilitation counselor can be of great assistance.

Other professionals who may contribute to the care and rehabilitation of the head and neck cancer patient are *nurses, dietitians, occupational therapists, physical therapists, speech pathologists,* and *dental hygienists.* Nurses can provide support and comfort for the patient, give instruction on the care of the surgical defect or tracheostomy, and arrange for visiting nurse support when the patient returns home. The dietitian advises the patient on his or her changing dietary requirements. Occupational and physical therapists help retrain altered muscular systems, and the speech pathologist can help the patient to adapt the speech mechanism to a new prosthesis or to altered physiology.

The dental hygienist is an important member of the team because maintenance of dentition is a vital factor in successful maxillofacial rehabilitation. A thorough prophylaxis and instruction in plaque control before and periodically after cancer therapy is essential to avoid severe dental disease.

The services of these clinicians broaden a maxillofacial rehabilitation program so that the entire scope of problems faced by these handicapped patients can be treated.

CLASSIFICATION

Head and neck cancer patients who require maxillofacial rehabilitation may be arbitrarily classified according to their posttreatment surgical defects and morbidities.

Maxillary defects. These patients present with defects of the maxilla and adjacent soft tissues. Maxillary defects range from small perforations of the hard or soft palate to extensive resections of the maxilla, soft palate, and paranasal sinuses, often including adjacent structures such as the orbit and cheek.

Mandibular defects. These patients have undergone resections confined to the mandible and adjacent soft tissues. Mandibular defects range from limited resections of the alveolar ridge and adjacent soft tissue, with mandibular continuity maintained, to extensive resections resulting in disarticulation of the mandible along with resection of portions of the tongue and floor of the mouth in continuity with the lymphatics of the neck.

Facial defects. These patients have defects ranging from orbital exenteration to excision of all or a portion of the nose, ear, or cheek. Also included in this category are patients with combination oral and facial defects.

Radiation therapy. These patients have been treated with a cancericidal dose of ionizing radiation. This mode of therapy produces changes in the volume and consistency of saliva, along with changes in bone and soft tissues, which must be considered in both surgical and prosthodontic rehabilitation.

MAXILLARY DEFECTS

Most tumors requiring maxillary resection arise either from paranasal sinus or palatal epithelium or from the minor salivary glands present in the submucosa. Resection of many of these tumors requires either a partial or a total maxillectomy. A radical maxillectomy entails resection of the entire maxilla to the midline, usually with exposure gained by reflection of a lip and cheek flap (Weber-Fergusson incision). A partial maxillectomy is less encompassing and may be performed transorally. The amount of soft palate included in these resections is variable and depends on the need to obtain tumor-free margins.

DISABILITIES

Defects of the hard or soft palate produce a variety of problems. Hypernasality makes speech unintelligible; mastication is difficult, particularly for the edentulous patient, because dental structures or denture-bearing tissue surfaces are lost; swallowing is awkward since food and liquids may be forced up into the nasal cavity and out the nose; the nasal mucous membranes become dessicated by abnormal exposure to the oral environment; nasal and sinus secretions collect in the defect area and may be difficult to control; and facial disfigurement can result from lack of midface bony support or resection of a branch of the facial nerve. In some cases, tumor invasion requires exenteration of the orbital contents.

Rehabilitation after resection of the hard or soft palate is best accomplished prosthodontically. Customarily, a temporary prosthesis, known as an immediate surgical obturator, is placed at the time of surgery or soon after. During the healing period, this prosthesis is relined periodically with temporary denture reliners to compensate for tissue changes secondary to organization and contracture of the wound. When the defect becomes well healed and dimensionally stable (usually three to four months after surgery), the definitive prosthesis is made.

Compromised retention, stability, and support are the main problems in fabricating a useful obturator prosthesis. The remaining teeth, therefore, become extremely valuable in providing support, retention, and stability for these restorations. Unilateral prostheses are particularly difficult because movement of the prosthesis may accelerate resorption of alveolar bone and subject abutment teeth to excessive lateral stress. The purpose of these prostheses is to restore the physical separation between the oral and nasal cavities, thereby restoring speech and swallowing to normal and providing support for the lip and cheek.

TREATMENT

It is essential that the prosthodontist examine and consult with the patient before surgery. The sequence of treatment should be explained to the patient, and diagnostic casts and appropriate radiographs should be obtained. With this information, the prosthodontist is ready to consult with the surgeon about the design and fabrication of the surgical obturator. Modifications in the surgical plan that may improve the prosthetic prognosis without adversely affecting tumor removal should be discussed at this time.

The surgeon can improve the prosthetic prognosis by considering the following modifications:

1. A split-thickness skin graft should be used to line the raw cheek surface of the defect. The skin graft provides a keratinized surface to support the prosthesis and forms a scar

band at the junction of the skin graft and oral mucosa that can be engaged prosthodontically to improve retention, stability, and support (Fig. 10-1).

2. If the surgeon can save some of the palatal mucosa normally included in the palatal resection and reflect this tissue during the bony resection of the palate, it can later be used to cover the medial cut margin of the palatal bone. If this palatal margin of the defect is covered with keratinized mucosa, the prosthesis may engage this surface more completely, thus improving its lateral stability.

3. An attempt should be made to save as much of the maxilla as possible, consistent with tumor control. The more palatal shelf area that remains, the more support will be provided for an obturator prosthesis. Retaining the premaxillary segment is particularly advantageous.

4. The transalveolar bony resection should be made as far from the tooth adjacent to the proposed defect as feasible. This practice leaves more bone around this tooth, improving its prognosis as a partial denture abutment.

5. If the soft palate does not retain the ability to effect palatopharyngeal closure, it should be resected. If a posterior, nonfunctioning band of soft palate remains after surgery, it often prevents proper placement of the palatopharyngeal obturator (Fig. 10-2).[2]

6. In edentulous patients the placement of osseointegrated implants into appropriate maxillary or mandibular bone sites should be considered. These implants can be used later to facilitate the retention, stability, and support for the future obturator prosthesis (Fig. 10-3).[3]

Immediate Surgical Obturator

Immediate or early coverage of a palatal defect with an obturator will greatly simplify the patient's postoperative course.[4] The obturator provides a matrix upon which the surgical packing can be placed, minimizes contamination of the wound in the immediate postoperative period, and enables the patient to speak and swallow effectively immediately after surgery. The immediate surgical obturator is useful in both dentulous and edentulous patients.

Making the prosthesis is simple. An irreversible hydrocolloid impression is obtained of the maxillary arch and the anterior portion of the soft palate, and the cast is retrieved. The obturator's size is determined by the surgical boundaries of the resection, as indicated by the surgeon. In the dentulous patient, teeth in the path of the surgical resection are removed from the cast (Figs. 10-4A and 10-4B). Care should be taken to extend the surgical obturator posteriorly past the proposed posterior soft palatal resection line to effectively seal off the defect. These prostheses are processed in autopolymerizing methyl methacrylate resin. They can be altered at surgery by trimming or by adding a temporary denture reliner. The prosthesis is wired to remaining teeth, alveolar ridge, or other available structures (zygomatic arch, anterior nasal spine, etc.) (Figs. 10-4C–10-4F).

After the surgical packing is removed (six to ten days after surgery), the prosthesis is relined with a temporary denture reliner. As healing progresses, the obturator is periodically relined and extended further into the defect and adaptation is improved. Three to five months after surgery, and after ini-

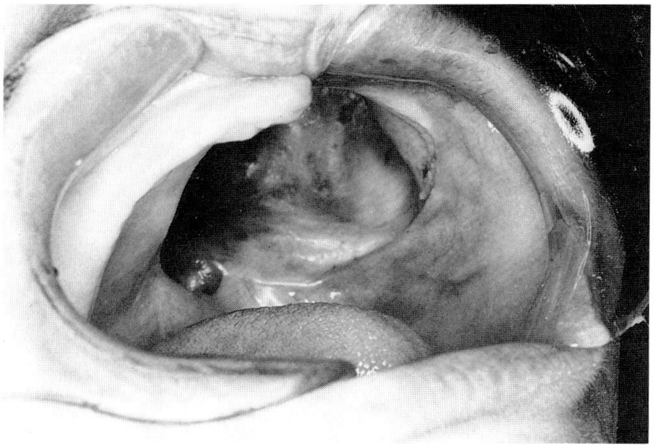

Fig. 10-1. Split-thickness skin graft lining lateral wall of radical maxillectomy defect.

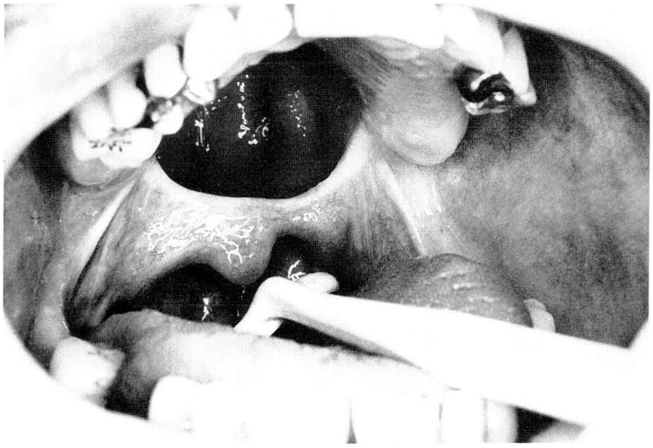

Fig. 10-2. Nonfunctional posterior band of soft palate prevents optimal placement of pharyngeal obturator.[2]

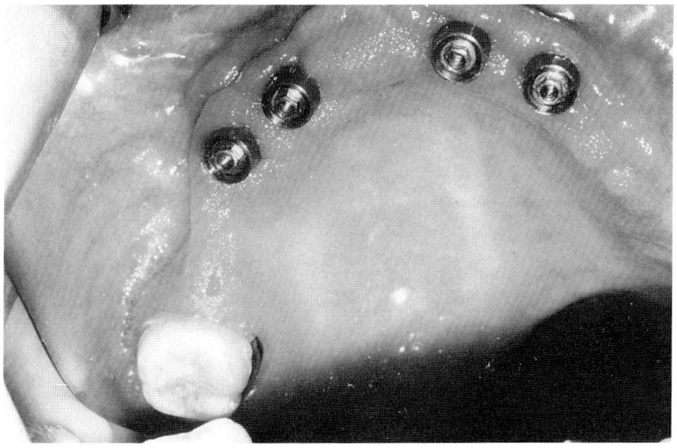

Fig. 10-3. This patient has undergone resection of the soft palate and a portion of hard palate. Osseointegrated implants have been positioned to retain, support, and stabilize the obturator prosthesis.

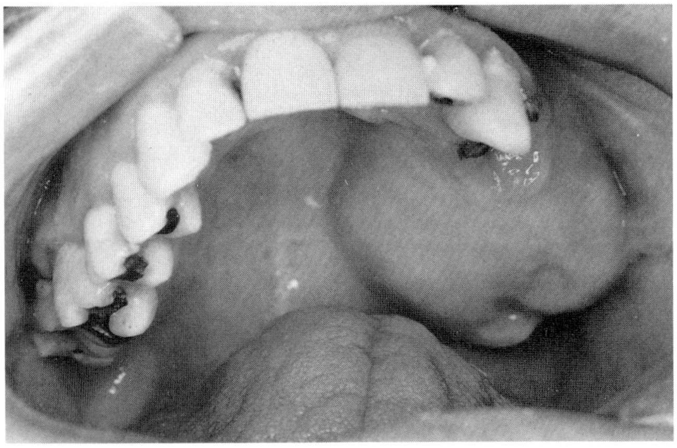

A

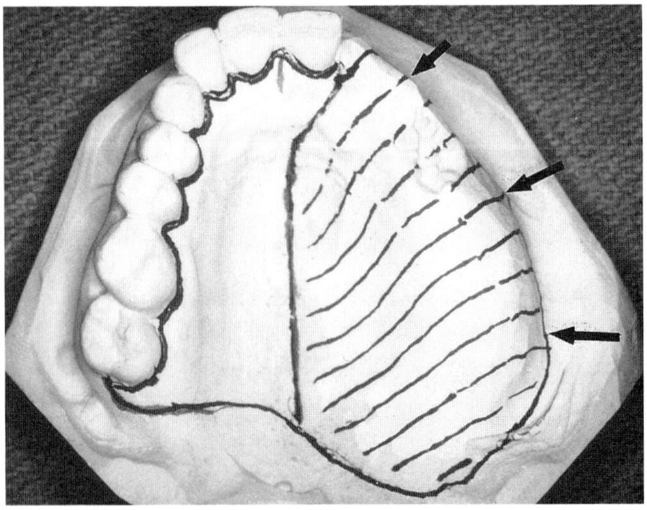

B

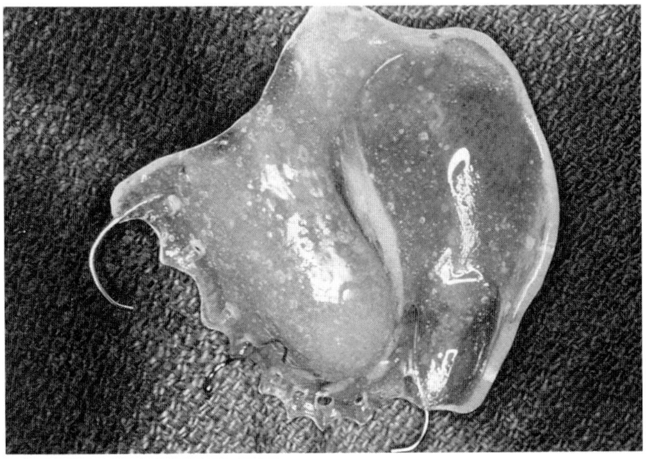

C

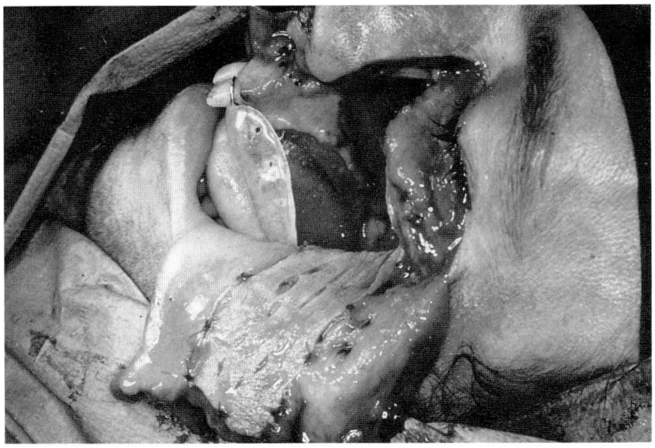

D

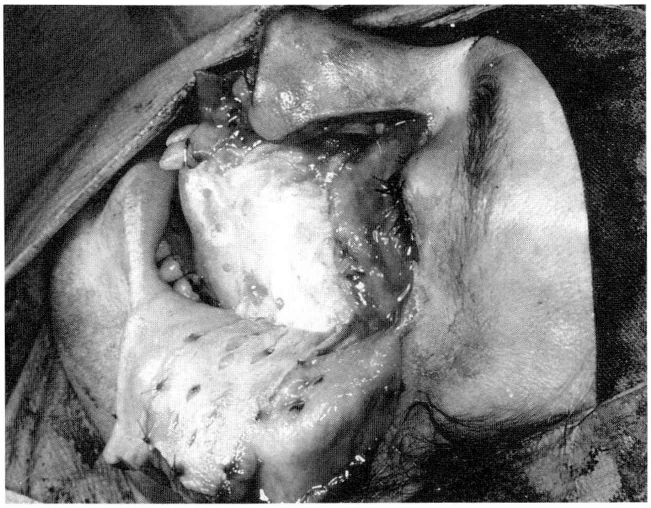

E

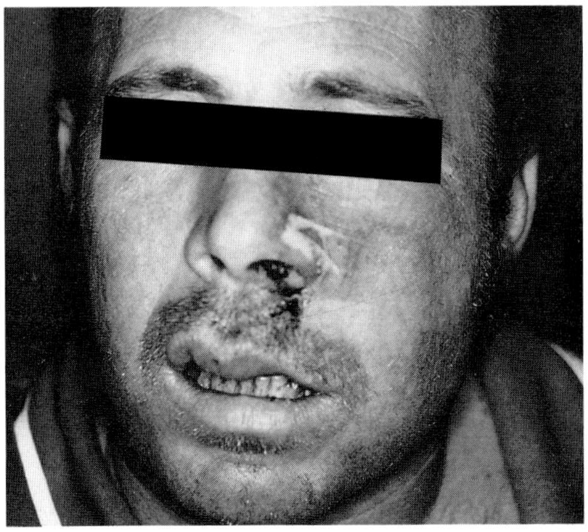

F

Fig. 10-4. Immediate surgical obturator. **A.** Palatal tumor requiring maxillectomy. **B.** Margins of proposed surgical resection trimmed appropriately for fabrication of immediate surgical obturator. Teeth included in resection were removed and alveolar ridge area was modestly reduced laterally and distolaterally (arrows). Vestibular depth on side of resection determines superior extension. **C.** Interproximal extensions of completed immediate surgical obturator are perforated to facilitate retention at surgery. **D.** Immediate surgical obturator in position and retained to remaining teeth and palate with wire ligation. Note that Weber-Fergusson surgical approach was used. Tension on cheek flap was adjusted before prosthesis was retained and defect packed with gauze. **E.** Prosthesis serves as platform for placement of surgical packing. **F.** Patient 6 days after surgery. Facial contours are nearly normal.

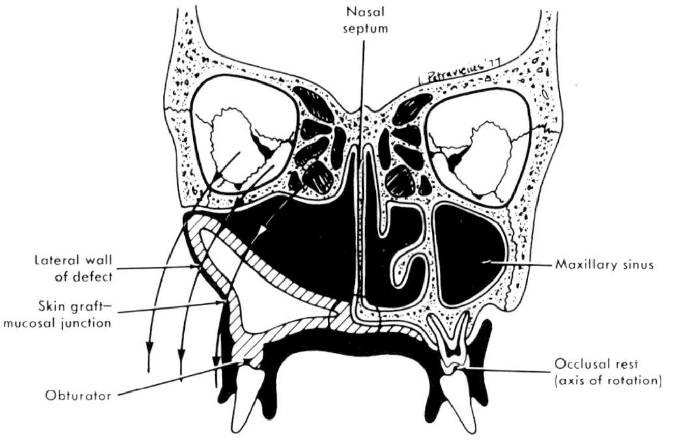

A

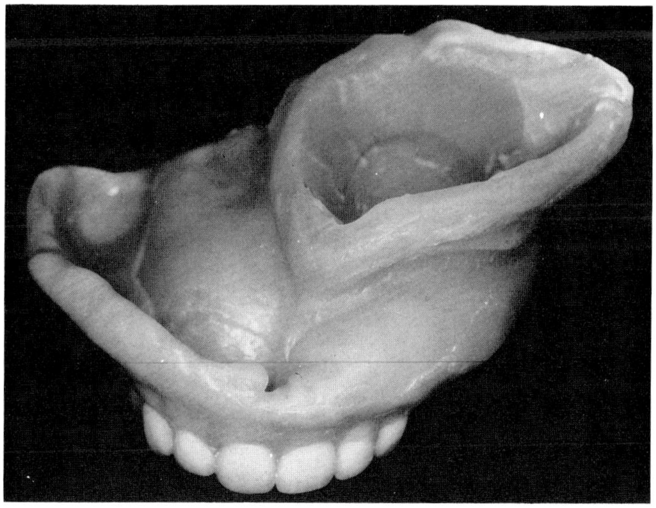

B

Fig. 10-5. Definitive obturator prosthesis. **A.** Diagrammatic frontal section of a radical maxillectomy with obturator prosthesis in position. **B.** Typical obturator of methyl methacrylate resin.[2]

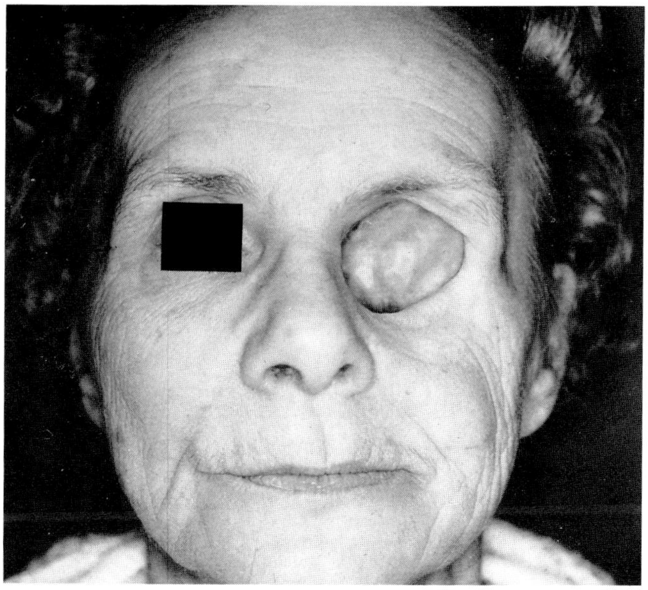

A

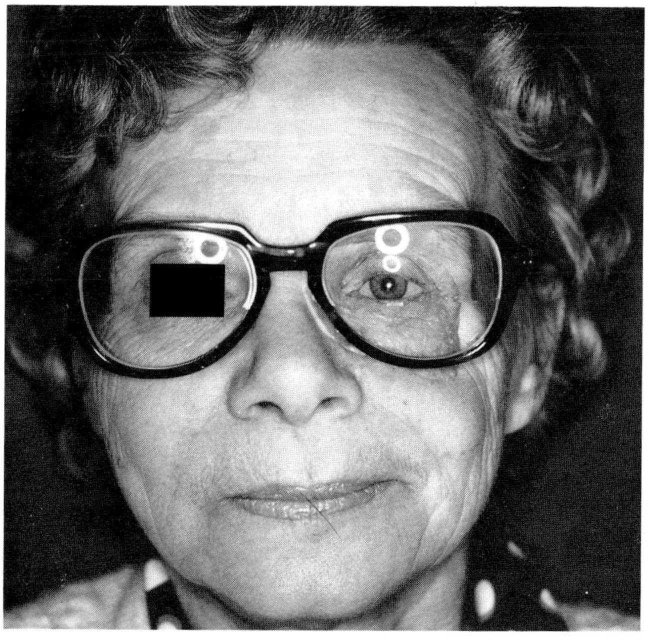

B

Fig. 10-6. Facial contours (**A**) without obturator prosthesis, (**B**) with obturator prosthesis. Note improved contours of left cheek area. Patient is also wearing an orbital prosthesis.

tial wound contracture is essentially complete, the definitive prosthesis is begun. Edentulous patients with maxillary defects often require a longer period of healing because the defect must be engaged more aggressively so as to maximize stability, support, and retention.

Definitive Obturator Prosthesis

Defects of the hard palate are restored most effectively with a prosthesis. Surgical reconstruction is usually neither possible nor desirable after resection in this region. If teeth are present, they greatly improve denture retention and stability. Speech, swallowing, mastication, and facial contour can be restored with proper extensions and obturation.[5] The obturator should extend maximally along the lateral wall of the defect (Fig. 10-5). This high lateral extension increases retention and lateral stability and provides support for the lip and cheek. The movement of the coronoid process into the distolateral area of the defect must be accounted for during border molding and final impression procedures. The extension superiorly along the medial margin of the defect should not exceed the level of the repositioned palatal mucosa. If it does, it provides little benefit and may result in unnecessary and painful ulceration of the respiratory mucosa lining the nasal septum. In some patients, extension across the nasal surface of the soft palate or into the nasal aperture may be necessary to provide acceptable retention.

When the prosthesis is completed, speech and swallowing are restored to normal limits and appearance is greatly improved (Fig. 10-6). The patient should be recalled periodi-

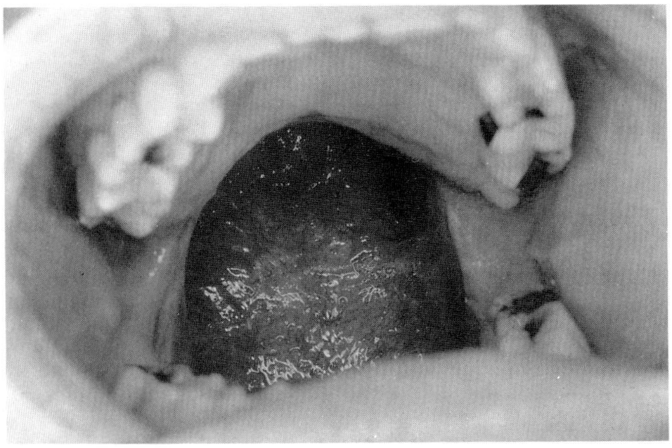

A

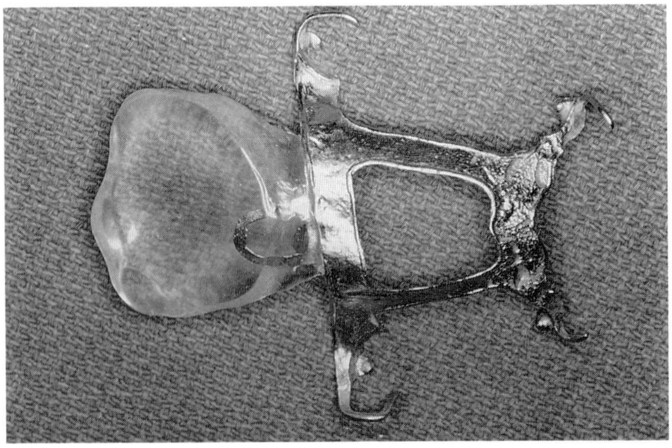

B

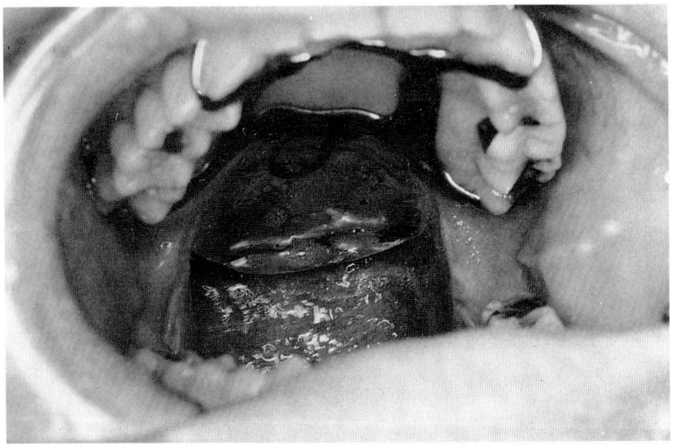

C

Fig. 10-7. Definitive soft palate prosthesis. **A.** Soft palate defect after resection of adenoidcystic carcinoma of soft palate. Residual palatopharyngeal mechanism continues to function adequately. **B.** Pharyngeal obturator attached to partial denture. **C.** Obturator in position. Note space between lateral pharyngeal wall and obturator. During closure required for speech and swallowing, residual pharyngeal musculature contracts and contacts the obturator.

cally for adjustments and examination for recurrent disease. Most prostheses require relining within the first year because of slow but continuous tissue changes on the periphery of the surgical defect.

Definitive Soft Palate Prosthesis

Defects of the soft palate require different and more complex prosthetic treatment. Palatopharyngeal closure normally occurs when the soft palate elevates and contacts the contracting lateral and posterior pharyngeal walls of the nasopharynx. When a portion of the soft palate is excised or when the soft palate is perforated, scarred, or neurologically impaired, complete palatopharyngeal closure cannot occur. Speech becomes hypernasal, and normal swallowing is not possible. With a pharyngeal obturator, the patient may be able to reestablish palatopharyngeal closure if the residual portion of the palatopharyngeal mechanism still exhibits normal movements (Fig. 10-7). The obturator must not interfere with breathing, impinge upon soft tissues during postural movements, or hamper the tongue during swallowing and speech.

The soft palate obturator remains in a fixed position in the nasopharynx and does not attempt to duplicate normal movements of the soft palate. The inferior surface of the obturator remains level with the hard palate contour, which in most patients is approximately the level of the anterior tubercle of the atlas. The inferior margin of the posterior surface of the obturator contacts Passavant's pad, if present, and extends approximately 10 mm superiorly into the nasopharynx. During breathing and the production of nasal speech sounds, the space around the obturator reflects the potential for muscular contraction. During swallowing and the production of other speech sounds, this sphincteric muscular network moves into contact with the stationary acrylic resin obturator, establishing palatopharyngeal closure. A correctly constructed obturator will usually result in the return of normal speech and swallowing for patients with acquired soft palate defects. There are instances, however, when speech therapy can help correct distortions associated with articulation that will not be adequately corrected by the obturator prosthesis.

MANDIBULAR DEFECTS

The management of malignant tumors associated with the tongue, the mandible, and adjacent structures represents a difficult challenge for the surgeon, the radiation oncologist, and the prosthodontist relative both to control of the primary disease and to rehabilitation after treatment. Common intraoral sites for squamous cell carcinoma are the lateral margin of the tongue and the floor of the mouth. Both locations predispose the mandible to the invasion of tumor, often necessitating its resection along with large portions of the tongue, the floor of the mouth, and the regional lymphatics.

DISABILITIES

Disabilities resulting from such resections include impaired speech articulation, difficulty in swallowing, deviation of the mandible during functional movements, and poor control of salivary secretions. There is also severe cosmetic disfigurement. These patients present a far more difficult rehabilitation problem than do patients with maxillary surgical defects, particularly if significant portions of the tongue are involved in the resection. It is usually not possible to restore function to presurgical levels in patients after mandibular resection, and permanent cosmetic disfigurement is inevitable. Consequently these patients experience many frustrations, and fewer return to presurgical levels of social function. Rehabilitation frequently requires the coordinated efforts of several disciplines, including social services, psychiatry, prosthodontics, surgery, speech therapy, and dietetics.

Advanced tumors of the anterior two thirds of the tongue and floor of the mouth often require extensive resection of bone and soft tissue. The degree of speech impairment after such resections depends on the extent to which tongue function is affected. In most of these lesions, large amounts of the tongue are resected and what remains is occasionally used for primary closure of the surgical wound (Fig. 10-8). The loss of large portions of the tongue prevents appropriate "valving" and/or interaction with other oral structures. This loss, combined with the loss of motor and sensory innervation plus impaired mobility, leads to misarticulation of many speech sounds. Other articulators such as the lower lip may also be affected by the structures removed during the radical neck dissection. Deglutition is less impaired, and most patients learn to swallow fairly efficiently.

The degree to which mastication is affected depends somewhat on the amount of mandible removed, but primarily on the status of tongue function. If much of the mandible is segmented and removed, the remaining functional mandibular segment(s) will be retruded and deviated towards the surgical site at the vertical dimension of rest. When the mouth is opened this deviation increases, leading to an angular path of opening and closing. In addition, loss of the proprioceptive sense of occlusion leads to uncoordinated, less precise movement of the mandible. Loss of attachment of the muscles of mastication on the surgical side also makes the mandible rotate upon forceful closure. Viewed from the frontal plane, teeth in the mandible on the surgical side move away from their opposing maxillary teeth after initial contact has been made on the nonsurgical side and as the force of closure is increased (Fig. 10-9). These factors, combined with impaired tongue function, may prevent effective mastication in some patients. The severity and permanence of mandibular deviation varies, depending on a number of complex factors. Some patients soon attain an acceptable interocclusal relationship without adjunctive therapy, while others are never able to do so.

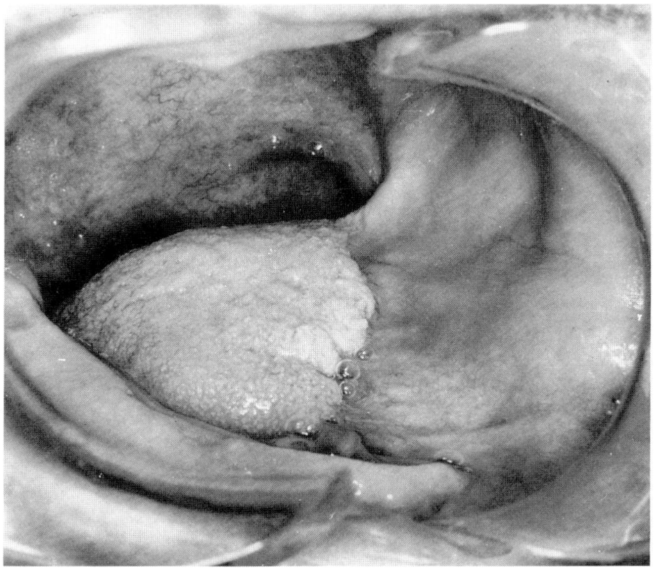

Fig. 10-8. Tongue sutured to buccal mucosa.

Control of saliva is adversely affected by most resections of the tongue and mandible. These resections often obliterate portions of the lingual and buccal sulci so that a means of collecting and channeling secretions posteriorly no longer exists. In addition, the motor and sensory innervation of the lower lip on the resected side is often lost, impairing oral competency and preventing the patient from detecting secretions escaping from the mouth. Impaired tongue control and mobility and drooping of the corner of the mouth on the defect side also contribute to poor saliva control.

When removal of tumors in the anterior floor of the mouth requires that the mandible be resected anteriorly, the disabilities are very severe unless mandibular continuity is restored at the time of initial tumor resection. If it is not restored, the two remaining posterior fragments are pulled medially by the residual mylohyoid muscles and superiorly by the muscles of mastication. This displacement of the mandibular remnants severely disfigures the face (Fig. 10-10), prevents intercuspation of teeth in dentulous patients, and precludes use of complete dentures in edentulous patients. In addition, with its anterior mandibular attachment lost, the tongue retrudes posteriorly and may occlude the oral airway. Many of these difficulties are partially alleviated if the missing portion of the mandible is replaced with an alloplastic implant at the time of resection, thereby maintaining mandibular continuity (Fig. 10-11). The intrinsic and extrinsic muscles of the tongue may be sutured to the implant, ensuring a more anterior tongue position and less risk of airway obstruction. Such implants result in little distortion of the tissue bed and allow for easy visualization and recognition of recurrent disease.

The nature and degree of the disabilities secondary to impaired tongue function after resection of lesions in the anterior floor of the mouth are proportional to the amount of tissue resected and to the nature of surgical closure (Fig. 10-12). In most cases, motor control is usually unimpaired and the functional deficits depend on the degree of tongue mobility. The resection of primary tumor and the required oral closure, however, often lead to excessive drooling. Sensory and motor innervation of the lower lip may be bilaterally impaired, affecting oral competency and precluding saliva control in some patients.

In tumors confined within the mandible or to the alveolar ridge, resection of the primary tumor results in only minimal loss of soft tissue, and the resulting disabilities are less severe. A simple marginal resection that retains bony continuity results in little morbidity other than alteration of sulci and denture-bearing surfaces. In discontinuity defects, some

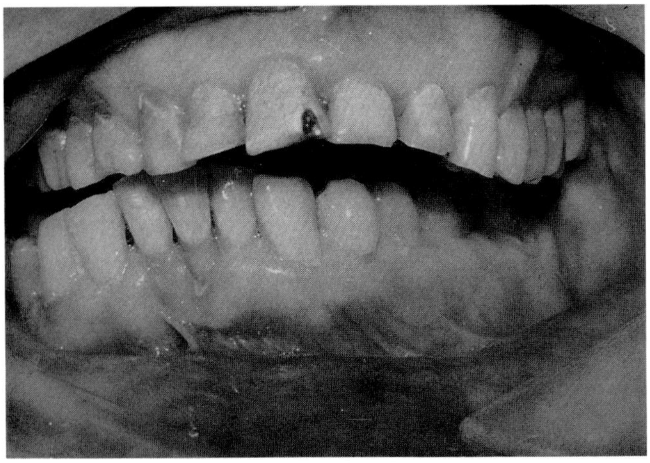

A

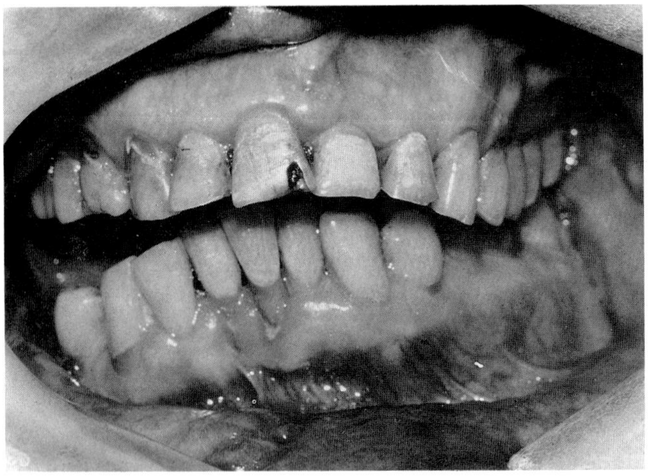

B

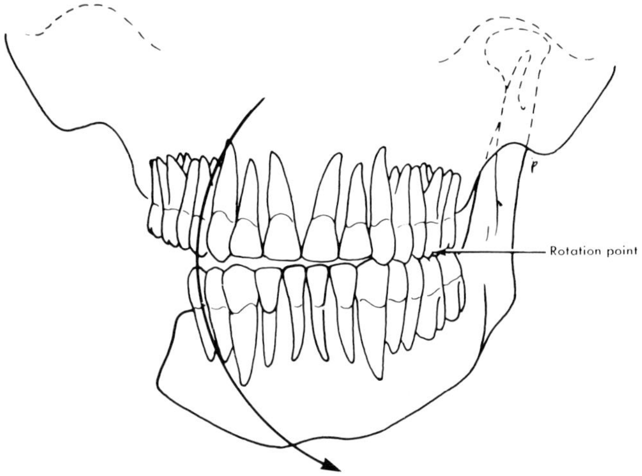

C

Fig. 10-9. Frontal plane rotation. **A.** Initial occlusal contact after right lateral mandibulectomy. Note degree of mandibular deviation and loss of cuspal interdigitation due to altered occlusal proprioception. **B.** Lateral terminus of mandible rotates inferiorly with forceful closure. **C.** Diagram of frontal plane rotation.[2]

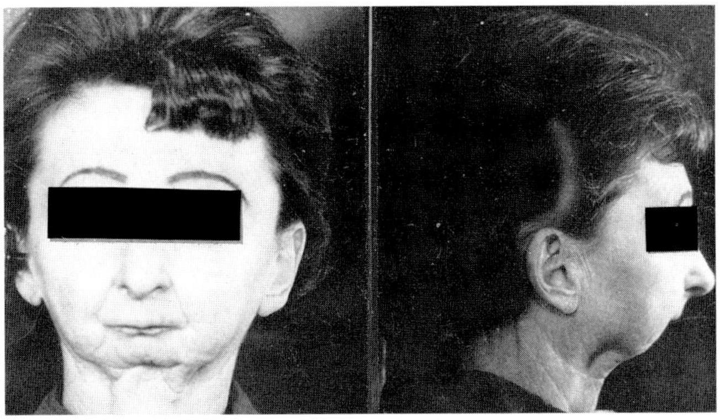

Fig. 10-10. Facial contours after resection of anterior portion of mandible.[2]

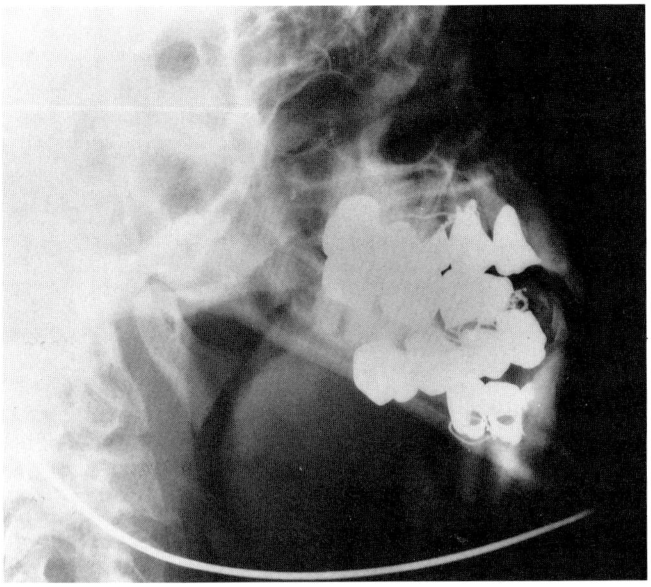

Fig. 10-11. Stainless steel wire used to maintain mandibular continuity.

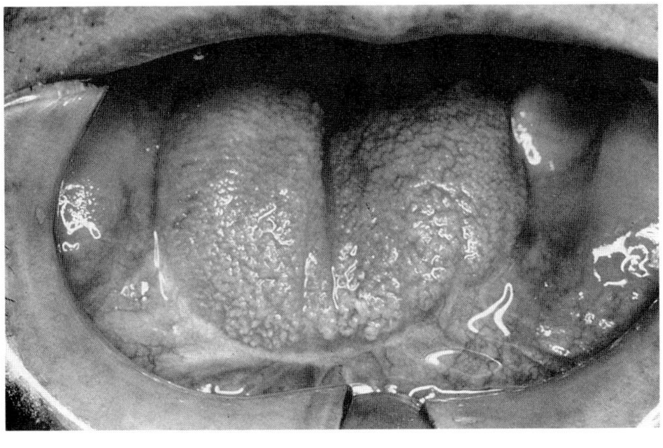

Fig. 10-12. Tongue sutured to labial mucosa to close the wound after anterior mandibular resection.[2]

deviation of the mandible results from scar contracture and muscle imbalances. Tongue function, however, is rarely affected. In these lesions, the tongue may be used for closure of the surgical wound, but little of the tongue is resected and the hypoglossal nerve on the resected side remains intact. With normal bulk and unimpaired motor control, the slight loss of tongue mobility secondary to surgical closure does not seriously affect saliva control, speech, or swallowing. If control of saliva is affected, it is primarily due to impaired innervation of the lower lip on the resected side, resulting from the radical neck dissection. Mandibular deviation is less profound than that seen in resections resulting in more extensive soft tissue loss.

From a prosthodontic point of view, it is far more desirable to close large oral composite resection defects in soft tissue with distant flaps rather than with local flaps. The myocutaneous flap based on the pectoralis major muscle is particularly useful (Fig. 10-13). The numerous advantages include the following: (1) Mandibular deviation is less evident than with primary closures or when tongue flaps are used for closure, and mandibular guidance therapy is more effective. (2) If primary closure or tongue flaps are employed, larger segments of the mandible must often be sacrificed, particularly in irradiated patients. (3) Less compromise of tongue function results with the use of distant flaps.

The recent development of myocutaneous flaps, which can be done in one stage, has made it possible to close many wounds without the cosmetic deformity associated with the use of forehead or nasolabial flaps. The large bulk of tissue that can be brought to the resected area minimizes mandibular deviation and provides additional bulk for restoration of facial contours. With less deviation of the mandible, mandibular guidance therapy is more effective, resulting in improved maxillomandibular relationships and more normal tooth placement when fabricating complete or partial dentures. Optimal levels of tongue function are retained, giving the edentulous patient the best chance of functioning with a mandibular complete denture. In addition, the need for subsequent tongue release and vestibuloplasty is often eliminated since the mandibular denture often can be extended onto the surface of the flap. Also, mandibular opening and closing movements, and therefore forces generated during mastication, are more vertical, resulting in more efficient mastication and a more stable prosthesis.

SECONDARY SURGICAL PROCEDURES

Vestibuloplasty, Tongue Release, and Skin Grafts

Vestibuloplasty and tongue release are of particular value when mandibular continuity has been maintained or restored. The creation of vestibules enables the patient to pool saliva more efficiently and allows for extension of denture flanges (Fig. 10-14). Creation of an attached keratinized mucosa on the ridge surface with either a skin graft or a palatal graft improves stability, support, and retention of a partial or complete denture. The patient's appearance may also be improved because a prosthodontic restoration can now be molded to provide contour and support for the lower lip and cheek portions of the resected area. Improvement of speech is less noticeable, except in patients with anterior soft tissue defects. In these patients, the motor and sensory innervations of the tongue are usually intact and the tongue dysfunctions result from its immobility. Tongue release and vestibuloplasty may also aid selected patients with unrestored mandibular discontinuity defects.

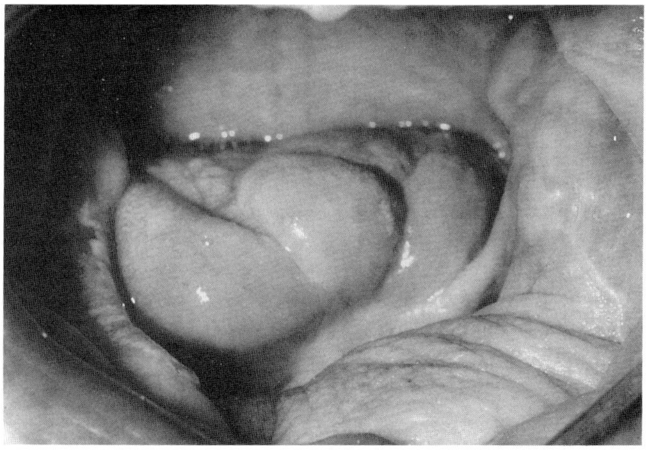

Fig. 10-13. Myocutaneous flap used to restore the soft tissue bed.

At surgery, posttreatment adhesions must be incised and the tongue recontoured at the same time as the sulci are deepened. These procedures leave large areas of exposed periosteum and submucosal tissue. To reduce subsequent postsurgical scar contracture, split-thickness skin grafts or palatal grafts are applied to cover the denuded areas. Skin grafts are obtained from a relatively hairless area of the patient's body, such as the upper thigh, buttocks, or abdomen. It has been

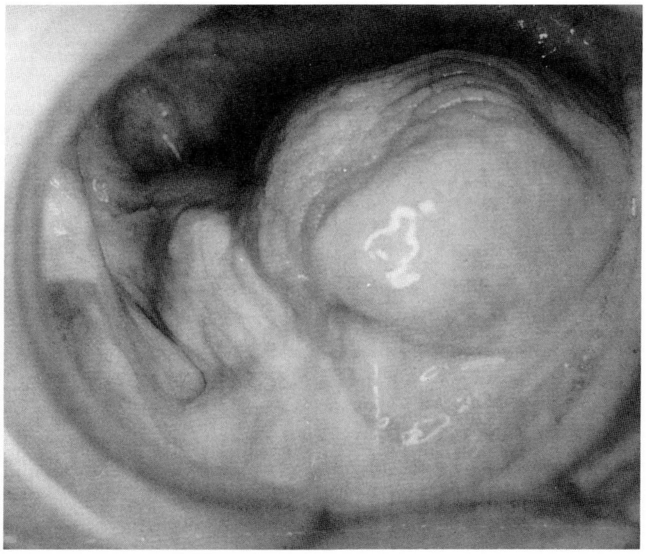

Fig. 10-14. Tongue release and vestibuloplasty. These procedures improve tongue mobility and permit construction of dentures. A split-thickness skin graft was placed at surgery to line the new vestibule and raw surface of the tongue.[2]

observed that the successful "take" of skin grafts relates inversely to the thickness of the graft, but successful thick grafts result in less subsequent scar contracture than do thin grafts. The thicker the graft, however, the greater the chance that skin appendages will be retained. Usually an attempt is made to secure a graft of moderate thickness, from 14- to 20-thousandths of an inch. The graft is either sutured in place covering the denuded areas or applied to a surgical stent which, in turn, is secured in place by circumferentially wiring the stent to the mandible. Regardless of the method used to develop or increase the depth of the alveolar sulci, scar contracture tends to cause shrinkage and loss of alveolar height.

Bony Augmentation

When alveolar bone has been reduced to a degree precluding a sulcus procedure, the size of the body of the mandible can be increased with bony augmentation procedures. Onlay grafts to the superior or inferior border have been successfully performed by intraoral and extraoral approaches and by using either rib or iliac crest bone. However, remodeling and resorption of up to 50% of the original graft should be anticipated. When bone grafts appear to have taken well, a sulcus extension operation may be performed in four to six months if deemed necessary for prosthetic treatment (Fig. 10-15).

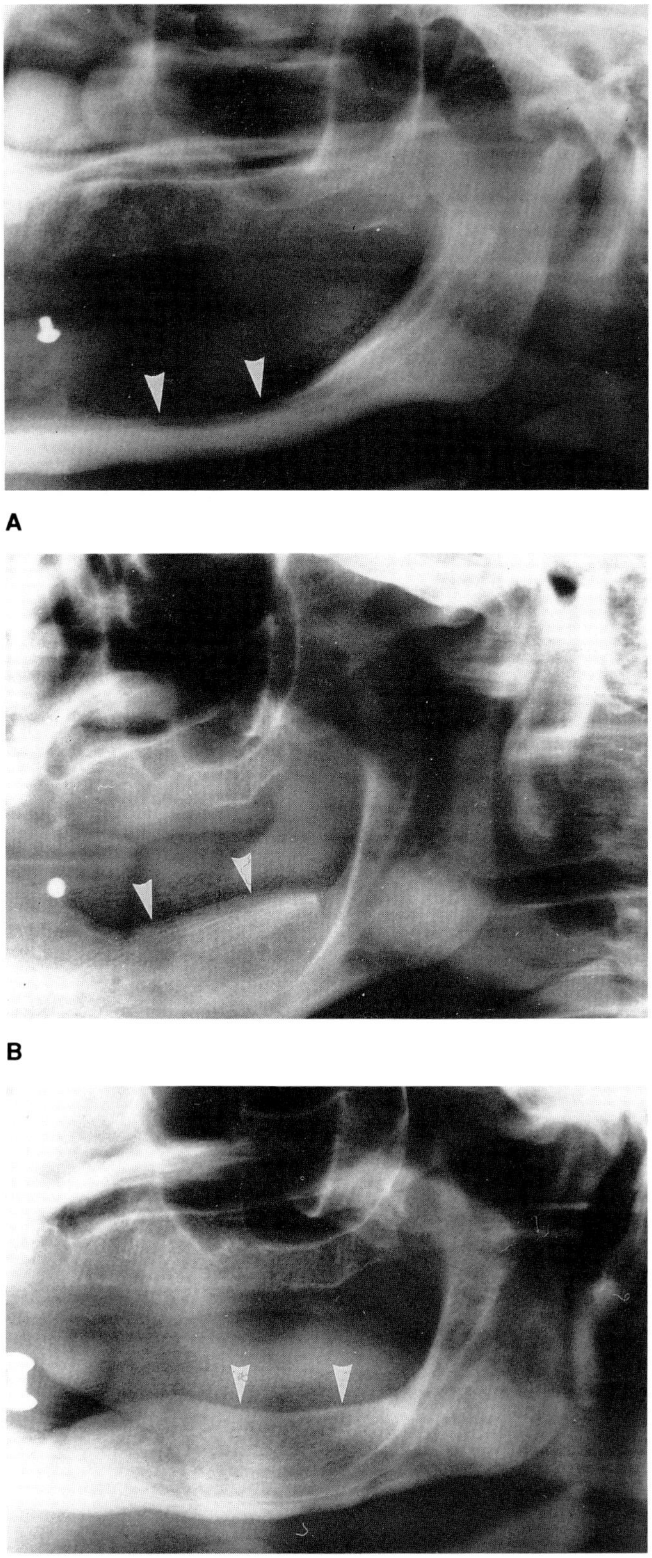

A

B

C

Fig. 10-15. Bony augmentation. **A.** Loss of alveolar bone (arrows), leaving inadequate ridge to retain a prosthesis. **B.** Increase in ridge height (arrows) achieved by grafting with iliac crest bone via submandibular resection. **C.** Two years after surgery, graft resorption is apparent (arrows) but ridge is sufficient to support a prosthesis.

Restoration of Mandibular Continuity

Significant benefits are derived from surgically restoring mandibular discontinuity defects. Reestablishing the bilateral function of the mandible results in more-normal mandibular movement patterns that enable an edentulous patient to exert force on both sides of the dental arch, thus increasing the stability of complete dentures. In dentulous patients, a properly proportioned implant will restore dental occlusion to normal and it will partially alleviate deviation of the mandible. This improves facial appearance and also provides support for soft tissues at the previously resected surgical site. This is not to imply that facial appearance can be restored to normal. Soft tissue asymmetries secondary to the primary resection are difficult to account for, and disfigurement usually persists.

Reconstruction after extensive resection of oral malignancies is difficult because of the lack of sufficient soft tissue to receive the graft, the decreased vascularity of the tissue bed secondary to radiation therapy and/or radical neck dissection, and the difficulty in achieving proper fixation of the graft during the healing period. A variety of methods has been employed.[6] Autogenous graft sources include iliac crest, rib, and clavicle. Rib grafts have not proven to be as successful as iliac crest grafts in these patients, and clavicular grafts have been used only sparingly. Most defects are restored either with particulate autogenous marrow housed in a metal tray (Fig. 10-16) or with a block of bone, both usually obtained from the iliac crest (Fig. 10-17). The use of myocutaneous flaps for closure of the initial wound should facilitate bone grafting of continuity defects.

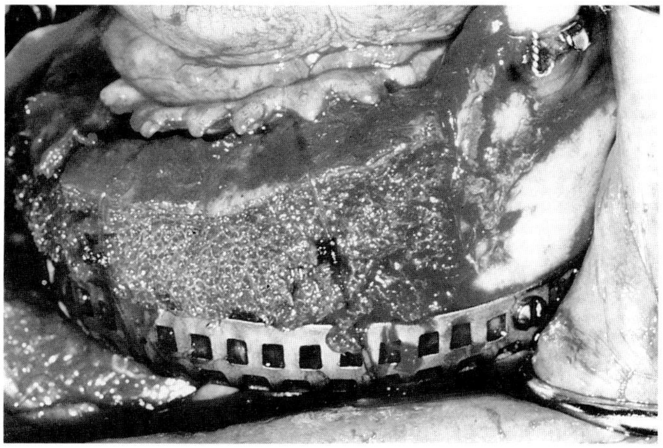

Fig. 10-16. Particulate marrow graft housed in titanium tray.[2]

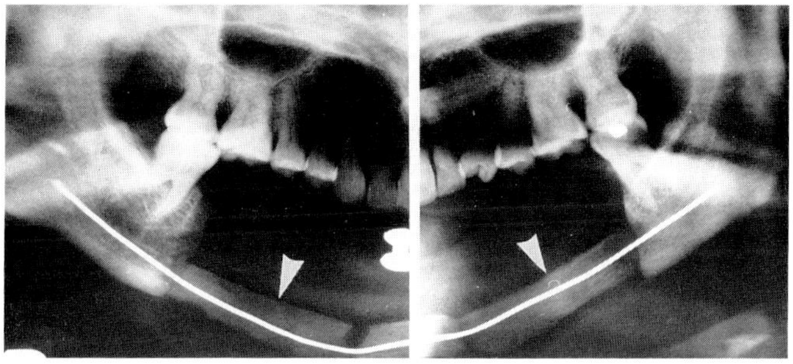

A

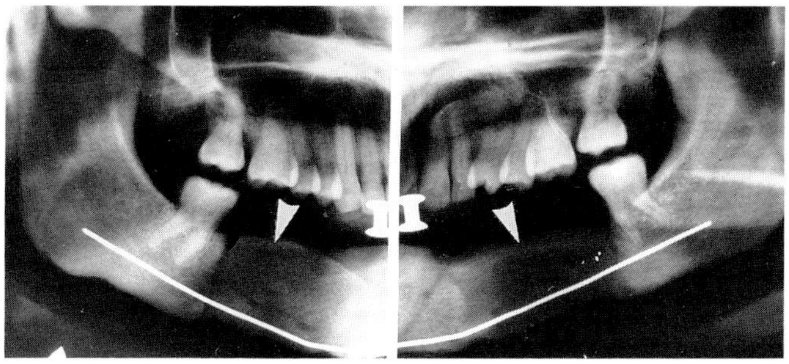

B

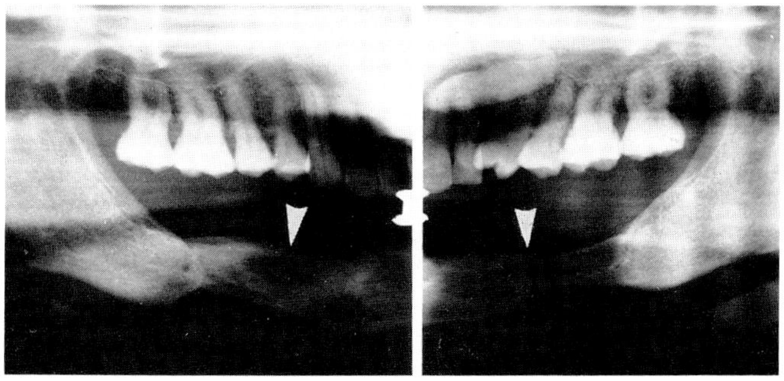

C

Fig. 10-17. Surgical mandibular reconstruction. **A.** Anterior mandibular defect was restored initially (at time of tumor resection) with a rib graft skewered on a stainless steel wire. **B.** Ten months later, iliac crest bone grafts were lashed to the stainless steel wire and remaining rib graft. **C.** One year later, moderate resorption of the graft is evident.

MANDIBULAR GUIDANCE RESTORATIONS

If mandibular continuity is not restored, there are a number of methods which will reduce the degree of mandibular deviation. These include intermaxillary fixation, mandibularly based guidance restorations, and palatally based guidance restorations. The method of choice depends on many factors and should be combined with a well-organized mandibular exercise regime.

One approach is to place the patient immediately into intermaxillary fixation, using arch bars and elastics, and to maintain fixation for five to seven weeks after surgery. Although no controlled studies have been performed to evaluate this approach, some clinicians feel that it is beneficial.[7] It appears most useful in patients with resections confined to the mandible with little associated soft tissue loss. In these patients scar contracture is minimal and, since ample soft tissue is available for surgical closure, mandibular deviation is actually due to muscle imbalances and impaired proprioception. Using intermaxillary fixation in these patients maintains the proprioceptive sense of occlusion and enables most patients to assume appropriate intercuspal positions after fixation is removed.

If intermaxillary fixation is not employed, the patient should be placed on an exercise program as early as possible after surgery. Upon maximum opening, the mandible is displaced by hand as forcefully as possible towards the nonsurgical side. These movements tend to lessen scar contracture, reduce trismus, and improve maxillomandibular relationships. Exercises should be carefully demonstrated to the patient and notes made periodically to record the degree of progress.

The earlier mandibular guidance therapy is initiated, the more successful the result. If the patient has undergone an extensive bony and soft tissue resection, a classical radical neck dissection, and radiation therapy, and if a considerable period of time has elapsed since the surgical procedure, guidance procedures are more difficult and a compromised occlusal relationship may result. Unfortunately, those patients suffering the most severe deviations of the mandible because of extensive soft-tissue loss, tight-wound closure, radiation therapy, and/or a classical radical neck dissection are most susceptible to those complications (fistula formation, flap necrosis, and other postsurgical morbidities) that delay the beginning of mandibular guidance therapy.

If the mandible can be manipulated into an acceptable maxillomandibular relationship, a cast mandibular resection prosthesis[8] is appropriate. This prosthesis consists of a removable partial denture framework with a metal flange extending 7 to 10 mm laterally and superiorly on the buccal aspect of the bicuspids and molars on the unresected side. This flange engages the maxillary teeth during mandibular closure, thereby directing the mandible into an appropriate intercuspal position (Fig. 10-18). The partial denture framework must be stable and retentive to counteract the lateral forces generated on the flange during closure. The guidance flange is constructed of cast chrome-cobalt metal, and modifications are made with acrylic resin.

A second design confines the guidance ramp and index to a maxillary prosthesis. This form of guidance prosthesis is indicated for patients whose severe deviation prevents ma-

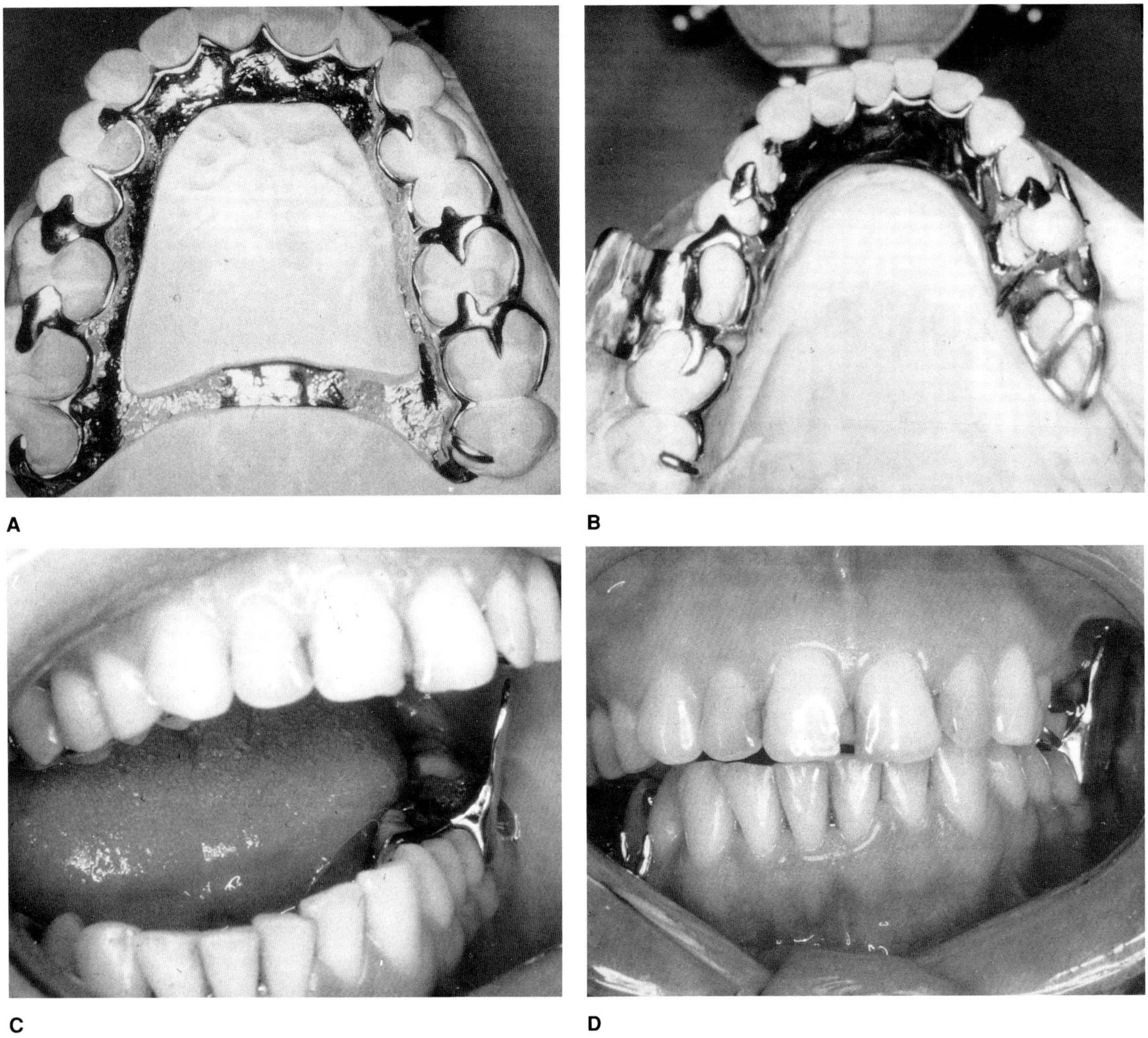

Fig. 10-18. Mandibular guidance prosthesis. A-B. Mandible from tooth #31 up to and including the condyle was resected. A cast partial denture framework was fabricated for both the maxilla and the mandible. Castings engage residual dentition to prevent movement of the individual teeth during mandibular guidance therapy. C-D. Note angular path of closure.[2]

nipulation of the mandible into any form of acceptable occlusal contact. Maxillary guidance ramps are more adjustable than mandibular guidance ramps. They are usually constructed of acrylic resin with either cast or wrought-wire retainers since they usually serve only temporarily until an acceptable occlusion can be established (Fig. 10-19).

The success of mandibular guidance therapy depends on the nature of the surgical defect, early initiation of guidance therapy, cooperation of the patient, and other factors. Patients with extensive posterior base-of-tongue lesions requiring significant soft tissue resection and radiation therapy are often unable to achieve useful intercuspal relationships. Mandibular guidance therapy is most successful when the resection involves bony structures only, with minimal sacrifice of tongue, floor of mouth, and adjacent soft tissues. The prognosis for mandibular guidance therapy is also improved when patients have not had a radical neck dissection or have not been irradiated.

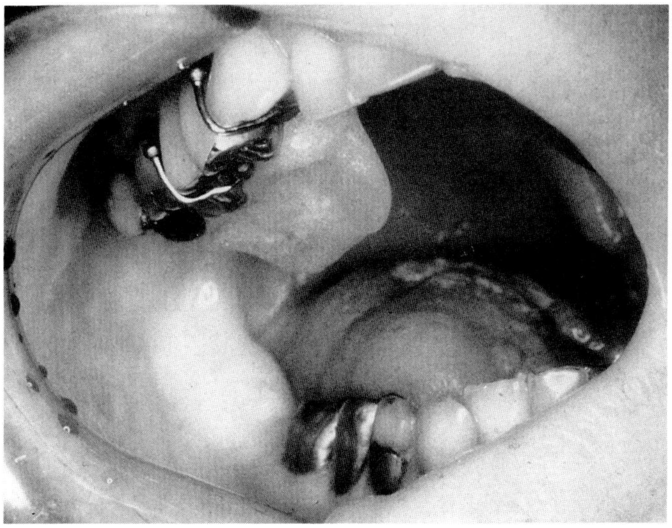

A

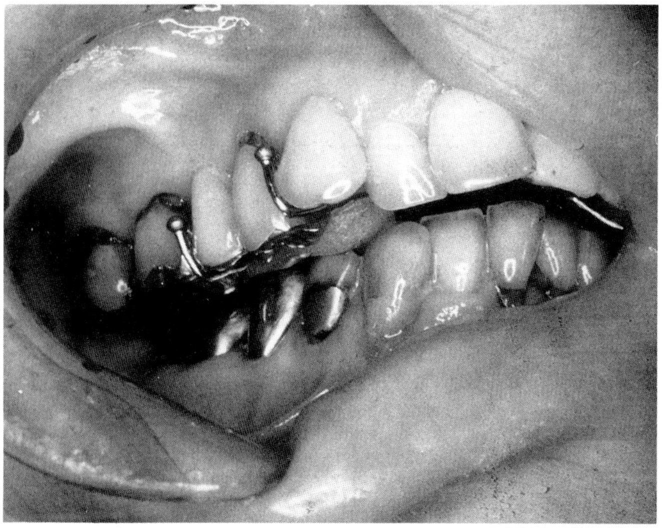

B

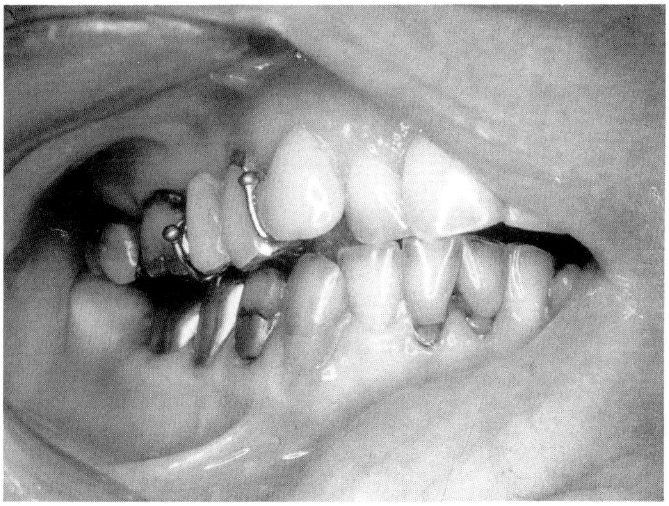

C

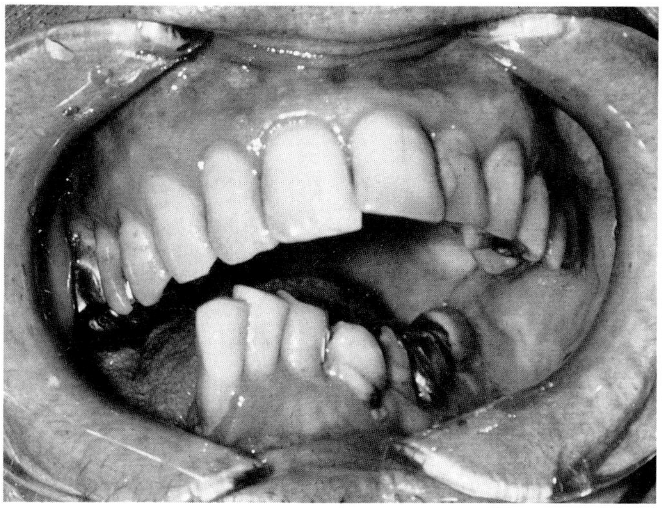

D

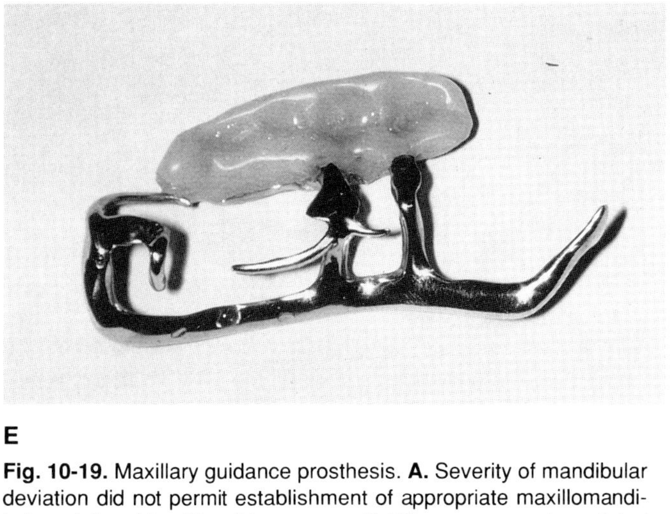

E

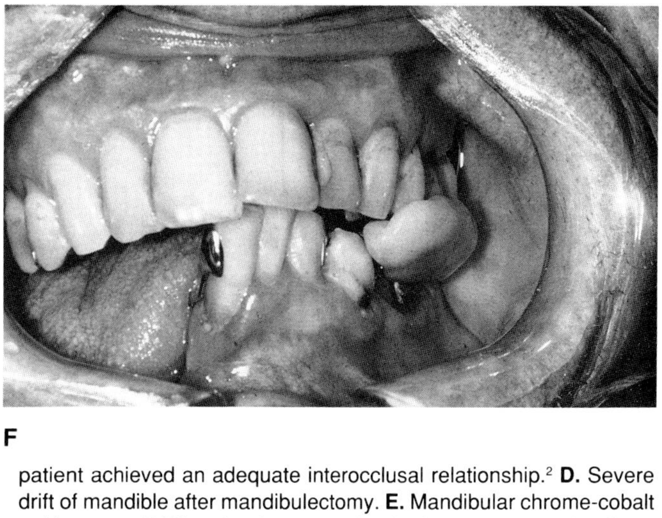

F

Fig. 10-19. Maxillary guidance prosthesis. **A.** Severity of mandibular deviation did not permit establishment of appropriate maxillomandibular relationship with guidance ramp. **B.** When ramp was formulated and delivered, mandibular teeth occluded lingual to the desired position. **C.** As scar contracture loosened, ramp was adjusted so that patient achieved an adequate interocclusal relationship.[2] **D.** Severe drift of mandible after mandibulectomy. **E.** Mandibular chrome-cobalt guide ramp. **F.** When in place, prosthesis decreases lateral shift towards defect. There are no denture teeth on distal extension because tongue has been sutured to cheek and there is no bony support.

DEFINITIVE PROSTHESES

The prognosis of removable prostheses for patients with resections of the tongue and mandible is dependent upon the function of the residual tongue. In some patients with poor tongue function, only appearance can be improved, while in others with good tongue function, mastication is a reasonable objective. In patients with mandibular defects, placement of the definitive prosthesis is not as urgent and the prosthetic prognosis is not as favorable as in patients with maxillary defects. Most mandibulectomy patients are not dependent upon their prosthesis for oral functions. If anterior teeth are not involved in the resection, some patients will prefer not to wear a removable prosthesis. Sometimes it is possible to use the cast framework constructed as a guidance prosthesis in the fabrication of the definitive mandibular prosthesis. In edentulous patients who have undergone partial mandibular resection and have reasonable tongue function, the placement of osseointegrated implants can improve mastication dramatically.

Partial Dentures

The usual principles of partial denture design and fabrication should be followed. Major connectors should be rigid, occlusal rests must direct occlusal forces along the long axis of teeth, guiding planes should be employed to increase stability and bracing, retention must be within the limits of physiologic tolerance of the periodontal ligament, and maximum support should be gained from the adjacent soft tissues. Retainers, minor connectors, and proximal plates should be designed so that they do not subject the remaining teeth to excessive lateral forces during function. The design should also consider the need for cleaning in view of the problems head and neck cancer patients have in maintaining oral hygiene and controlling plaque.

In patients with lateral discontinuity defects, it may not be possible to design a framework with retainers that disengage during function because of the altered patterns of force upon the prosthesis. Viewed from the frontal plane, the arc of closure of the mandible is angular rather than vertical, with unilateral forces of occlusion confined to the nonresected side. Rotation of the mandible in the frontal plane causes the resected side to drop down out of occlusion as the force of contracture on the unresected side is increased. The location of the fulcrum line of a partial denture is not easily determined because of the difficulty in predicting movement patterns of the prosthesis during function. A typical lateral mandibulectomy defect with a suggested design is shown in Fig. 10-20. The forces of occlusion are unilateral, so the axis of rotation (fulcrum line) of the partial denture deviates from the norm. By placing the occlusal rest on the mesial of the bicuspid, it is possible to place a retainer on the bicuspid that disengages during expression of an occlusal load. However, a retainer cannot be positioned in a retentive area on the opposite cuspid which disengages during occlusal function. Consequently, this retainer must either be placed on the height of contour or it must be flexible enough that an occlusal load will not expose the cuspid to undue pathologic stress. All partial denture frameworks should be physiologically relieved.[9]

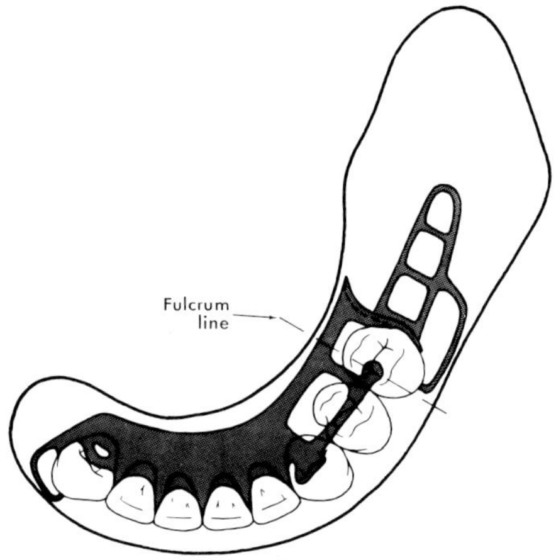

A

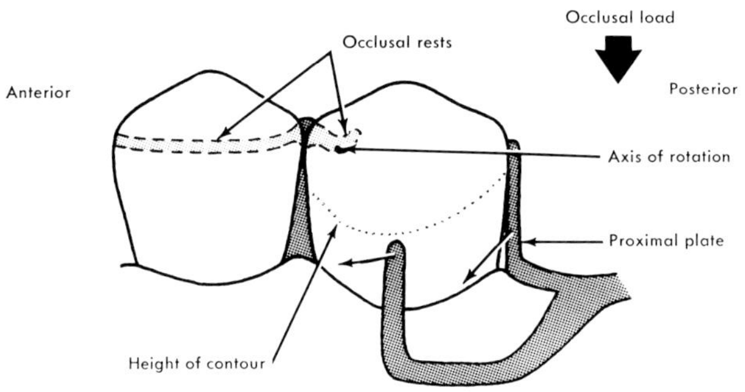

B

Fig. 10-20. Suggested design for partial denture. **A.** Occlusal view. **B.** Buccal view, "I" bar retainer on left side disengages with occlusal pressure. Similar retainer on right side is placed at height of contour to avoid applying torque to this abutment.[2]

After the partial denture casting has been fabricated, verified, and adjusted, an altered cast impression is obtained of the edentulous areas. Particular attention should be paid to the lingual extension on the unresected side, especially the polished surfaces. This extension, when suitably developed, provides additional retention and stability (Fig. 10-21). Maximum extension of the denture base is always attempted. Coverage of the buccal shelf on the unresected side is essential to maximize support. Centric relation records are made and occlusal schemes developed that are consistent with the unilateral mandibular movement patterns of mandibulectomy patients. The partial denture prostheses are delivered, adjusted, and periodically monitored in the usual way.

Complete Dentures

Before the introduction of osseointegrated implants, only a small percentage of edentulous patients with lateral discontinuity defects of the mandible had any hope of ever being

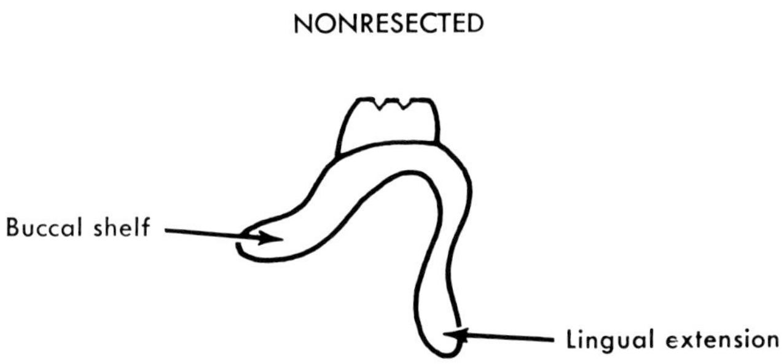

Fig. 10-21. Cross-section through molar area of mandibular partial denture. Lingual extension on nonrestricted side improves stability and retention.[2]

able to masticate as efficiently as before surgery. However, when these implants are used, mastication can actually be improved over that achieved prior to surgery and the implant-retained-and-supported restorations may improve saliva control, appearance, and in some cases, the ability to articulate certain speech sounds (Fig. 10-22).

A number of factors affect the patient's ability to function with resection dentures:

1. With only one half or two thirds of the mandible remaining, stability, support, and retention of the mandibular denture are compromised.
2. Since most patients will have received radiation therapy either before or after surgery, the oral mucosa is atrophic and fragile, predisposing it to soft-tissue irritation. Chronic alcohol abuse and poor nutrition may further compromise the health of the oral mucous membranes. The diminished output and thick mucinous nature of the saliva that remains after radiation impairs retention and may be inadequate to lubricate the denture-mucosa interface.
3. The angular pathway of mandibular closure induces lateral forces upon the dentures that tend to dislodge them.
4. The deviation of the mandible creates abnormal maxillomandibular relationships that may prevent ideal placement of the denture teeth over their supporting structures.
5. The impairment of motor and/or sensory control of the tongue, lip, and cheek limits the ability of the patient to control dentures during function. The integrated neuromuscular balance between tongue, lips, and cheeks which serves to stabilize complete mandibular dentures in healthy patients is disrupted in patients with mandibular discontinuity defects.
6. Unilateral forces of occlusion tend to tip and dislodge both maxillary and mandibular dentures during function.

As one can readily appreciate, implant-supported resection dentures can overcome many of the difficulties referred to above, particularly those associated with compromised retention, stability, or support.

The prosthetic prognosis depends upon many complex factors, including the amount of mandible remaining, severity of mandibular deviation, character of mandibular movements, postsurgical lip posture and control, tongue control and mobility, and previous radiation therapy. The status of the remaining tongue is probably the most important prognostic factor. If motor or sensory control, or both, have been significantly impaired, the prosthetic prognosis becomes extremely guarded even if implants are placed in the anterior mandible. The mobility of the tongue is less important. If the patient can move his tongue in several directions, he will probably be able to stabilize a resection denture and control the bolus during function. Obviously, patients who have lost

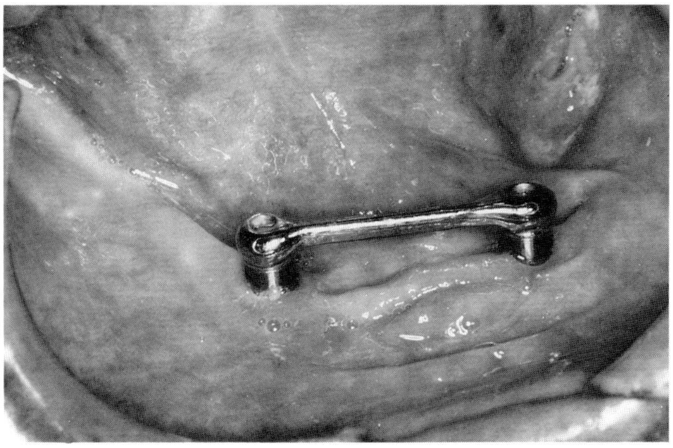

A

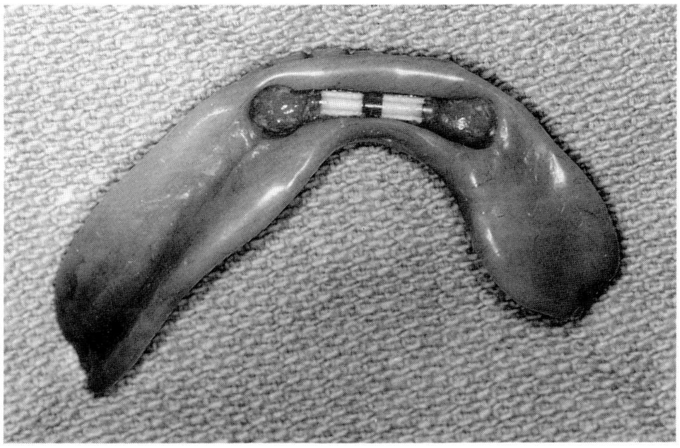

B

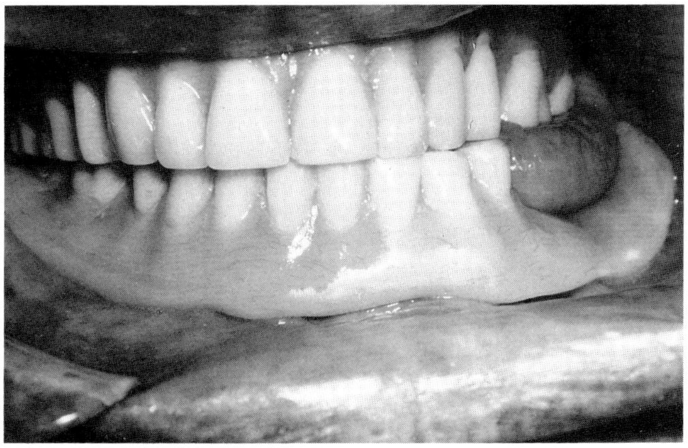

C

Fig. 10-22. A. Two implants placed anteriorly in a patient having undergone a partial mandibulectomy. **B.** Note resection denture with clip retention. **C.** The prosthesis positioned intraorally.

significant amounts of tongue in combination with resection of one of the hypoglossal nerves accompanied by considerable local paresthesia, have the poorest prosthetic prognosis. Paradoxically, immobility of the tongue creates a minor anatomic advantage in that it often permits a more aggressive extension of the lingual flange on the nonsurgical side, thus facilitating stability and retention. As in normal patients, the position of the tongue is also an important prosthodontic prognosticator. Resection of a base-of-tongue lesion often results in a retruded tongue position, making it difficult to obtain peripheral seal. However, more lateral and anterior resections of the mandible and tongue often leave it in a more favorable position.

Impressions are developed using conventional prosthodontic principles and techniques. Centric and lateral registrations and occlusal schemes should take into consideration the altered pattern of mandibular movements (Fig. 10-23). Delivery and follow-up are accomplished in the usual way. Denture extensions can be verified with a disclosing wax and excessive tissue displacement eliminated with the aid of pressure-indicating paste. These patients require continued encouragement and support during the prolonged adjustment period to help them adapt to their new prosthesis. Those with normal tongue control and mobility, surprisingly, often are able to masticate quite efficiently, particularly if the post-resection denture is implant-retained and supported.

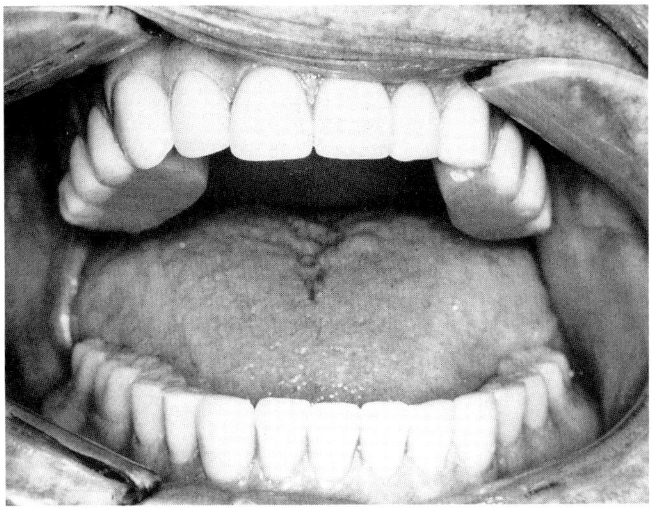

A

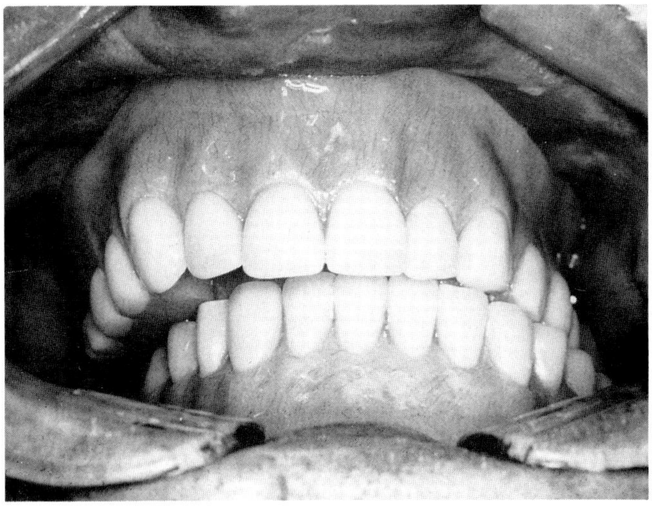

B

Fig. 10-23. Complete dentures. **A.** Occlusal ramps are provided to extend the occlusal table. **B.** Bilateral occlusal contact is maintained with the occlusal ramps. During forceful closure, mandible slides further to the right along the functional pathway.

FACIAL DEFECTS

Restoration of facial defects is a difficult challenge for both the surgeon and the prosthodontist. Surgical reconstruction and prosthodontic restoration both have distinct limitations. The surgeon is limited by the availability of tissue, the damage to the local vascular bed in tumor patients, the need for periodic visual inspection of an oncologic defect, and the physical condition of the patient. The prosthodontist is limited by the materials available for facial restoration, the movable tissue beds, the difficulty in retaining large prostheses, and the patient's willingness to accept the result. Whatever the mode of rehabilitation, the patient should be fully informed about future problems and of the expected quality of the final result. In patients with extensive facial tumors requiring resection, the method of facial restoration should be considered before surgery. The patient should be involved in this discussion and should participate in the decision-making process. A well-informed patient with realistic expectations is the objective to be achieved before surgical resection of large facial tumors.

SURGICAL RECONSTRUCTION VERSUS PROSTHETIC RESTORATION

The choice between surgical reconstruction versus prosthetic restoration of large facial defects is difficult and complex and depends on the size and etiology of the defect as well as the wishes of the patient. Surgical reconstruction of small facial defects is possible in most cases and is preferable. Many patients prefer masking a defect with their own tissue rather than with a prosthetic restoration. It is safe to say that it is difficult, if not impossible, for the surgeon to fabricate a facial part that is as successful in appearance as a well-made prosthesis. However, not everyone will accept an artificial part, and many would rather have a permanent, even if less esthetic, nose or ear. In general, younger patients prefer to have a permanent reconstructed facial part rather than an artificial one. The application of osseointegrated implants in facial defects has, in part, changed patient perceptions about facial prostheses because of the effectiveness of retention achieved.

A variety of circumstances may dictate prosthetic restoration of large facial defects:

1. When a large resection is necessary and recurrence of tumor is likely, it is advantageous to be able to monitor the surgical site closely. A prosthesis permits such observation, whereas primary surgical reconstruction may make it impossible.

2. Surgical restoration of large defects is technically difficult and requires multiple procedures and hospitalizations. Patients confronted with this type of defect are usually older and less able or willing to tolerate the multiple procedures required for surgical reconstruction.

3. Increasing numbers of these types of tumors are being treated with radiation. Reduced vascularity, increased fibrosis, and scarring of tissue bed bordering the defect increases the risk of complications associated with reconstruction. In many patients, full-course radiation therapy precludes successful surgical reconstruction.

Even when surgical reconstruction is deemed possible, significant delay may be necessary to ensure control of the tumor. Most surgeons prefer to wait at least one year after a large resection before beginning surgical reconstruction of a facial defect resulting from removal of a malignant tumor.

PROSTHETIC FACIAL RESTORATIONS

The challenge to the prosthodontist is to fabricate an esthetically pleasing restoration (Figs. 10-24 and 10-25). A conspicuous prosthesis may produce more anxiety and permit less social readjustment than a simple facial bandage or eye patch. Since successful use of the restoration may depend upon the patient's psychological acceptance of it, it is beneficial to have the patient seen by a social worker during the rehabilitation period. The most critical period is the first two to three days after delivery of the prosthesis. The conflicting emotional responses of the patient should be anticipated and discussed before delivery. In some cases, a patient will not wear a facial prosthesis because of unrealistic expectations. Since all facial restorations are detectable under close scrutiny, the patient must understand that the prosthesis has two different roles. For family, close friends, or business associates, it can only cosmetically replace the tissues excised. For the public at large, however, it generally provides enough concealment to render the reconstructed defect inconspicuous.

Materials Used for Facial Prostheses

A number of materials have been used for facial prostheses. These include wood, wax, metals and, recently, polymers. Current materials exhibit some excellent properties, but also some frustrating deficiencies, and all possess some undesirable characteristics. The materials most often used today are the silicone elastomers. The newest silicone elastomer, MDX-4-4210, has been shown to be the most clinically acceptable material and has achieved wide acceptance.

Retention

A major development in recent years has been the use of osseointegrated implants for retention. In eligible patients with sufficient bone at the desired sites, the result is an extremely well-retained prosthesis, allowing for vigorous physical activities. The tissue adhesive systems used during the last 40 years are rapidly being discarded in favor of these new implant systems (Fig. 10-25).[10]

Design Considerations

While the details concerning fabrication of facial prostheses are beyond the scope of this review, a few basic principles should be mentioned. A presurgical moulage can be very helpful, especially if a total rhinectomy or auriculectomy is anticipated. Impressions of the defect are usually obtained with elastic impression materials, taking care not to displace the tissues being recorded. The contours of the prostheses are sculpted in wax, both on the cast and on the patient. Surface characteristics, appropriate contour, coloration, and margin placement are equally important factors to be considered. Processing the materials used in facial restoration is complicated and requires special instrumentation. Special large flasks are necessary for processing large prostheses.

Coloration

Coloration of the prosthesis varies with the materials used and the preference of the clinician. Basic skin tones should be developed into a shade guide for each material. The base shade selected for a patient should be slightly lighter than the lightest skin tones of the patient, because as color is added the prosthesis will darken. Color may be applied either intrinsically or extrinsically. Intrinsic coloration is longer-lasting and is therefore preferred, but is more difficult to accomplish than extrinsic coloration.

Combined Oral and Facial Defects

Large combination defects of the oral cavity and the external face create innumerable problems for the patient and the prosthodontist. When the integrity of the oral cavity has been destroyed, food and air escape during swallowing, speech is often unintelligible, and saliva control is difficult. It is extremely difficult to adapt the margins of the prosthesis so that tissue contact will be maintained during facial and mandibular movements. Successful adjustment depends on the patient's having a realistic understanding of the degree of potential rehabilitation afforded by the future restoration.

Surgical reconstruction is usually not considered in patients with large defects because of the size of the defects, previous radiation therapy, and the probability of recurrence. Retention of maxillary teeth or a portion of the hard palate improves the prosthetic prognosis. Surgical modifications such as skin grafts to decrease tissue contraction and creation of undercut areas for retention improve the prosthetic prognosis.

Patients will experience less depression if as many functions as possible are restored immediately after surgery with a temporary prosthesis. These functions include the ability to swallow food (thereby eliminating the need for a nasogastric tube), the ability to control saliva, and the ability to speak intelligibly. The oral portion of the temporary prosthesis is constructed of acrylic resin and formed so that contact is established with healthy tissues adjacent to the defect. Functional contact with the remaining portions of the lips allows the patient to effectively seal the oral cavity. Tissue-bearing surfaces of the prosthesis are relined with temporary denture reliner at frequent intervals to accommodate tissue changes.

In constructing a definitive midface prosthesis, a custom tray is used for the master impression. Movable portions of the defect are recorded with a thermoplastic material. Record bases are fabricated, and centric relation records enable casts to be mounted on an articulator. Osseointegrated implants, eyeglass frames, adhesives, straps, teeth, and engagement of defect undercuts supply retention. The finished restoration usually provides the patient with acceptable appearance and function (Fig. 10-26).

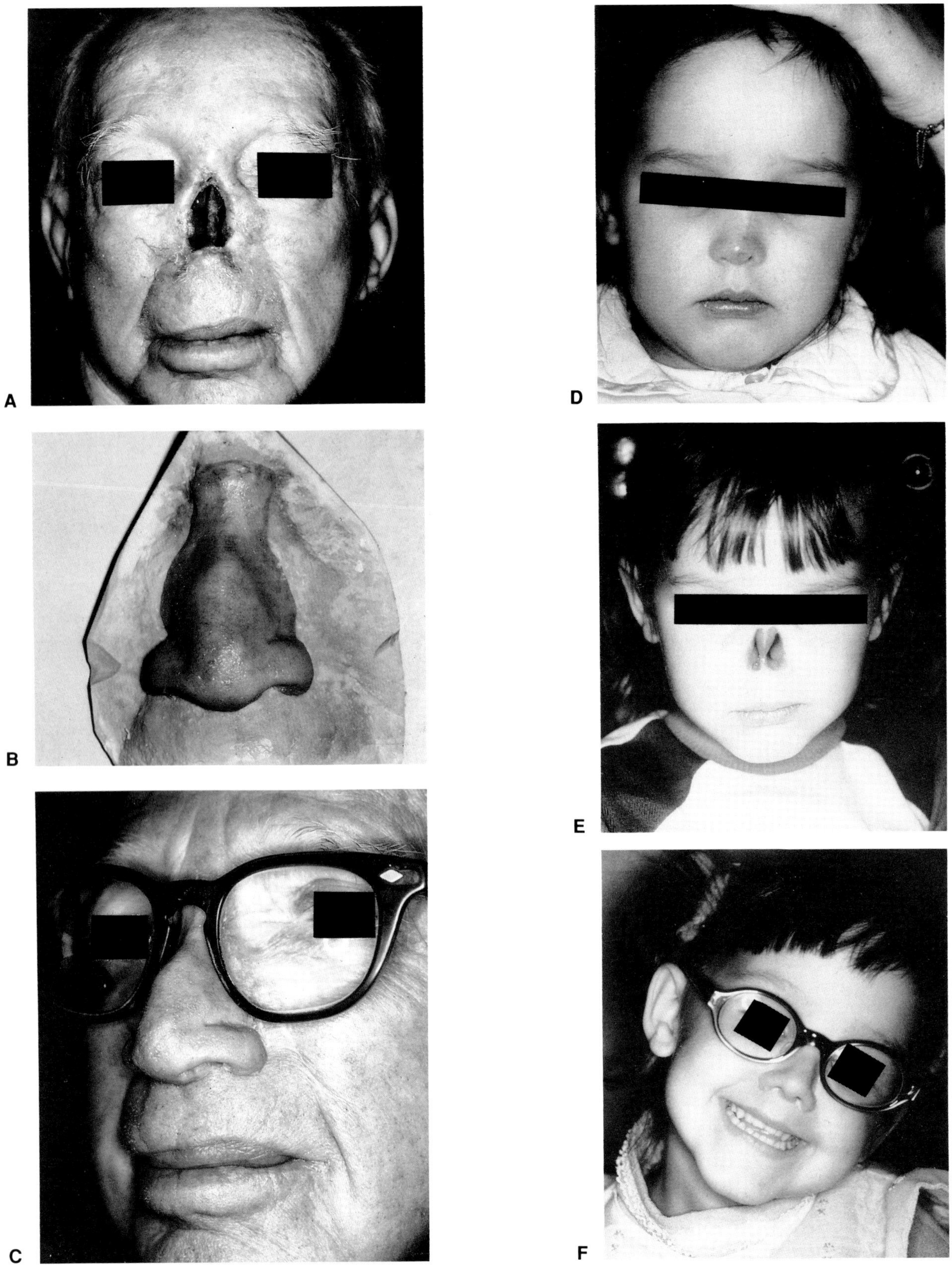

Fig. 10-24. Prosthetic restoration of the nose. **A.** Postrhinectomy defect secondary to a recurrent squamous carcinoma of skin. **B.** Prosthesis on the cast. **C.** Nasal prosthesis in position. **D.** Rhabdomyosarcoma of the nose, necessitating a total rhinectomy. **E.** The defect. **F.** The prosthesis.

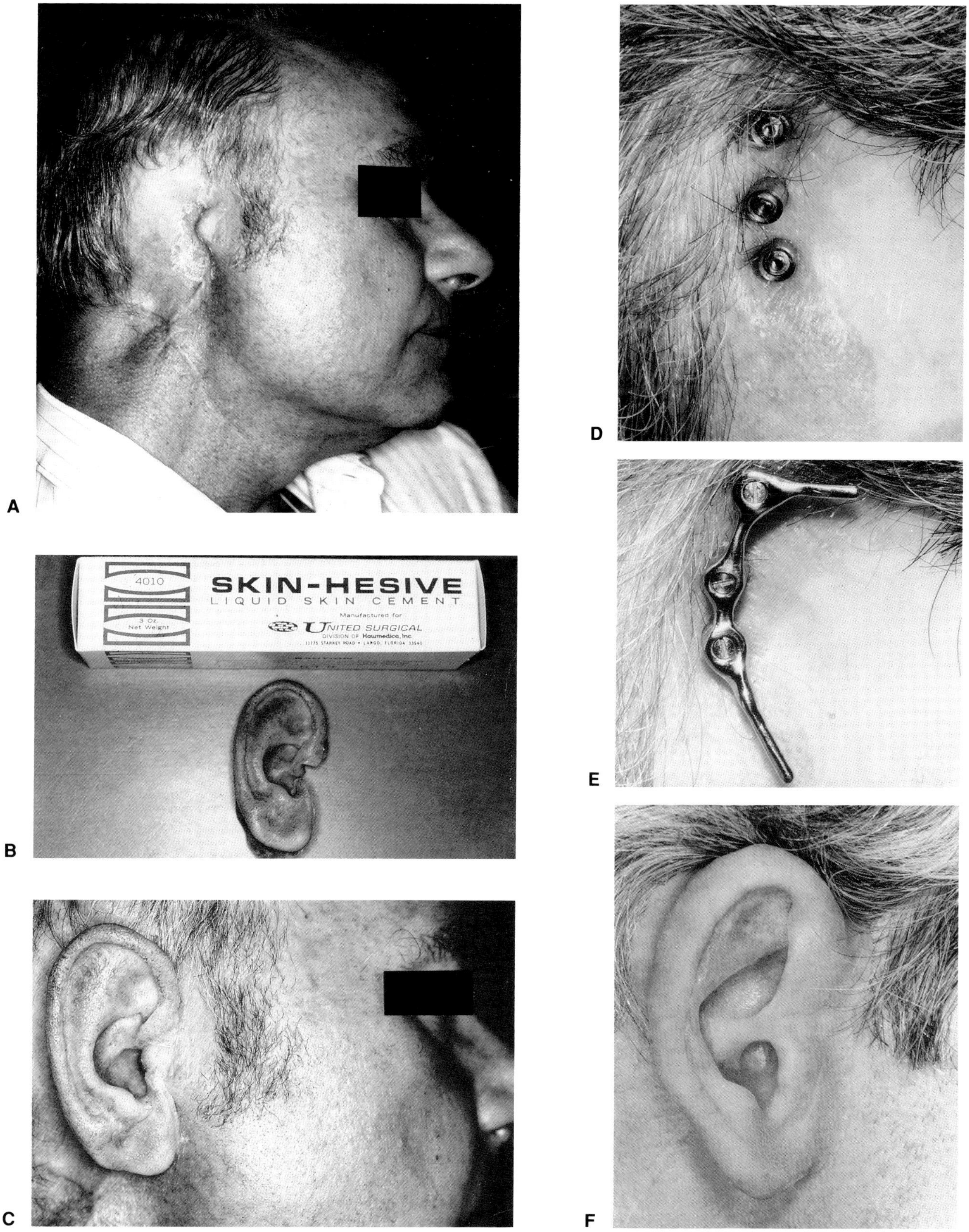

Fig. 10-25. Prosthetic restoration of the ear. **A.** Postauriculectomy defect. **B.** Prosthesis with adhesive. **C.** Ear prosthesis in position. **D.** Postauriculectomy defect with osseointegrated implants. **E.** Ear prosthesis bar clip retention. **F.** Prosthesis in position.

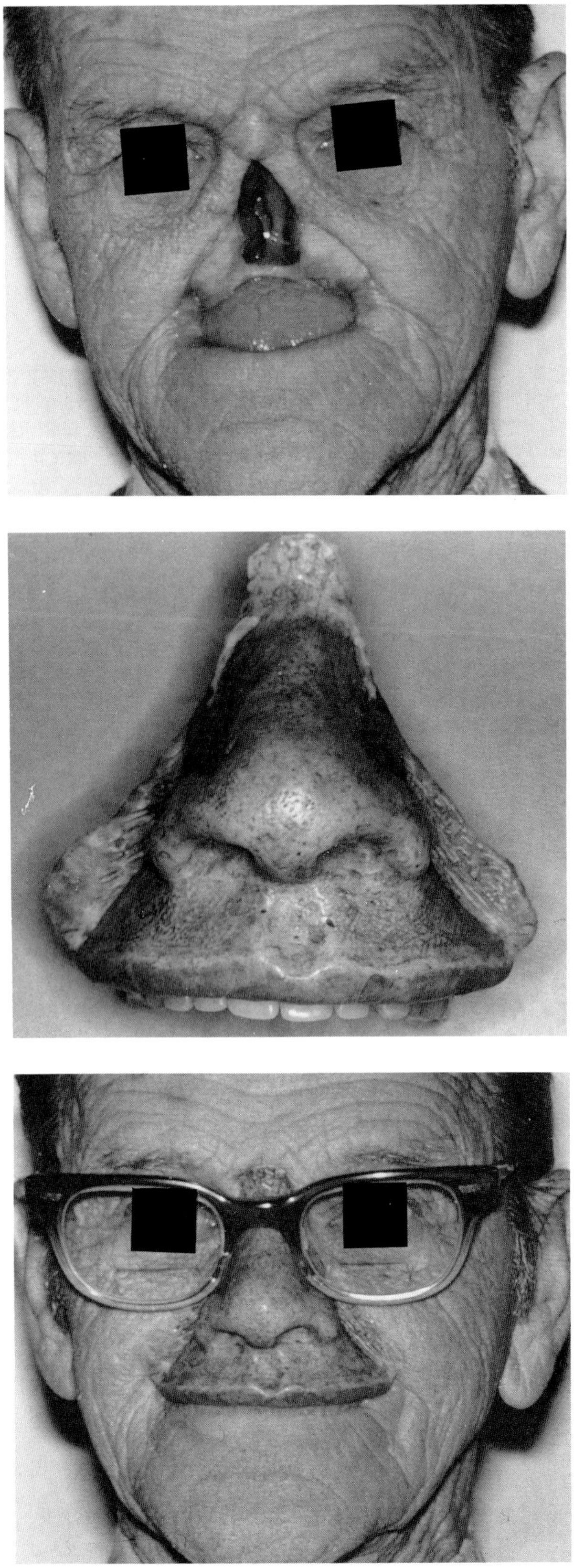

A B C

Fig. 10-26. Prosthetic restoration of a midface defect. **A.** Large midfacial defect secondary to removal of extensive tumor. **B.** Prosthesis. **C.** Prosthesis in position.

RADIATION THERAPY

RISK FACTOR

The histopathologic changes in the oral mucous membranes and bone and the changes in the amount, physical properties, and biologic effectiveness of saliva have caused some radiotherapists and dentists to be uncertain whether irradiated patients should ever wear dentures. However, recent studies reveal that the risk of developing an osteoradionecrosis is minimal in patients who had been edentulous for some time before undergoing radiation therapy which included denture-bearing surfaces (See Chapter 6). A University of California study[11] found that no bone exposures developed in 92 such patients who received complete maxillary and mandibular dentures. In 87 of these patients, the bearing surface of the mandibular denture was within the radiation field. The risk of bone necrosis is significant, however, in those patients who have had teeth removed just before or after radiotherapy. In the same report, three cases of bone necrosis attributed to dentures developed (all in extraction sites) in a group of 36 patients rendered edentulous by preradiation or postradiation extractions. All three healed within six months without surgical intervention.

The literature reveals few cases of bone necrosis associated with dentures leading to resection of the mandible. Investigators in Texas reported five cases of osteoradionecrosis among 82 patients receiving intraoral prostheses after radiotherapy to the head and neck region.[12] Sixty-four patients received complete dentures and 18 received removable partial dentures. Four healed by conservative treatment and one was still unhealed at publication. It was not stated whether these cases were related to recent extraction.

PLACEMENT OF DENTURES—TIMING

Some controversy exists as to when dentures can be safely constructed for irradiated patients who have completed therapy. Recommended insertion times have ranged from one to three years after surgery.[12–15] The University of California study[11] sheds some light on this clinical dilemma. In the 92 patients who were edentulous before onset of disease (87 of whom reported previous experience with complete dentures), prostheses were inserted an average of 15.4 months after radiation was completed. Eliminating nine patients who waited longer than 50 months from the end of therapy to delivery reduces the average to 8.9 months. Forty-five patients received dentures within six months after radiation therapy. None in the group of 92 developed an osteoradionecrosis associated with the use of their dentures.

Those patients who have had teeth extracted in conjunction with radical alveolectomies before radiotherapy seem to need a more conservative approach. In the same report, 23 such patients received dentures an average of 22.2 months after completion of therapy. Two patients in this group developed bone necroses.

The efficacy of the alveolectomies and the status of the residual ridge are also important clinical factors to appraise. An irregular mandibular ridge in which the entire body of the mandible was within the radiation field may prompt the clinician to defer dentures indefinitely. On the other hand, a smooth, well-contoured mandibular bearing surface may permit the clinician to insert dentures soon after therapy.

As to when dentures should be placed for the irradiated patient, the data differ for those who were edentulous and experienced denture wearers before therapy and for those who had teeth extracted within the radiation field before therapy but who were not experienced denture wearers. The former showed little risk of developing significant complications from denture wear, and it seems justified in most instances to place dentures in these patients 6 to 12 months after radiation therapy. In the latter group the risk of bone necrosis is higher, and placement of dentures should depend on the status of the mucosal and bony bearing surfaces, the amount and fields of radiation, and the degree of patient cooperation. Some patients in this group may never be candidates for complete dentures.

Prosthodontic Procedures—Complete Dentures

Clinical manifestations of radiation treatments important to note include (1) appearance of oral mucous membranes, (2) scarring and fibrosis at the tumor site, (3) degree of trismus, and (4) status of salivary function. Translucent, boggy mucosa with prominent telangiectasia implies that prosthodontic restorations will be poorly tolerated and mucosal integrity is at risk. Where there are severe mucosal changes, dentures may be postponed or precluded altogether. Scarring at the tumor site may be prominent, especially if interstitial therapy was employed. In the case of floor-of-mouth lesions, it may be prudent to somewhat limit extension of the lingual flange of the mandibular denture at the former tumor site. Such scar tissue is most unyielding, and the slightest overextension can result in a mucosal perforation and perhaps lead to an osteonecrosis or soft tissue necrosis. Excessive trismus is occasionally observed in patients whose radiation field includes the temporomandibular joint and muscles of mastication. If there is severe trismus, it may be necessary to reduce the vertical dimension of occlusion of the complete dentures. This will make intake of food easier and may reduce the forces exerted on the supporting mucosa during closure. The amount and viscosity of saliva is an important determinant of prosthodontic success. Impaired salivary function leads to more friction at the denture-mucosa interface, increasing the chance of mucosal irritation. The less saliva, the more difficult it is for the patient to tolerate dentures.

Any condition that clouds the prosthetic prognosis in nonirradiated patients is even more significant in irradiated patients. For example, mandibular ridges in patients with severe bilateral undercuts or excessive ridge resorption with little attached mucosa make them poor candidates for complete dentures after radiation therapy.

Impressions. Conventional border molding using a custom tray and modeling plastic is advocated. If xerostomia is particularly profound, a thin coating of petroleum may be applied over the soft modeling plastic to prevent its sticking to dry mucosa. Displacement of the tissues of the floor of the mouth in an attempt to obtain peripheral seal is not advocated. Efforts in developing the lingual flange should be directed toward gaining stability and support rather than retention. In all other extension areas, attention should be paid to attaining maximum stability and support. The elastic impression materials are most suitable in refining the impression.

Vertical dimension. The completed impressions are boxed and poured in dental stone. Conventional record bases are prepared and used to determine the vertical dimension of occlusion. The usual methods of determining vertical dimension apply: phonetics, closest speaking distance, swallowing, neuromuscular perception, and recording vertical dimension of rest. Centric relation records are obtained in the usual manner. Wax, plaster, and zinc oxide paste are suitable media for obtaining the final registrations. Graphic recording devices can likewise be employed successfully.

Occlusal forms. On a theoretical basis, we have come to favor monoplane occlusal schemes with bilateral balance obtained with posteriorly situated balancing ramps. In arranging posterior teeth, careful attention should be given to attaining proper buccal horizontal overlap; in some patients edema of the tongue and buccal mucosa is prominent, predisposing them to tongue and cheek biting. In dentures constructed with anatomic posterior teeth, bilateral balance during function is mandatory.

Delivery and postinsertion care. Occlusal discrepancies due to processing errors should be eliminated before dentures are removed from the cast. Pressure-indicating paste is used to identify areas of excessive pressure, and disclosing wax is useful in verifying extension of denture flanges. Remounting on a suitable articulator with new maxillomandibular records taken at the time of delivery is mandatory.

The patient is given an instruction sheet detailing possible problems and precautions. Instructions are provided about the need to remove the dentures if soreness develops, to return for periodic visits, and initially to limit use of the prosthesis for mastication. Such restorations should never be worn during sleeping hours. The care rendered after delivery of dentures is critical and requires an understanding patient if untoward complications are to be avoided. During the first week, 24- and 48-hour recall appointments are recommended regardless of how well the patient is tolerating his dentures.

It must be emphasized that the risk of serious postradiation sequelae in denture wearers is small. At the same time, it must not be forgotten that individual reactions to radiotherapy can vary greatly, and good judgment and sound techniques are factors that can never be ignored in placing prostheses. Cooperation of the patient is a necessity. Without it, the best intentions of the dentist may result in bone or soft tissue necrosis. The patient must understand the tissue changes resulting from radiation treatment and be available for close follow-up.

REFERENCES

1. Ordway D: The crisis of cancer—challenge to change. *J Prosthet Dent* 37:184, 1977.
2. Beumer J III, Curtis T, Firtell D (eds): *Maxillofacial Rehabilitation—Prosthodontic and Surgical Considerations.* St. Louis: CV Mosby, 1979.
3. Brånmark P-I: Osseointegration and its experimental background. *J Prosthet Dent* 50:399. 1983.
4. Lang BR, Bruce RA: Presurgical maxillectomy prosthesis. *J Prosthet Dent* 17:613, 1967.
5. Desjardins RP: Obturator prosthesis design for acquired maxillary defects. *J Prosthet Dent* 39:424, 1978.
6. Parel SM, Drane JB, Williams EO: Mandibular replacements: A review of the literature. *J Am Dent Assoc* 94:120, 1977.

7. Aramany M, Myers E: Dental occlusion and arch relationship in segmental resection of the mandible. *In* GA Sisson, ME Tardy (eds): *Plastic and Reconstructive Surgery of the Face and Neck,* Proceedings of the Second International Symposium. New York: Grune & Stratton, 1977.
8. Robinson J, Rubright WC: Use of a guide plane for maintaining the residual fragment in partial or hemimandibulectomy. *J Prosthet Dent* 14:922, 1964.
9. Schwartzman B, Caputo A, Beumer J III: Occlusal force transfer by removable partial denture designs for a radical maxillectomy. *J Prosthet Dent* 54:397, 1985.
10. Hamada M, Lee R, Beumer J III, Moy P: Restoring facial defects with osseointegrated implants (in preparation) 1989.
11. Beumer J III, Curtis TA, Morrish RB Jr: Radiation complications in edentulous patients. *J Prosthet Dent* 36:193, 1976.
12. Daley TE, Drane JB: *Management of Dental Problems in Irradiated Patients.* Austin: University of Texas Press, 1972.
13. Krajicek DD: Oral radiation in prosthodontics. *J Am Dent Assoc* 78:320, 1969.
14. Rahn AO, Matalon V, Drane JB: Prosthetic evaluation of patients who have received irradiation to the head and neck regions. *J Prosthet Dent* 19:174, 1968.
15. King RE, Elzay RP, Prentiss MD: Effects of ionizing radiation in the human oral cavity and oropharynx. *Radiology* 91:1001, 1968.

PICTURE CREDITS

Fig. 10-5A. Redrawn from Brown KE: Peripheral considerations in improving obturator retention. *J Prosthet Dent* 20:176, 1968.

Fig. 10-9A. Courtesy Dr. Gary Laine.

Fig. 10-10. Originally printed in Curtis T, Cantor R: The forgotten patient in maxillofacial prosthetics. *J Prosthet Dent* 31:662, 1974.

Figs. 10-15, 10-17. Courtesy Dr. William Ware.

Figs. 10-16. Courtesy Dr. Bruce Sanders.